Lifetime Encyclopedia of Natural Remedies

Myra Cameron

PARKER PUBLISHING COMPANY
West Nyack, New York 10995

© 1993 by

PARKER PUBLISHING COMPANY, INC.
West Nyack, NY

This book is a reference work based on research by the author. The opinions
expressed herein are not necessarily those of or endorsed by the publisher. The
directions stated in this book are in no way to be considered as a substitute for
consultation with a duly licensed doctor.

10 9 8 7 6 5 4

Library of Congress Cataloging-in-Publication Data

Cameron, Myra
  Lifetime encyclopedia of natural remedies / Myra Cameron
      p.   cm.
  Rev. and expanded ed. of: Treasury of home remedies. 1987.
  Includes index.
  ISBN 0-13-535220-7; —ISBN 0-13-535212-6
    1. Herbs—therapeutic use. 2. Medicine—Formulae, receipts, prescriptions.
3. Traditional medicine—formulae, receipts, prescriptions. 4. Therapeutics,
Physiological. I. Cameron, Myra. Treasury of home remedies. II. Title.
RM666.H33C36 1993
615.8′82—dc20   93-1957
                                                                                  CIP

ISBN   0-13-535220-7

ISBN   0-13-535212-6 (PBK)

Parker Publishing Company
Career & Personal Development
West Nyack, NY 10995

Simon & Schuster, A Paramount Communications Company

Printed in the United States of America

Other Books by Myra Cameron:

HOME-STYLE MICROWAVE COOKING
THE G.N.C. GOURMET VITAMIN COOKBOOK
TREASURY OF HOME REMEDIES
MOTHER NATURE'S GUIDE TO VIBRANT BEAUTY AND HEALTH

Author's Note

Welcome to the newly revised and expanded edition. Hundreds of readers have written to offer thanks for the original version of this *Lifetime Encyclopedia of Natural Remedies*. This encouraging response urged me to devote more time and energy to discovering new health tips, emergency first-aid measures, and forgotten remedies for common ailments. The happy result is this new work, packed with new findings and the latest information from current health periodicals, 120 books published after the first *Treasury of Home Remedies* was completed, and personal interviews for anecdotal remedies.

No other book on the market encompasses Lifetime's variety of self-help options for so many different health problems. Home medical encyclopedias offer definitions and descriptions of orthodox procedures. Most health books are limited to one disease or to one facet of health care (exercise, foods, reflexology, stress management, vitamins and minerals). Home remedy collections are specialized—allopathic, naturopathic, or folklore. This compendium has it all in one volume.

I've reorganized this work for the reader's convenience. For example, Fever and Infections are incorporated with other comparable maladies; Senility is replaced with specific problems such as Dry Skin, Wrinkles, and Hair Loss; Trichinosis is included with Food Poisoning; and the remaining, rarely encountered Worms omitted. I've also expanded the book from seventy four to one hundred sections, many of which cover several related ailments, plus the first "First-Aid Supplies and Tips" in the longer Introduction.

At the same time I've retained the virtues of the original. The entries are easy to read and understand. Health advice from folk healers, biochemists, nutritionists, and holistic physicians is correlated and presented without technical or biased verbiage. Nostrums from ancient cultures, folklore from the Middle Ages, commonsense cures from both colonial and contemporary America, and current case histories add interest and authenticity.

All ingredients and supplies can be obtained from supermarkets and health food stores. The folk recipies do not call for archaic or dangerous substances—no lark's tongues, herbals gathered by the light of the moon, Indian hemp (marijuana), or laudanum (opium)—and they are "translated" for modern measurements and preperation methods. No potentially harmful treatments such as moxibustion (burning an herb directly on the skin at an acupuncture point) or lengthy fasts are offered. Precise quantities and directions are given so that every remedy and treatment can be tried—and nothing requires the assistance of another individual.

Preventive tips, emergency first-aid measures, treatments for common colds, etc. save unneccessary office calls. There are remedies that have proven successful for everything from acne, allergy and arthritis to varicose veins and yeast infections. But this book does not promise "snake oil cures." It recommends professional attention when indicated, and the suggested supplements (taken with the doctor's approval) often augment medical treatment to reduce or eliminate prescribed medications (and their side effects) while speeding recovery.

I hope *Lifetime Encyclopedia of Natural Remedies* will be useful as well as informative, and will be as interesting to read as it was to compile.

Myra Cameron

Contents

Introduction

More than just a collection of remedies, this comprehensive manual offers "abouts" (brief explanations and possible preventives) and first-aid tips as well as "how-to" suggestions. To encompass the many facets of personal health maintenance, information provided by doctors (allopathic, holistic, homeopathic, naturopathic, orthomolecular), research scientists, folk healers, herbalists, nutritionists, reflexologists, and acupressure therapists has been synthesized, condensed, and combined with anecdotal home remedies. With the exception of references from periodicals, the sources are listed numerically in the Bibliography and referred to by number within the text and at the conclusion of each segment. By definition, any treatment not initiated by medical professionals qualifies as "folk medicine," but for convenience, each type of self-help is delineated in this Introduction and grouped accordingly in the alphabetically arranged sections for specific ailments.

Home remedies are invaluable for coping with common mishaps and self-limiting maladies, for preventing minor ailments from becoming major illnesses, and for augmenting necessary medical care. Although individual differences and reactions preclude the possibility of every suggestion working for everyone, there are many options, and all have been successful for some people.

Note: People with any physical or mental disorder should consult their physicians before making drastic changes in diet, supplements, or exercise regimens, and before attempting any form of self-treatment. The therapeutic quantities of nutrients shown in this book are for adults and represent research findings, not prescriptive amounts. Individual dosages should be determined by a health care professional; tolerances and requirements vary according to age, ailment, body size, and metabolism. People who are taking anticoagulant medications or who have diabetes, high blood pressure, hypothyroidism, or rheumatic heart disease should take no more than 100 IU of vitamin E for several weeks, then gradually increase the dosage after consultation with a doctor.

Diet and Supplements

Government guidelines for a healthful diet are formulated to provide the RDA (recommended daily dietary allowance) or RDI (reference daily intake) of nutrients essential for preventing known deficiency diseases in healthy adults. Consuming 2,000 to 2,800 calories daily from the suggested six to eleven servings of bread, cereals, and grains, five to nine servings of vegetables and fruits, and two or three servings each of milk products and protein foods (meats, poultry, fish, legumes) can accomplish this goal as long as fats and sweets are used sparingly.

As explained in *Longevity* (July 1992), however, factors such as illness or lifestyle (smoking destroys at least twice the RDA of vitamin C) increases the body's nutritional requirements. Eating a serving of acidophilus yogurt each day while taking antibiotics assists in replacing helpful intestinal flora annihilated along with the harmful bacteria. Other foods and dietary adjustments can be beneficial for certain disorders. Supplements cannot replace wholesome food, but they are the most feasible means of ingesting therapeutic amounts of specific nutrients to help the body heal itself. For instance, acquiring enough vitamin C to squelch an incipient cold would require eating a dozen oranges each hour. Vitamins, minerals, and the enzymes in food all work in concert. Unless otherwise directed, supplements should be taken with meals and especially whenever therapeutic dosages of individual nutrients are used, a multivitamin-mineral formula should be taken daily.

Vitamin A/Beta Carotene Preformed vitamin A (from fish liver oil) is stored in the liver and can have toxic effects if more than 15,000 to 25,000 IU are taken daily for long periods of time. Women who are pregnant or who are taking oral contraceptives are advised to limit preformed vitamin A to 5,000 IU daily. Beta carotene (water-soluble provitamin A, from dark-green, yellow, and orange plant foods) is converted to vitamin A within the body and does not interact adversely with birth control pills, but is not recommended for diabetics because they may not be able to convert it to vitamin A. [17, 98] Some doctors and nutritionists advise taking half the vitamin A dosage in beta carotene and half in preformed vitamin A. Other nutritional experts prefer beta carotene, the form suggested in this book, to avoid potential toxicity. Beta carotene is reported to produce the same benefits as preformed vitamin A and has been found nontoxic even when extremely high doses were administered for prolonged periods.[151]

B Complex These vitamins include B_1 (thiamine), B_2 (riboflavin), B_3 (niacin, nicotinic acid, and a synthetic form called niacinamide), pantothenic acid (B_5), B_6 (pyridoxine), folic acid (folate), B_{12} (cobalamin), biotin, choline, inositol, and PABA (para-aminobenzoic acid). Although all are water soluble and considered nontoxic because excesses are excreted rather than stored, B vitamins are so interrelated that high doses of individual members of the group can create deficiencies of the others unless a comprehensive B-complex supplement is taken as a daily accompaniment.[17, 189, 190] Lecithin contains choline and inositol; brewer's yeast (especially if B_{12} has been added) is an excellent source of the B complex.

Vitamin C and Bioflavonoids Vitamin C (ascorbic acid) and Bioflavonoids, (formerly called vitamin P, now include citrus bioflavonoids, hesperidin, quercetin, and rutin) function synergistically, are water soluble, and are considered nontoxic. Individual tolerance levels should be accommodated to avoid side effects of intestinal gas or diarrhea. Persons with ulcers or digestive difficulties may need to take vitamin C in the form of calcium ascorbate or accompany each dose with ¼ teaspoon of baking soda to neutralize the acid. When massive amounts of vitamin C have been taken to combat a cold or infection, gradually reducing the dosage allows the body to readjust and avoids a rebound effect of susceptibility to illness.

Vitamin D Actually a hormone produced by the action of the sun's ultraviolet rays on the skin, vitamin D can be acquired in minuscule amounts from egg yolks, fatty fish, liver, and milk fat. Since vitamin D is essential for the assimilation of calcium as well as for many bodily functions, it is used to "fortify" milk and is included in multivitamin supplements. Although excess amounts of this fat-soluble vitamin are stored in the liver and can be toxic, doses of less than 1,000 IU daily are unlikely to cause adverse effects.[151]

Vitamin E Supplemental vitamin E is available as D- or DL-alpha tocopherol alone or in combination with beta, delta, and gamma tocopherols. The initial D indicates natural vitamin E; DL, a synthetic form.

Minerals The body's thirty-some minerals function interactively as partners, assistants, and/or competitors. To avoid upsetting this balance when using individual minerals therapeutically, a multi-mineral supplement should be taken unless the minerals are included in a daily multivitamin formula. Calcium, for instance, requires phosphorus, magnesium, and other minerals plus vitamins A, C, and D in order to be properly utilized. Although phosphorus and calcium cooperate in building and maintaining sturdy bones and teeth, supplementary phosphorus is rarely necessary because it is so abundant in foods that an excess (which can obstruct calcium assimilation and lead to osteoporosis) is common.[190] Copper and zinc compete for absorption by the body, so copper supplements may be needed when high doses of zinc are taken. Other supplemental minerals include chromium, and selenium.

Amino Acids Twenty of these organic compounds must be present in the proper proportions in order for the body to biosynthesize the proteins essential for the maintenance of life. The body can manufacture twelve of the amino acids but the remainder must be obtained from the diet. Animal products, including milk and eggs, are complete proteins that provide all the essential amino acids; plant foods are incomplete proteins, lacking in one or more amino acids, but they can be combined to rectify these deficiencies.[17, 98]

Antioxidants Besides performing their basic functions, certain vitamins, minerals, and amino acids assist the immune system by protecting the body from self-produced oxidation and free radicals acquired from external contaminants in air, food, and water. When not kept in check by antioxidants, free radicals damage the basic structure of cells, can contribute to the development of practically any malady from arthritis to varicose veins, and are prime suspects in cancer and heart disease. The principal antioxidants are vitamins A (especially beta carotene), C and bioflavonoids, and E. Others are B_2, niacin, pantothenic acid, B_6, folic acid, B_{12}, and PABA; the minerals magnesium, manganese, selenium, and zinc; and the amino acids L-cysteine and L-glutathione. According to a report in *Natural Health* (October 1992), Coenzyme Q10 and garlic (from food sources or supplements), and SOD (superoxide dismutase, an enzyme) are recommended as antioxidants by an increasing number of orthomolecular and naturopathic doctors.

Essential Fatty Acids Once called vitamin F and often referred to as UFA, unsaturated fatty acids are essential for many bodily functions.

They are available from vegatable oils (except for coconut or palm kernel oil) and fish, or supplements of Omega-3 (EPA—eiosapentaenoic acid—primarily found in cold-water fish) and Omega-6 (GLA—gamma-linoleic acid—from primrose oil or black current seed oil).

Tissue Salts Also called biochemic cell salts, these are inorganic components of the body's tissues. First isolated by a German doctor in the 1870s for use in homeopathic medicine, tissue salt tablets are produced by the "trituration" of natural minerals and milk sugar to a dilution of 1 to 1 million for 6X, the most generally used potency. The third-trituration 3X tablets are less potent. One or more of the tiny tissue salt tablets may be dissolved under the tongue or in a little water for immediate assimilation. Only the twelve original tissue salts that have been used for over a century and are available in health food stores are mentioned in this book. They are shown in the remedies by the abbreviations under which they are sold.

Calc. Fluor. = Calcarea Flurica = Calcium Fluoride = Fluoride of Lime

Calc. Phos. = Calcarea Phosphorica = Calcium Phosphate = Phosphate of Lime

Calc. Sulph. = Calcarea Sulphurica = Calcium Sulphate = Sulphate of Lime

Ferr. Phos. = Ferrum Phosphoricum = Iron Phosphate

Kali. Mur. = Kali Muriaticum = Potassium Chloride = Phosphate of Potash

Kali. Phos. = Kali Phosphoricum = Potassium Phosphate = Phosphate of Potash

Kali. Sulph. = Kali Sulphuricum = Potassium Sulphate = Sulphate of Potash

Mag. Phos. = Magnesia Phosphorica = Magnesium Phosphate

Nat. Mur. = Natrum Muriaticum = Sodium Chloride = Chloride of Soda

Nat. Phos. = Natrum Phosphoricum = Sodium Phosphate = Phosphate of Soda

Nat. Sulph. = Natrum Sulpuricum = Sodium Sulphate = Sulphate of Soda

Silicea = Silicon Oxide or Dioxide = Silicic Acid

First-Aid Supplies

A well-stocked medicine chest should include a first-aid pamphlet containing instructions for procedures to be followed in case of serious injuries and a list of emergency telephone numbers if there is no community wide emergency medical services system with a three-digit phone number. Keeping basic first-aid items together saves time when attending to minor mishaps. A preassembled kit is convenient for boating, camping, or motor trips; a zip-close plastic bag packed with emergency supplies can be stored in a suitcase as an auxiliary kit for travelers.

Bandaging Materials These include adhesive tape (roll, box of assorted strips, plus "butterflies" to hold the edges of a cut together to minimize scarring) and gauze (2- or 3-inch roll and individually wrapped square pads). In lieu of a bandage, clear nail polish can be used to coat a clean paper cut to protect it from irritation. To stop bleeding, direct pressure can be applied with one of the gauze pads. If blood soaks through the pad, it should be left in place and another applied over it to avoid dislodging the coagulating blood cells. Clean cloth may be substituted for the gauze pads, but absorbent cotton should not be used because its fibers can adhere to the wound. Elevating the injured part and/or applying ice help slow the flow of blood. Medical help should be obtained for large cuts, deep puncture wounds, bleeding that cannot be stopped, and arterial bleeding that is bright red and spurting.

Ice Packs Freezing a mixture of 2 cups water and 1 cup rubbing alcohol in zip-close plastic bags provides flexible ice packs in assorted sizes; a package of frozen fruit or vegetables can be substituted in emergencies. To avoid the risk of frostbite, cloth should be placed between the ice bags and the skin. For small bumps and scrapes, little screw-top plastic bottles can be filled with water and stored in the freezer; for larger areas, a wet sponge or towel can be chilled in the freezing unit. Sports doctors suggest freezing water in styrofoam cups, which can be torn off as the ice is used to massage muscle aches and sprains for 10 or 15 minutes at a time. For this treatment, the ice should be kept in constant motion and removed if there is a burning sensation or if the skin turns red.[291]

Soap and Antiseptics To minimize the possibility of infection, cuts, scratches, and abrasions should be cleansed by swabbing with wet sterile gauze or clean cloth, or by holding the injury under running water. Washing the wound with soap is often recommended, but the *Berkeley Wellness Letter* (March 1992) warns that soap can damage tissue. Antiseptics, which kill certain microorganisms, can also damage the skin. When a disinfectant is desired, hydrogen peroxide is usually advised because it is less irritating than iodine or isopropyl alcohol.[322] However, a pain-relieving antiseptic to spray on small cuts, skinned knees, and other abrasions can be prepared by combining 1 tablespoon of iodine with ½ cup of rubbing alcohol in a spray bottle.[32]

Skin Soothers Aloe vera gel and petroleum jelly are suggested for irritation from dry air, sun exposure, or wind chapping. Aloe vera gel speeds healing and is a proven remedy for burns but should not be applied to open wounds. Petroleum jelly both soothes and helps restore damaged skin.

Basic Supplies These include thermometers (disposable, for travel kits), scissors (to cut bandages and to help remove clothing from burns), elastic bandages (for applying compression to ice packs or for wrapping sprained ankles or wrists), and a 40-inch square of cloth for slings. When over-the-counter painkillers are used, aspirin should not be given to children or teenagers, or to adults with ulcers; ibuprofen should not be taken by persons who are allergic to aspirin or who have kidney disease.[76]

Herbalists, holistic doctors, and naturopaths recommend including vitamin C (chewable tablets or crystals for rapid assimilation), cayenne pepper or powdered yellow dock (for topical application to staunch bleeding), and capsules of powdered ginger for nausea or motion sickness. The tissue salt Ferr. Phos. may help control bleeding when tablets are crushed and applied to a wound and when the tablets are dissolved in water and sponged over the injury may alleviate the pain of abrasions and contusions.

Folk practitioners suggest papain-containing meat tenderizer for bee or sea creature stings; a paste of baking soda for skin irritations; a solution of sugar and water for relief from insect bites, rashes, and minor burns; and the fumes from burning sugar for painful mishaps. When Madge O. slammed the car door on her finger as she was rushing to a luncheon meeting, she remembered witnessing a horse with a crushed hoof being calmed by having the leg held in the smoke from sugar burning in a bucket. In excruciating pain, Madge went directly to the restaurant chef and asked him to burn some sugar. The chef complied, using his steak-braising, blowtorchlike tool to ignite some sugar in a coffee can. The pain eased immediately, but Madge held her hand in the billowing smoke for several minutes as a precautionary measure before having lunch and making her pain-free presentation.

First-aid tips for animal bites, asthma, bitten tongue, black eyes, blisters, burns, diarrhea, frostbite, heat exhaustion, injured teeth, insects in the ear, nosebleeds, sea scrapes, snakebite, spider bite, sprains, stings (bees, hornets, wasps, yellow jackets, scorpions, jellyfish, and sea anemones), sunburn, and toothache are included in the text and listed in the Index.

Herbs and Folk Remedies

Many modern pharmaceuticals are based on ancient herbal curatives. For example, salicylic acid (the main component of aspirin) was first isolated from willow bark. Although the Federal Drug Administration regards herbs as foods safe for human consumption, several have been removed from the market and others are being studied. Herbs can have pronounced effects and can adversely interact with medications; therapeutic use of more than one or two capsules or cups of tea a day should be under the guidance of a professional. Anyone with severe symptoms or a serious illness should have the approval of a doctor before experimenting with herbs or folk cures. Some of the old remedies have been substantiated by scientific studies; others are shared here simply because people have found them helpful. Quantities and instructions for all of the remedies included in this book are adapted for modern usage, and all of the herbs, spices, and miscellaneous ingredients are obtainable from supermarkets, pharmacies, or health food stores.

Nerve Pressure and Massage

Acupressure, finger pressure, reflexology, reflex balance, jin shin jyut-su, shiatsu, and zone therapy are pressure and massage therapies used to relieve pain and to promote healing by stimulating points often far removed from the site of the disturbance. Sometimes described as acupuncture without needles, all the variations are based on the theory that invisible currents run throughout the body in longitudinal energy lines, meridian paths, or zones. Professional therapists advocate using finger or thumb pressure on the charted pressure points (buttons or neural receptors), identifying the precise location by a sensation of tenderness or tingling. Pressure can then be exerted steadily or as a pressing–rolling massage for 20 seconds to 5 minutes in alternating intervals of 10 seconds on and 10 seconds off, for 30 seconds of pressure; or as a series of seven to fourteen applications of pressure that gradually increases in intensity without being completely released. According to one theory, massaging the pressure points in a clockwise motion energizes the body; counterclockwise massage is relaxing.

Relaxation Techniques and Guided Imagery

The human body reacts to stressful situations with the same fight-or-flight response essential for survival in prehistoric times. It releases hormones that increase blood pressure, heart rate, and metabolism, and sends extra blood to the muscles by slowing other bodily functions such as digestion. The stress reaction is useful in a crisis, but since the body is unable to discriminate between the dangerous approach of a sabertoothed tiger and the frustration of a traffic snarl, this autonomic response usually must be reversed by a "relaxation response" rather than by clubbing an unreasonable employer or running away from a tax deadline. If not burned off by fighting or fleeing, the accumulation of stress hormones can bring about feelings of anxiety and depression; increase sensitivity to pain; and cause, contribute to, or worsen any disorder from acne to a yeast infection. According to a report in *American Health* (December 1992), stress-related complaints are responsible for 75 to 90 percent of all visits to physicians.

The relaxation response, first defined by Dr. Herbert Benson,[24, 25] can be elicited by stress-management techniques. Biofeedback, transcendental meditation, yoga, and Zen require professional assistance and training. Detailed instructions for the Benson system, progressive relaxation, the Silva method, autosuggestion, and other techniques for self-induced relaxation and healing through guided imagery are available in books and on tapes. Experimentation with these self-help approaches can determine the most effective program for each individual.

> **Controlled Breathing** Breathing in a controlled manner is the cornerstone of many relaxation disciplines. Taking a few deep breaths from the diaphragm (letting the stomach expand with each inhalation for a count of three, then exhaling for a count of six) can help offset immediate tension or anger and pave the way for complete relaxation.

Exercise A regular program of aerobic exercise may reduce susceptibility to stress. Physical exertion not only burns off the hormones released during the fight-or-flight response the way they were meant to be dissipated but can also produce natural opiates to elicit calm and even a euphoria in some instances. Muscles tensed from repressed irritation and frustration can be relaxed by a few minutes of gentle stretching exercises before bedtime. Walking briskly for 5 minutes during a break in a business meeting or between classes dissipates stress responses if tension-creating thoughts are pushed aside and concentration is focused on the cadence of breathing and the repetitiveness of feet meeting the floor or pavement.[49]

Progressive Relaxation (PR) First described in the 1930s by Dr. Edmond Jacobson, progressive relaxation now encompasses elements from several disciplines and can be used in conjunction with healing techniques.

○ Sit or recline comfortably with eyes closed in a quiet room. Take a few deep breaths and, starting with either the feet or the face, tense and relax each muscle group in sequence.

○ Visualize a peaceful place, such as a private beach, and become immersed in the surroundings by imagining the feel of the sand, the warmth of the sun, the salty aroma of the ocean, and the sounds of the soaring sea gulls and the waves lapping on the shore.

○ Select a word such as "peace" or "salaam" that conveys relaxing connotations and repeat it mentally with each breath for 10 to 20 minutes. If distracting sounds or thoughts intrude, they should be passively ignored and the mind refocused on repetition of the mantra. Daily practice may make it possible to use the chosen focus word as a cue for achieving complete relaxation by simply closing the eyes and concentrating on deep breathing for a minute or two in any surrounding.

○ Emerge from the relaxed state gradually before opening the eyes and returning to normal activity.

Guided Imagery and **Positive Affirmations** These help reprogram the body for healing and better health. Both may be used while relaxing with PR or may be substituted for mantra repetitions.

Slowly counting backward from ten to one while picturing each number and mentally saying, "Nine, I am growing more relaxed; eight, I am growing more relaxed . . ." may encourage communication between both hemispheres of the brain and help establish the physiological state in which the body can use its energy for repair and healing as it normally does for short periods during deep sleep.[112, 113]

Positive self-suggestions to augment more orthodox methods of treatment may be generalized ("the pain is fading") or specific ("my elbow is comfortable"). Reinforcing verbal phrases with visual imagery increases the benefits. Mentally picturing the elbow in perfect condition or vividly imagining rubbing a magically curative salve over it provides show-and-tell instructions for the subconscious. Other options include fanciful visualizations such as painting uncomfortable areas with white light or imagining a row of miniature robots knitting a broken bone together.

After a few minutes of autosuggestion and images, further benefits may be derived by adding affirmations such as, "When I open my eyes at the count of five, I will feel better than before," reaffirming at the count of three, and concluding with, "Five, I am wide awake and feeling better."

Sources (see Bibliography)

17, 19, 24, 25, 32, 47, 49, 58, 64, 65, 76, 86, 98, 111, 112, 113, 117, 149, 150, 151, 177, 186, 189, 190, 265, 270, 271, 291, 293, 294, 295, 308, 319, 321, 322

Aching, Burning Feet; Blisters; and Ingrown Toenails

The average person walks 45,000 miles by the age of 35, and each step concentrates a force one-third greater than full body weight on each foot.[232] Even when provided with correctly fitted shoes, feet may rebel unless treated with consideration. Their covering of skin and nerves close to the surface reflect internal deficiencies as well as external pressures by tingling, burning, and blistering. Their bones (28 per foot) and musculature (107 ligaments, 31 tendons, 18 muscles)[112] require nutritional nourishing from a well-balanced diet, as well as occasional release from confinement for care and exercise.

Foot Baths for Aching Feet

Lorna C. sits on the side of her bathtub and utilizes a hand-held shower spray for a 2-minute foot freshener between shopping expeditions. For truly weary feet, 15-minute soaks are more effective. Ralph R. credits his improvised foot tub with saving his job. He was well enough to return to work at the machine shop, but months of enforced idleness had left his feet unable to cope with steel-toed safety shoes and concrete floors. Their agonizing aching forced him to head for home and a restorative foot bath an hour before quitting time on the first day. The next morning, Ralph took along a small ice chest half-filled with water so he could give his feet a midday break while he ate lunch in his car. After 2 weeks of this pampering, his feet could make it through the days with only nighttime soaks.

For Stiff, Aching Feet Add a handful of epsom salts or table salt to a warm-water footbath, or use diluted camomile or oak bark tea, then rinse with cool water.

For Sore or Swollen Feet Alternate 5 minutes of comfortably hot saltwater soaking with 2 minutes in cool water. Repeat the sequence and rinse with cold water.

Exercise and Massage

Standing up or sitting down for extended periods can cause feet to swell, ache, and cramp unless they are moved every few minutes. Alternating heel heights from day to day can prevent the aching arches and shortened tendons that engender foot and leg pain for lovely ladies in 3-inch heels and macho men in cowboy boots.

- **Calf and heel stretches** relieve plantar fasciitis (pain along the bottom of the foot in the fibrous bands connecting heels and toes) and strengthen Achilles tendons. (1) Sitting with bare feet elevated, rotate both feet from the ankles ten times in both directions, then point toes down and up ten times. (2) Standing in bare feet, rise up on the toes and down on the heels ten times. (3) With hands at shoulder level flat against a wall, step back about 30 inches, then lean forward while keeping heels in contact with the floor.

- **Foot relaxing and revitalizing exercises.** (1) While sitting down, roll bare feet over tennis balls, 12-ounce beverage cans, or a rolling pin. (2) Either sitting or standing, scrunch up a terry cloth towel or try to pick up marbles or pencils with only the toes.

- **Foot massage,** besides abolishing the tired-all-over feeling emanating from weary feet, can intercept pain impulses being relayed along the nerves between feet and brain. (1) Smooth lotion over each foot, then use the thumbs to rub with circular movements from the soles, over the insteps, and around the ankles. If the skin is chafed or irritated, substitute aloe vera gel, castor oil, or garlic oil for the lotion. (2) To alleviate swollen feet, massage each toe and apply firm pressure on the cuticle, the knuckle, and the base of each toe.

Burning Feet

Temporarily fiery feet may be caused by air-excluding shoes or perspiration-retaining cotton or wool socks—orlon and spun acrylic draw moisture away from the feet; natural leather and "breathable" shoes allow perspiration to evaporate. Other possible causes are allergic reactions to the dye in new hosiery, the chemicals used in tanning leather, or the rubber compounds in athletic shoes.

Persistently scorching soles and tingling toes may be caused by nerve inflammation which can be relieved by supplementing the diet with B vitamins. During World War II, B_1, B_2, and pantothenic acid cleared up the painfully burning feet of returning prisoners; including B_6 and B_{12} abolished pins-and-needles sensations as well.[3, 87] Stirring a tablespoon of brewer's yeast into a glass of juice or milk for breakfast and taking a B-complex tablet each day often solves the problem in a few weeks. Recovery may be speeded by taking three 6X tablets *each* of the tissue salts Ferr. Phos. and Silicea 3 times a day.

Foot baths are folk healers' solutions for burning feet. To a basin of cool water they advise adding one of the following remedies: (1) 2 tablespoons *each* ammonia and rubbing alcohol; ¼ cup *each* baking soda and table salt; 2 cups of brewed camomile, comfrey, horsetail, lavender, mint, oak bark, or sage tea; 1 cup apple cider vinegar and ⅓ cup lemon juice. (2) two cups of water boiled with 1 cup of used coffee grounds, then cooled and strained. Follow with a rinse of cold water, thorough drying, and a dusting of cornstarch or talc.

Burning feet that do not respond to home remedies should be checked by a physician—they could harbor a fungal infection (see "Athlete's Foot") or a neuroma (a benign tumor composed of nerve cells), or they might be an early warning of diabetes, or atherosclerosis.

Hot Spots and Blisters

First-Aid Tip Whether initiated by ill-fitting shoes or socks, or by not wearing hose, reddened, chafed skin on the feet portends blisters unless immediate action is taken. Lightly rubbing the area with an ice cube deadens the pain. Applying a piece of adhesive tape over the irritated spot or padding around the tender areas with foam or felt reduces further friction. So does a sprinkling of powder or a coating of petroleum jelly, or donning two pairs of lightweight socks instead of one thick pair when wearing athletic shoes or hiking boots.

If a blister does develop, twentieth-century treatment is less painful and less likely to cause complications than the old-fashioned practice of drawing a needle with worsted thread through the blister, clipping both ends, and leaving it until the skin peeled off. The liquid inside a blister is an ideal growth medium for bacteria that can cause infection. Prompt puncturing removes this threat and speeds healing by allowing the covering skin to adhere to the raw flesh. After washing with soap and water or swabbing with alcohol or hydrogen peroxide, prick the blister with a needle sterilized in alcohol or over a match flame. Blot the fluid with sterile gauze, then apply a small bandage with an air-vented center. Coating the pierced blister with aloe vera gel or the oil from a garlic perle hastens healing, as does removing the bandage whenever possible to allow the free flow of air. A blister that breaks by itself should be treated the same as a punctured one but warrants even closer observation for signs of infection requiring medical care.

Ingrown Toenails

Although ingrown nails can result from stubbed toes or blows to the nails, the usual causes are improper toenail trimming and shoe pressure. Obesity may be a contributing factor if flabby tissue engulfs the nail. Cutting a V-shaped notch in the center does not prevent or correct ingrown nails and can be hazardous to the health of the toe. Toenails should be clipped straight across and smoothed with an emery board or nail file, not rounded to an oval.

People who are prone to ingrown toenails may benefit from daily doses of the tissue salt Silicea, plus an application of vitamin E oil over the nails at least once a month. Traditional treatment calls for a softening soak in warm water, then gentle insertion of a wisp of cotton between nail and skin. Adding Epsom salts to the water and saturating the cotton with castor oil or oil squeezed from capsules of vitamin A or vitamin E enhances the treatment's effectiveness. A badly ingrown nail may require the assistance of a podiatrist to prevent infection from developing.

Sources (see Bibliography)

3, 43, 46, 47, 53, 65, 85, 86, 87, 109, 111, 112, 159, 165, 177, 186, 190, 202, 203, 206, 232, 233, 256, 283, 284, 289, 291, 292, 293, 300, 304

Acre

Genetically inherited pore defects, not food preferences or sexual practices, are the determining factor in acne's selection of victims.
Nutritious foods are important for good health—only in the case of allergy
or overindulgence are junk foods considered responsible for the onset of
acne. As production of sebum (a skin-lubricating substance secreted by the
sebaceous glands) surges during adolescence, pore openings can become
clogged and comedones develop—"whiteheads" when enclosed with skin;
"blackheads" if open and oxidized to a dark color. The pustules of acne
vulgaris result from bacterial growth within the comedones. Mental stress
often triggers before-the-prom zits and outbreaks of adult acne; allergic
reactions to cosmetics, foods, or medications are other potential instigators.

Gently removing the droplet of pus from a pimple may speed its healing, but
vigorous squeezing contributes to scarring and can force bacteria into surrounding
tissue, spreading the acne. Shaving presents special problems for acne-beset men.
Vito L., who is barbering his third generation of customers, volunteers these words
of wisdom: "Don't shave if you don't have to. When you do have to, shave with
the grain—not against it—'smooth' isn't that important. If you shave with a blade
razor, lather up with your hands—the bristles of a shaving brush will hang onto
those pimply germs and spread them around so your face will never clear up."

Diet

A natural low-fat diet accentuating fresh fruits, vegetables, and whole
grains aids acne control. Two servings of beets or beet juice weekly, and/or
two glasses of carrot juice daily (blended with the juice from cucumber,
lettuce, or spinach, if desired) reportedly have improved acne within a few
weeks.[36, 144, 218] Avoiding certain foods brings relief to many acne sufferers.
Common offenders are chocolate, refined sugar, saturated fats, alcohol, and

caffeine. Eliminating all the possible offenders for 2 weeks then reintroducing them one at a time may identify individual culprits.

Herbal specifics for acne include burdock, chickweed, dandelion, echinacea, red clover, white oak bark, valerian, and yellow dock. One or two capsules of any one of those herbs can be taken daily, or one or two cups of the tea may be sipped and some of the liquid sponged over acne lesions. Chaparral and comfrey tea are considered excellent facial rinses.

Supplements (see note on page xii)

Vitamin A   In the form of beta carotene, 10,000 to 25,000 IU once or twice a day (under medical supervision, up to 100,000 IU daily for 1 month).

B Complex   One comprehensive tablet daily plus up to 300 milligrams each B_6, niacin, and pantothenic acid in divided doses each day for no longer than a month. Vitamin B_6, taken in small doses throughout the month, is especially effective for acne that flares up during menstrual periods.

Vitamin C and Bioflavonoids   1,000 to 3,000 milligrams of vitamin C and 200 to 1,000 milligrams of bioflavonoids in divided daily doses speed healing and retard spreading.

Vitamin E   100 to 800 IU daily to protect vitamin A from destruction within the body.

Calcium   If milk and dairy products are restricted, calcium supplements totaling 800 milligrams a day will help maintain the acid/alkali balance necessary for a clear complexion.[98]

Zinc   30 to 50 milligrams, daily during outbreaks. Besides being an effective bacterial suppressor, zinc aids healing and is essential for oil gland efficiency.

Acidophilus   One or two capsules or a serving of acidophilus yogurt with each meal—particularly important if antibiotics have been prescribed.

Brewer's Yeast   One or two tablespoons a day. Stirring the yeast into skim milk and accompanying the mixture with two lecithin capsules has cleared many cases of acne.[58]

Charcoal Taking two activated charcoal tablets after each meal for 2 weeks, then two tablets daily, thereafter, has accomplished astounding results in clinical tests[143] but should not be continued for extended periods because charcoal can interfere with nutrient absorption.

Tissue Salts Three tablets of 6X Calc. Phos. three or four times daily is the suggested remedy for adolescent acne. If skin is inflamed, alternating doses of Calc. Sulph., Ferr. Phos., Kali. Sulph., Nat. Phos., and Silicea may be added. When acne is slow to heal, Nat. Sulph. may be of benefit.[55, 64, 65]

Cleansing and Treating

Gentle cleansing is a vital component of acne treatment. Frequent shampooing helps prevent acne from spreading to the scalp. For acne-affected skin; washing twice daily with mild soap, rinsing thoroughly with warm water, then pat-drying with a soft towel is the generally accepted method. For those who would rather not use soap, optional washing liquids are milk (buttermilk can be blotted dry without rinsing), diluted lemon juice, a solution of one part alcohol to ten parts water, or double-strength papaya-mint tea.

Herbalists suggest facial saunas. Cover the head with a towel and lean over a bowl of steaming tea prepared from a blend of red clover, lavender, and strawberry leaf; or from two parts elder flowers to one part eucalyptus leaves. As an option, a poultice of ground chaparral, dandelion, or yellow dock root mixed with hot water and cooled can be applied to the affected areas and allowed to remain for several hours, then rinsed off with tepid water.

Nutrient-laden foods can be used as external treatments when patted over affected areas and allowed to penetrate for 20 minutes before being rinsed off.

Carrots Cook in as little water as possible, then mash and cool.

Cucumber Peel if coated with wax, then grate or slice very thin and soak in rum.

Egg Yolk Whisk with a spoonful of water.

Oatmeal Cook in milk until thickened; cool before applying.

Tomato-Oatmeal Whir a chopped ripe tomato in an electric blender with a tablespoon of dry oatmeal and a teaspoon of lemon juice.

Nonedible Options As suggested by folk healers; apply a paste of baking soda mixed with water, rinse immediately with water, follow with a rinse or spray of diluted apple cider vinegar, then conclude with a clear-water rinse. Or smooth on the oil from a vitamin E capsule, wait 30 minutes, then apply a coating of lightly whisked egg white and let it dry before rinsing off.

Spot Treatments

The old-fashioned practice of rubbing acne lesions with fresh garlic several times a day is believed safe and is undoubtedly effective—at least it prohibits anyone from coming close enough to notice the blemishes! Barbara B. prefers milk of magnesia, the home remedy she credits with clearing her teenage acne, as a before-bed coating for each adult-acne pimple that appears. An overnight coating of toothpaste is another option. Gerald and Jerry T., an acne-prone father and son duo, concoct their own medication to dab on and leave overnight: a spoonful of cornstarch mixed to a paste with rubbing alcohol.

Nerve Pressure and Massage

For acne control, reflexologists advise stimulating any or all of the following points once each day.

- On each shoulder, press and massage the outer edge of the hollow just beneath the collarbone.
- Bend the left arm at a 45-degree angle. Use the right thumb to press the point where the elbow crease ends on the outer arm. Repeat with the right arm.
- Clench the left fist, leaving thumb extended against the index finger. With the right thumb, press or massage the mound formed between the thumb and index finger. Repeat with the other hand.

Sources (see Bibliography)

6, 13, 17, 32, 36, 41, 42, 44, 53, 55, 57, 58, 64, 65, 75, 80, 81, 82, 86, 87, 89, 98, 111, 112, 121, 122, 137, 143, 144, 156, 159, 161, 166, 176, 190, 193, 205, 218, 226, 233, 234, 256, 260, 278, 281, 282, 283, 286

Allergy

The American Medical Association describes allergies as inappropriate or exaggerated reactions of the immune system. Researchers believe that a genetic tendency to produce greater than normal amounts of a histamine-producing antibody accounts for abnormal responses to ordinarily harmless substances. Stress, insufficient sleep, infections, or poor diet can predispose the body to allergic reactions. For susceptible people, anything from inhaling airborne pollens to being zapped by an insect can trigger responses manifested as any affliction from asthma to pimples.

Identification and avoidance are the basics of allergy management. Life-threatening reactions such as heart irregularities or severe breathing difficulties warrant tests and treatment by an allergist. Lesser irritations often can be self-helped. Easily detected allergens create obvious responses, for example, breaking out in a rash after eating strawberries or becoming sneezy and itchy-eyed while petting a puppy. More detective effort is required for pinpointing subtle allergens. They may lurk in customary cosmetics or laundry detergents—and even in hypoallergenic products. Switching brands may be the solution. The formaldehyde incorporated in permanent-press material to prevent wrinkling can cause problems when released by body warmth and moisture—linen, silk, pure synthetics, and Sanforized fabrics are formaldehyde-free options. Symptom-instigating dust mites (microscopic animals that thrive in household fabrics) can be minimized by replacing carpets with bare floors and washable rugs.

Temperature extremes are tricky allergens that can trigger asthmatic attacks. Cold allergy is more common in children; heat allergy in adults. To test for cold: place an ice cube on the skin for a minute or two. If inflammation or hives appear, a cold allergy is indicated. Heat allergy is confirmed if red bumps develop after soaking the hands in 100-degree water for a few minutes.

Food Allergies

Allergic reactions to edibles have long beset mortals. Lucretius' first-century-B.C. declaration: "What is food for some may be fierce poison for others," holds true, but the Babylonian Talmud's advice for curing food allergies by building up tolerance through ingestion of small amounts (2 grains per day of an offending substance such as wheat) is no longer considered viable. The immunotherapy of periodically injecting a drop or two of an allergen has been found to reinforce rather than desensitize in many cases of food allergy[204] but usually is effective against cat allergies. And according to a report in the June 1991 issue of *In Health*, professional insect venom therapy almost always works.

Gastrointestinal distress experienced after ingesting milk products may not be an allergy. If the difficulty is due to a genetic lack of the enzyme lactase, which is essential for digestion of the milk sugar lactose, taking lactase supplements can correct the problem without having to eliminate the milk. Besides chemical colorings and preservatives, the most common allergens among foodstuffs are chocolate, citrus, corn, eggs, peanuts, peas, shrimp, strawberries, tomatoes, and wheat. Self-testing usually identifies specific culprits.

- ○ If one food is suspect, avoid it for a week or 2, then try it again to see if the symptoms reappear. For precise testing, allergists recommend checking the pulse rate before eating the food and again 20 minutes afterward—an increase of 10 beats per minute indicates an allergic response.[17] The food should be reintroduced as part of a meal; eating it by itself on an empty stomach could turn a mild reaction into a severe one.

- ○ If no particular food is suspected, test favorite foods first. A craving for allergenic foods can be a form of addiction—the subconscious compulsion is for the temporary "high" produced before unpleasant reactions appear.

- ○ Super-sleuthing may be necessary when mild allergies are caused by an amalgamation of foods. Mabel J. discovered that her occasional allergic reaction of immediate diarrhea after a meal was not a response to any one food but to any combination of several foods to which she was only marginally allergic, for instance, eggs and oranges. A breakfast egg was fine with a glass of cranberry juice; orange juice with a bowl of oatmeal was acceptable; but an egg plus orange juice had her off and running. Peas, shrimp, and tomatoes were other foods she could not tolerate two at a time.

Diet and Supplements (see note on page xii)

Taking a teaspoon or two of bee pollen granules every day has prevented or corrected allergic disturbances for some people. Accompanying each meal with two acidophilus capsules, a serving of yogurt, or a glass of water blended with 2 teaspoons *each* apple cider vinegar and honey has relieved symptoms for others. Herbs with antihistamine properties include burdock, comfrey, dandelion, eyebright, fenugreek, goldenseal (unless allergic to ragweed), lobelia, and St. Mary's thistle.

B Vitamins Taking 50 to 100 milligrams of pantothenic acid three times a day for a few days stimulates the production of allergy-fighting cortisone within the body. A daily B-complex tablet plus sublingual B_{12} may also be helpful.

Vitamin C This vitamin acts as a detoxifying agent and antihistamine and helps regulate immune system responses. Most effective when taken before exposure or when combined with B-vitamin therapy after symptoms are present, up to 1,000 milligrams of vitamin C each hour can be used during severe attacks.[87]

Vitamin E Essential for proper immune function, vitamin E's antiallergenic properties are most efficient when 100 to 800 IU are taken for several days prior to anticipated exposure to allergens.[234]

Sources (see Bibliography)

6, 17, 33, 41, 44, 45, 46, 62, 72, 75, 87, 89, 98, 109, 111, 112, 122, 148, 159, 162, 172, 176, 183, 204, 207, 234, 239, 256, 264, 278, 281, 282, 283, 293, 302, 316, 317

Anemia

Iron is an essential component of the hemoglobin molecules necessary for the blood's transport of oxygen to all parts of the body. Insufficient hemoglobin or a reduction in the number of red blood cells results in symptoms of anemia: fatigue, loss of appetite, pallor, cold hands. Severe anemia can weaken the immune system, impair wound healing, and cause poor coordination and mental fuzziness.

Diet

The RDAs for iron are 10 milligrams for men of all ages and women over 51; 15 milligrams for women during their childbearing years. The average American diet provides 6 milligrams of iron per 1,000 calories, yet iron deficiency is common—largely due to the vagaries of absorption.

Fifteen to 30 percent of the organic heme iron in meat, poultry, and seafood is assimilated by the body; only about 5 percent of the inorganic nonheme iron in dairy products, fruits, vegetables, and grains (and the substances used to enrich them) is assimilated. Although all grains, vegetables, and fruits contain nonheme iron, they also contain substances that hinder its assimilation. The phytates are substances in high-fiber foods which can bind with some of the iron so the body cannot absorb it. Iron-rich spinach (3.2 milligrams per fresh-cooked half cup), cashews (4.1 milligrams per dry-roasted half cup), and other nuts and grains harbor oxalic acid, which interferes with iron absorption. Phosphate additives used in bakery goods, beer, soft drinks, candy, ice cream, and many packaged foods reduce the absorption of iron, as does the cadmium from smoking. Studies reported in *Longevity* (February 1991) show that polyphenols in coffee and tannins in tea lower the amount of iron assimilated from foods by 40 to 90 percent if they are sipped with a meal (drinking either beverage between meals has no effect on iron). To increase iron absorption:

○ Accompany meals, especially meatless ones, with foods that are high in vitamin C, such as tomatoes and citrus fruits. Drinking a glass of orange juice with breakfast cereal doubles or triples the amount of iron absorbed.

○ Include heme-iron-containing foods with otherwise meatless meals. Adding a few shrimp to a pasta salad, or bits of beef or chicken to chili beans, increases nonheme iron absorption up to tenfold.

Food Sources of Iron*			
Heme Iron per 3-oz. serving	mg	Nonheme Iron	mg
Clams	5.2	1 Tbs. blackstrap molasses	3.2
Raw oysters	4.8	½ cup baked beans	3.0
Lean pork	3.3	1 med. baked potato w/skin	2.8
Lean beef	3.0	1½ oz. dried apricots	2.0
Chicken, dark meat.	2.5	½ cup cooked lima beans	2.0
Fish	1.0	3 Tbs. peanut butter	0.9
*Compiled from *Nutritive Value of Foods*[130] and *Wellness Encyclopedia*.[300]			

Cholesterol conscious restriction of red meat and increased consumption of fiber for other facets of good health make adequate iron acquisition more complex than it once was, but it can be accomplished. In ancient times, physicians dipped a sword in water or wine, then had the anemic patient drink the liquid to absorb the strength of the sword. Folk healers advise sipping a glass of water combined with 1 teaspoon apple cider vinegar, or with 2 teaspoons *each* apple cider vinegar and blackstrap molasses, with each meal. For vegetarians, people on low-calorie diets, and others at high risk for anemia, nutritionists suggest 1 or 2 glasses daily of any combination of the following fruit and vegetable juices: apricot, beet (the juice from fresh red beets has been a remedy for anemic symptoms since the Middle Ages), blueberry, carrot, celery, cranberry, cucumber, grape, prune, or spinach. Herbalists recommend a cup or two daily of any of these teas: alfalfa, comfrey, dandelion, fenugreek, mullein, nettle, or red raspberry. Old-fashioned tea tonic is an intriguing option. Steep 1 ounce *each* camomile tea leaves and ground orange peel with ½ teaspoon ground ginger in 2 cups boiling water. Cool and strain, then add ½ cup brandy, and take half a cupful several times a day.

Supplements (see note on page xii)

Self-diagnosis and self-treatment with iron supplements is not recommended. Studies reported in *American Health* (December 1992) indicate that iron overload increases heart attack risk. If iron is prescribed, taking the supplements at night on an empty stomach with a glass of orange juice maximizes iron assimilation while minimizing stomach upset. Professional diagnosis is essential because iron-deficiency anemia can be caused by internal bleeding, which requires prompt medical attention; some people are susceptible to iron toxicity because their bodies cannot regulate iron absorption; and there are other forms of anemia that cannot be corrected by iron supplementation.

Pernicious anemia (macrocytic anemia) is a vitamin B_{12}-deficiency disease that usually occurs when the digestive system is unable to absorb B_{12} from foods. Standard treatment is a monthly injection of B_{12}. According to the July 1991 issue of *Longevity*, however, oral doses of 1,000 micrograms have been effective for 40 percent of the patients in one study. Strict vegetarians, alcoholics, and the elderly are targets for megaloblastic anemia from lack of B_{12} and/or folic acid. This type of anemia can be remedied with diet and oral supplements, but medical supervision is essential because large amounts of folic acid can mask pernicious anemia.

B Complex One comprehensive tablet daily, plus individual B vitamins as advised by a physician. Besides B_{12}/folic acid-deficiency anemias, there are others that respond only to 100 milligrams a day of either B_2 or B_6.

Vitamin C 500 to 1,500 milligrams in divided doses with meals to increase iron absorption.

Vitamin E 100 to 600 IU daily. Hemolytic anemia can result when a deficiency of vitamin E causes a reduction in red blood cells.

Bee Pollen For people who are not allergic to bee pollen, one teaspoon of granules or the equivalent in tablets each day. Tests have shown that bee pollen stimulates the body's production of hemoglobin.[302]

Tissue Salts To increase the number of red blood cells and their hemoglobin content, homeopathic doctors suggest taking 3 tablets, 3 times a day, of any or all of these 6X-potency tissue salts: Calc. Phos., Calc. Sulph., Ferr. Phos.

A combination of diet and supplements proved beneficial for Frieda G., who was still abed one afternoon when a neighbor came to call. "I'm not sick; I just didn't feel like getting up today," Frieda assured her worried friend, but she did agree to a medical checkup. The only problems indicated were low stomach acid (hydrochloric acid, necessary to dissolve iron so it can be assimilated) and borderline anemia. "Well, I haven't bothered with cooking meat-and-potato meals since Josh passed on," 78-year-old Frieda admitted when queried about her diet, "but I do eat. I have a snack and a cup of tea whenever I get hungry." Her new, easy-to-prepare regimen required several changes: cereal and juice instead of tea and toast for breakfast, sweet snacks replaced with light meals concocted from deli salads and frozen entrees, and supplements from the health food store—250 milligrams of vitamin C and one 324-milligram tablet of betaine hydrochloride after each meal, plus a daily multivitamin-mineral, 800 milligrams of folic acid, and 1,000 micrograms of B_{12}. Within a few weeks, Frieda's lethargy turned into energy, and she spends her afternoons visiting, not napping.

Nerve Pressure and Massage

Pressing and massaging the hollows on each side of the spine at the base of the skull; or massaging the outer edge of the left hand between the base of the little finger and the wrist, and/or the outer edge of the underside of the left foot between the center of the arch and the little toe is believed to help increase the production of red blood cells within the body.

Sources (see Bibliography)

2, 6, 17, 26, 39, 50, 59, 72, 75, 81, 86, 87, 92, 98, 106, 111, 126, 130, 138, 143, 148, 151, 156, 162, 163, 171, 173, 179, 186, 190, 204, 205, 218, 222, 226, 234, 262, 282, 283, 300, 302, 315

Arteriosclerosis and Atherosclerosis

Atherosclerosis (fatty deposits on artery walls) is the most common type of arteriosclerosis, a group of disorders that cause arterial thickening and loss of elasticity. Atherosclerosis begins when streaks of cholesterol stick to the interior of the arteries. As blood flows through the narrowed channels at greater pressure, platelets (particles in the blood that assist coagulation), additional lipids (fats), and cellular debris build up over the patches of fatty plaque. As circulation is impeded, calcium deposits can harden over the plaque to cause "hardening of the arteries," or a portion of the plaque may rupture to form a blood clot that further obstructs the flow of blood and can lead to a stroke or heart attack.

A family history of heart disease also increases the likelihood of developing atherosclerosis. Hypertension (high blood pressure); the inability to effectively metabolize sugar, refined carbohydrates, or fats; or familial hypercholesterolemia (abnormally high cholesterol) may be genetic in origin. Physical inactivity, smoking, unrelieved stress reactions, high cholesterol levels, dietary excesses or deficiencies, and obesity are risk factors that can be modified to reduce the probability of developing atherosclerosis and, in many cases, even clear partially clogged arteries. Exercise (30 minutes of brisk walking or its aerobic equivalent three times a week) strengthens the heart, improves circulation, and helps work off the adrenal hormones produced by stress. Anxiety, anger, and other types of stress use up nutrients needed for fat metabolization and when not alleviated by the relaxation techniques described in the Introduction, release hormones that can create minute injuries in the walls of the arteries and make them more susceptible to arterial plaque.[98]

17

Diet

The American Heart Association recommends limiting dietary fats to 30 percent of daily calories—with no more than one-third derived from the saturated fat in meats and dairy products, the remainder from polyunsaturated and monounsaturated vegetable fats. Coconut and palm oils (the most highly saturated of all natural fats) should be avoided. Cold pressed oils are advised (heat expressing alters their chemical structure), hydrogenating the oils for solid shortening or margarine produces a type of fat that can be more harmful than naturally saturated fat.[308] Polyunsaturated oils (such as corn, safflower, and soybean) contain linoleic acid, which is essential for the body's utilization of fat; monounsaturated canola or olive oil slightly improves the ratio of "good" HDL cholesterol to the "bad," artery-clogging LDL cholesterol.

As reported in the February 1990 issue of *Atherosclerosis*, researchers are now speculating that the low heart attack rate of Eskimos may be due as much to the high proportion (58 percent) of monounsaturates in whale and seal blubber as to the heart-healthy omega-3 fatty acids from the cod and herring in their high-fat diets. At 9 calories per gram of fat, the daily fat allowance from a 2,000-calorie diet equals 60 grams—1 tablespoon of vegetable oil contains 14 grams of fat, approximately 120 calories. By taking advantage of the array of fat- and cholesterol-free products, and by baking, broiling, microwaving, or steaming natural foods, a low-fat diet need not entail any deprivation.

Broccoli, brussels sprouts, cantaloupe, carrots, pumpkin, sweet potatoes, and spinach are considered especially beneficial in providing the nutrients needed for healthy arteries. All fresh vegetable and fruit juices—up to two glasses daily of any combination of beet, carrot, celery, citrus, parsley, and spinach—are helpful. Alcohol not utilized for immediate energy is transformed into saturated fat, as are excess amounts of sugar and refined carbohydrates, so these substances should be limited. As substitutes for caffeine-containing beverages, which may contribute to atherosclerosis, herbalists suggest cayenne, chickweed, comfrey, red clover, rose hip, and sage teas.

Supplements (see note on page xii)

Hardening and narrowing of the arteries is not a new ailment. The 2,100-year-old mummy of an Egyptian who died at the age of 40 shows atherosclerotic plaque.

And the disease is becoming more common. Autopsies performed on American soldiers killed in Korea and Vietnam showed that 77 percent of those healthy young men had some form of arteriosclerosis, while similar studies conducted during World Wars I and II revealed little or no signs of the malady. Since all the soldiers were physically active, ate approximately the same amounts of cholesterol and fat, and were subject to equal stress, an assortment of explanations for this change in arterial health have been investigated. Increased sugar consumption along with a lack of fiber in processed foods is considered partially responsible. Mounting scientific evidence, however, indicates that antioxidants may be the crucial clue to the secret of healthy arteries. Expanding on Dr. Passwater's theory[221] that obstructed arteries are caused by an accumulation of mutant cells from food additives and pesticides, the control of free radicals with vitamin antioxidants are the subject of ongoing clinical studies. Beta carotene and vitamins C and E (the major antioxidants) apparently help prevent fatty deposits on artery walls by scavenging the free radicals produced within the body or inhaled or ingested from outside sources.

Vitamin A   In the form of beta carotene 15,000 to 50,000 IU daily for its antioxidant properties.

B Complex   One comprehensive tablet once or twice daily. B vitamins assist in the metabolization of fat. Under medical supervision, 100 to 3,000 milligrams of niacin in divided doses have been used to dilate small arteries and lower cholesterol.

Vitamin C and Bioflavonoids   500 to 5,000 milligrams of vitamin C and 300 to 600 milligrams of bioflavonoids, in divided doses daily. Besides being a scavenger of free radicals, ascorbic acid and the bioflavonoids help preserve the health of artery walls so they are less susceptible to atherosclerotic lesions.

Vitamin E   100 IU daily, gradually increased to 400 to 1,000 IU. In addition to its antioxidant capability, vitamin E helps clear arterial scars to discourage atherosclerotic deposits, helps dissolve preexisting blood clots, and, as reported in *Journal of the American College of Nutrition* (October 1991), reduces 80 percent of the ability of blood platelets to stick to the plaque on artery walls.

Calcium and Magnesium   500 to 1,500 milligrams of calcium plus 300 to 750 milligrams of magnesium in divided daily doses. Calcium is essential for nerve and muscle function as well as for a sturdy skeleton. When there is a deficiency of calcium, the body withdraws it from the bones (which can lead to osteoporosis), and some of the withdrawn calcium clings to the artery walls before being delivered to the areas where it is needed.[151] Magnesium is necessary for the assimilation of calcium and the prevention of cell calcification. Although a two-to-one ratio of calcium to magnesium is generally advised,[190] some nutritional consultants believe the proportions should be reversed so that more magnesium than calcium is provided.

Selenium   100 to 200 micrograms daily. Selenium promotes the action of vitamins C and E to protect against arterial plaque.

Zinc   10 to 30 milligrams daily. Adequate amounts of zinc reduce the likelihood of fatty deposits on the arteries and assist the cleansing of already obstructed arteries.

Lecithin   Two capsules with each meal, or 1 to 2 tablespoons of granules daily. Lecithin emulsifies fats in the blood so they can be utilized by the body and is believed to help break up existing plaque on arterial walls.

Tissue Salts   To compensate for the reduced circulation caused by hardened or clogged arteries, three or four tablets of these 6X-potency tissue salts may be taken three or four times a day: Calc. Phos. if the hands and feet are always cold; Silicea for internal chilliness—if accompanied by cold extremities, add Nat. Mur.

Nerve Pressure and Massage

Once or twice each day, press and massage inward and upward against the hinge of the jawbone, just in front of the ears.

Sources (see Bibliography)

2, 14, 15, 17, 57, 64, 75, 78, 82, 87, 98, 105, 111, 151, 155, 157, 164, 177, 186, 190, 203, 205, 207, 215, 218, 223, 224, 228, 248, 254, 264, 268, 281, 283, 285, 293, 294, 300, 301, 303, 308, 314, 316, 317, 320

Arthritis

Prehistoric skeletons reveal that dinosaurs had arthritis; so did the Java man. In ancient Rome, arthritics were exempt from paying taxes—an impractical plan for the United States where more than 37 million people suffer from the disease.[174] Two forms of osteoarthritis are the most common of its over 100 different types. Primary osteoarthritis (degenerative joint disease) affects almost everyone over 40 to some degree as cartilage at frequently used joints and the lower spine gradually wears away to create stiffness, pain, and, sometimes, an overgrowth of bone. Secondary osteoarthritis can occur as a result of infections or a disease such as diabetes, or as a result of injury to a joint or the physical stress of obesity or poor posture. Rheumatoid arthritis, which usually strikes between the ages of 20 and 40, begins with inflammation of membranes lining the joints; gradually erodes cartilage; can involve blood vessels, muscles, and practically every organ of the body, and eventually can cause joint deformity.[281] Autoimmune disorders, bacterial infections, emotional stress, or reactions to certain foods are often associated with the onset of rheumatoid arthritis or its recurrence after a remission.

Medical diagnosis is essential, and, if anti-inflammatory agents and painkillers have been prescribed, the physician's approval should be obtained before experimenting with extensive alterations in diet or vitamin intake. The only "proven cure" for arthritis is surgical joint replacement, but much can be done at home to alleviate discomfort, improve flexibility, and, perhaps, slow progression of the disease.

Diet

For over 65 years, European clinics have treated arthritis with a diet of raw food and fresh juices. Even with the low-fat, low-sodium "normal" diet recommended by the Arthritis Foundation, drinking one or two glasses daily of any combination of the raw juices from alfalfa, beets, carrots, celery, cucumbers, parsley, or potatoes may be beneficial. Fresh pineapple contains bromelin, an enzyme thought to reduce swelling and inflammation in arthritic joints when eaten regularly. Increasing the consumption of oily saltwater fish such as mackerel, salmon, and sardines, which are rich in omega-3 fatty acids, or taking capsules of omega-3 fish oils effected improvement in 63 percent of the cases reported in one survey.[49] A bowl of cooked cabbage and onions daily has alleviated stiffness for other people.

Unsuspected food allergies may account for individual successes with restrictive diets such as Dr. Collin H. Dong's,[95] which allows no meat, no dairy products or egg yolks, and no fruits (including tomatoes) or their juices. Recent studies have shown that even taking capsules without knowing that they contain milk products, rice, or members of the nightshade family (bell peppers, eggplant, tomatoes, tobacco, white potatoes) triggers arthritic flareups in some people and that total abstinence from the offenders provides remission and apparent cures.[272]

For most arthritics, merely upgrading the diet with ample fruits, vegetables, and whole grains; cutting down on fats; limiting or eliminating alcohol and concentrated sweets; and incorporating appropriate supplements produces beneficial results.

Supplements (see note on page xii)

Arthritis, or drugs prescribed for its treatment, can interfere with the body's utilization of nutrients to cause deficiencies that instigate additional health problems such as those experienced by 70-year-old Dorothy W. She became listless and weepy, "rested" most of the time, and could not walk more than a few steps despite the arthritis medications she took. When her physician offered to prescribe an antidepressant, Dorothy opted for the dietary supplements suggested by a nutritionist. The doctor was skeptical but agreed that a daily multivitamin-mineral, a B-complex tablet, extra vitamins C and E, and a before-bed calcium capsule would do no harm. Within a few weeks Dorothy began to regain her vibrant energy and, with the doctor's cooperation, gradually tapered off the arthritis medications.

Nutritionally oriented experts frequently advise individual supplements such as the antioxidant vitamins A, C, and E, plus selenium, to reduce the cell damage that contributes to arthritis.

Vitamin A 10,000 to 35,000 IU (at least one-half in the form of beta carotene), especially if taking cortisone, aspirin, or other anti-inflammatory drugs that can increase the risk of infection and retard wound healing.

B Complex One comprehensive tablet daily, plus optional B vitamins, with medical supervision for the higher amounts. B_2 in the amount of 50 to 100 milligrams, or 15 to 600 milligrams of pantothenic acid stimulates the body's production of cortisone to combat arthritis.[87] Immunosuppressive drugs, and aspirin and other salicylates can create a deficiency of folic acid, which along with B_{12}, is needed for protection against nerve damage—with professional guidance, sublingual folic acid and B_{12} plus high doses of the other B vitamins have reduced pain and stiffness for some individuals.[17, 98]

Vitamin C and Bioflavonoids 500 to 5,000 milligrams of vitamin C plus 100 to 1,000 milligrams of bioflavonoids in divided daily doses. Inflammation and/or anti-inflammatory medications deplete the body's supply of vitamin C, which is necessary for the formation of cartilage and the prevention of capillary breakdown that allows swelling and pain in the joints.[294] Bioflavonoids encourage the absorption of vitamin C and strengthen capillaries.

Calcium and Magnesium These minerals have pain relieving attributes and help prevent the development of osteoporosis caused by calcium being withdrawn from the skeleton for enlargement of arthritic joints.[17, 98] Suggested amounts to be taken in divided daily doses range from 500 milligrams of each, to 1,500 milligrams of calcium plus 750 milligrams of magnesium, or 2,000 miligrams of magnesium and 1,000 milligrams of calcium. The attending physician should be consulted to determine the proper dosage for each individual.

Vitamin E 100 to 1,000 IU, plus 150 to 250 micrograms of selenium to act as scavengers of the free radicals that are a contributory factor in arthritis. Vitamin E is also believed to help stimulate cortisone production, have anti-inflammatory properties, and reduce pain—especially when accompanied by topical applications of vitamin E oil.

Less orthodox supplements also have been known to alleviate arthritis. Taking three yucca tablets with each meal, or two primrose oil capsules twice daily have been helpful in some instances. Nora J. swears by brewer's yeast. Her physician had explained that the painful knuckles were nothing to worry about—just a natural process of degenerative arthritis in overworked joints—so she accepted as inevitable the aching twinges that occasionally spread to her wrists, elbows, and shoulders. Then on the advice of a friend, Nora started drinking a glass of milk mixed with 2 tablespoons of brewer's yeast every morning. After 2 weeks, the pain and stiffness in her joints was much less noticeable. Off-and-on experimentation convinced Nora that the brewer's yeast was helping to relieve her arthritic discomfort.

Superoxide Dismutase (SOD)   200 to 800 milligrams daily. Tablets and sublingual forms of this enzyme are now available in lieu of injections to inactivate peroxide radicals and relieve stiffness, pain, and swollen joints, but the effectiveness of oral supplements is now being questioned.[17, 98]

Tissue Salts   For chronic conditions; three tablets of 3X Silicea twice daily. If worse in damp weather, add three tablets of Nat. Sulph. on rainy days. To restore flexibility; one tablet of 3X Calc. Fluor. each morning and evening, plus one tablet of 6X Silicea three times daily. If not improved in a few weeks, one 6X tablet of Nat. Phos. can be taken with each dose of Silicea.

Exercise

Inactivity weakens muscles supporting the joints and leads to more stiffness and arthritic pain. Regularly performed exercises help maintain, or partially restore, joint mobility. In a recent survey, 95 percent of the 836 arthritics who exercised reported increased flexibility in affected joints and noticeable pain relief.[272]

Gentle stretches limber up muscles, serve as a warmup for other exercises, and can be performed in bed or in a tub of warm water when joints are painful. Resistance exercises (with wrist, ankle, or other weights) strengthen muscles to compensate for damaged joints. Isometrics, which do not require joint movement, are an alternative during painful flareups. Aerobic exercise, such as walking, improves overall fitness; joint-jarring activities like jogging are not recommended. Swimming is excellent because the water supports body weight to reduce pain and permit exercises with a full range of motion. Medical approval should be obtained before embarking on any new exercise regimen, and persons with severe arthritis should follow the instructions of a physical therapist for individually designed exercises.

There are three basic guidelines for safe, effective exercise, whether it involves squeezing a foam ball, lifting weights, or swimming laps.

- ○ Start any program slowly and gradually increase repetitions.
- ○ Stop when it hurts, and rest between periods of activity, but exercise every day.
- ○ Warm up before and cool down after with slow movements.

Hot and Cold Therapy

A warm shower helps relieve morning stiffness and relaxes muscles both before and after exercising. Comfortably hot baths are one of the oldest methods for reducing pain. Practicing a relaxation technique (see Introduction) while soaking provides relief from the stress that not only triggers arthritic flareups but that can worsen pain by keeping the muscles tense. To increase water's therapeutic benefits, swish 1 cup of epsom salts or sea salt in the tub, soak for half an hour, then rinse off with a warm shower. For painful hands or feet: dissolve 1 pound of epsom salts in a large pan of hot water, soak for 5 minutes, rub hands or feet gently, then soak again for 10 minutes. After rinsing with warm water, massage peanut oil into the affected areas. Louisa L., a retired efficiency expert, has a practical solution for her morning stiff fingers. She saves the previous day's rinsed dishes to wash in hot, soapy water before breakfast.

Hot wax has been used for generations to relieve pain in arthritic hands. For at-home treatments; once each day, dip the hands in melted paraffin (never heated above 125 degrees) and allow the coating to remain for half an hour before peeling it off into the container for remelting. If desired, ½ cup of mineral oil may be added to each 2 cups of paraffin.

Cold is useful for relief of acute pain. A cloth-covered ice pack can be applied for 15 to 20 minutes, removed for 10 or 15 minutes, and the alternation of application and removal repeated as needed. Alternating heat with the cold sometimes maximizes the benefits of both. A hot-water bottle, heating pad, or a towel wrung out of hot water can be applied to the painful joint between cold applications.

Folk Remedies

Oliver Wendell Holmes is said to have carried a chestnut in one pocket of his greatcoat and a potato in the other to protect himself from rheumatism, the term with which most folk remedies for arthritis refer to the affliction.

Apple Cider Vinegar Four times a day, drink a glass of water containing from 1 teaspoon to 1 tablespoon of vinegar.

Blackstrap Molasses Once daily, drink a mixture of 1 tablespoon of molasses and ½ cup of apple juice or grape juice.

Garlic Eat minced raw garlic and rub the affected parts with garlic or garlic oil.

Herbal teas Drink two cups (or take two capsules) daily of alfalfa, angelica (dong quai), black cohosh, buckthorn, celery seed, comfrey, feverfew, nettle, parsley, peppermint, rosemary, sarsaparilla, skullcap, slippery elm, uva ursi, valerian, watermelon seed, or white willow. Taking two capsules of cayenne three times a day with milk or apple juice has diminished the pain of rheumatoid arthritis for some sufferers.[150]

Ointments Liquefy ½ cup of prepared horseradish in an electric blender, then mix with an equal amount of melted paraffin; or combine ⅓ cup *each* dry mustard and melted paraffin.

Poultices and compresses Apply packs of warmed castor oil, moistened comfrey tea leaves, or grated raw potato; or stir ¼ cup cayenne pepper and 4 teaspoons lightly crushed mustard seed into 1 pint of whiskey and simmer for a few minutes, then apply compresses of cloth saturated in the liquid.

Nerve Pressure and Massage

For arthritic arms; press and massage the tip of each shoulder where the bone ends, the tip of each elbow, and across the inside of each wrist. For arthritis of the legs, massage a circle around the outside of each kneecap, then press and massage the hollow behind and slightly below each anklebone.

Sources (see Bibliography)

2, 5, 6, 9, 13, 14, 17, 27, 30, 38, 42, 49, 57, 61, 62, 64, 72, 82, 86, 87, 89, 92, 95, 98, 105, 111, 112, 115, 116, 119, 135, 144, 150, 159, 162, 171, 174, 177, 182, 186, 190, 193, 200, 202, 204, 205, 207, 218, 221, 224, 225, 233, 257, 264, 266, 267, 272, 275, 281, 283, 284, 293, 294, 300, 304, 305, 306, 311, 317

Asthma and Emphysema

Genetic inheritance may be responsible for the supersensitive airways of asthmatics and for the easily weakened air sacs (alveoli) of individuals with emphysema. The two ailments often coexist in adults and are classified together as COPD (chronic obstructive pulmonary disease). Bronchial asthma can appear at any time but frequently starts in childhood and, in one-third of the cases, is outgrown by the age of 21. Asthmatic attacks can be precipitated by animal dander, disorders of the adrenal glands, dry or cold air, environmental pollutants, foods or other allergens, low blood sugar, physical or emotional stress, and respiratory infections. Emphysema seldom becomes obvious until after the age of 45, when the cilia (hairlike bronchial filters) grow overburdened and allow irritants to reach the alveoli and reduce their elasticity so the tiny sacs no longer expand with inhalations and contract with exhalations to eject carbon monoxide. Cigarette smoking, exposure to air pollution, various dusts, asthma, and bronchitis are factors that contribute to the onset of emphysema and breathlessness during exertion.

COPD is not a byproduct of modern civilization. Ephedrine and several other bronchodilators were developed from 2,000-year-old remedies used in China and India. Severe respiratory problems warrant medical evaluation and treatment. But besides refraining from smoking, there are many ways to augment professional care, reduce episodic recurrences and their severity, and slow or halt the progression of emphysema. Stress reactions can be modified through the relaxation methods described in the Introduction. Home air filters plus a profusion of plants help purify household air. Humidifiers help lubricate air passages and liquefy mucus for easy bronchial expulsion—inhaling steam from boiling potatoes is a Russian folk remedy. Some asthmatics have resorted to spending 8 hours zipped up in a tent with a vaporizer as a way to get a good night's sleep.

Diet

Orthomolecular physicians advise a diet similar to that for low blood sugar (see "Hypoglycemia"), high in complex carbohydrates and protein but devoid of sugar.[98] Even when allergies are involved, blood sugar levels may be the deciding factor in an asthmatic attack. The frequent small meals that are part of the diet for low blood sugar also preclude breathing difficulties resulting from a full stomach pressing against the diaphragm.

Specific foods recommended for those with respiratory ailments are apples, apricots, cabbage, carrots, celery, cherries, citrus, garlic, green beans, onions, peaches, peppers, turnips, and turnip greens. Eating fish twice a week and taking two fish oil capsules before meals has been known to mitigate the severe "second response" that often occurs several hours after exposure to an allergen and the initial asthmatic episode.[47] Horseradish, spread on sandwiches or mixed with honey or lemon juice and taken by the spoonful, helps dissolve accumulated mucus. Preservatives such as the sulfites used on restaurant vegetables and in beer, wine, pickles, potato chips, and many frozen foods are potential triggers to be avoided if possible. Even smelling the foods to which a person is allergic can bring on an asthma attack.[293]

Although extremely hot or cold beverages may initiate bronchospasms in very rare cases, imbibing generous amounts of liquid helps control mucus and moisten the air passages. Herbalists suggest a before-breakfast cup of warm tea prepared from anise seed, camomile, cayenne, comfrey, echinacea, fenugreek, ginger, ginseng, horsetail, juniper berry, licorice, lobelia, marjoram, mullein, rosemary, slippery elm, or thyme. Apple juice or clear soup may be equally effective in warding off breathing difficulties.

First-Aid Tip To help prevent airway constriction when prescribed medication is not available at the onset of an attack: drink a cup of hot strong regular tea or black coffee—theobromine, a natural chemical in tea and coffee plants, has bronchodilating effects similar to theophylline, one of the most commonly used drugs. Or put several drops of lobelia extract (available in pharmacies) in the mouth. Or take 750 milligrams of magnesium.[17, 112, 256]

Supplements (see note on page xii)

All the antioxidants (see Introduction) are recommended to help control the free radicals partially responsible for respiratory problems. Combinations of supplements are effective under individual circumstances. Kevin J.'s earliest memories are of struggling for breath, and his most embarrassing moments were those spent on the sidelines, gray-faced and gasping, while his teammates continued to play. Kevin accepted his physical limitations and, in his mid 40s, felt fortunate to have a teaching schedule that matched his seasonal attacks. When a fellow sufferer enthusiastically detailed the benefits of vitamin supplementation, Kevin was skeptical but willing to experiment. He switched to a higher-potency multivitamin-mineral, added a B-complex tablet and 400 IUs of vitamin E, and took 500 milligrams of vitamin C with bioflavonoids four times a day. By the end of the next school term, Kevin began to wonder if he had ever had asthma—there had been no more attacks.

Vitamin A   In the form of beta carotene, 10,000 to 35,000 IU daily to maintain healthy tissues in the respiratory tract and to diminish the symptoms of asthma and emphysema.

B Complex   One comprehensive tablet daily plus individual B vitamins as indicated. Asthmatics often benefit from 50 to 300 milligrams of B_6 per day.[190] Taking 100 milligrams of pantothenic acid, 30 micrograms of B_{12}, and 50 milligrams of B_{15} has relieved symptoms in many cases.[98]

Vitamin C and Bioflavonoids   500 to 5,000 milligrams of vitamin C and 200 to 1,000 milligrams of bioflavonoids in divided daily doses to strengthen fragile air sacs and help prevent allergic reactions.

Vitamin D   At least 400 IU daily to assure absorption of vitamin A and calcium.

Vitamin E   32 IU daily for children; 100 to 1,000 IU daily for adults. Vitamin E is an important ingredient of the fluid protecting the tiny air sacs in the lungs—an insufficiency can allow the alveoli to become scarred, lose their elasticity, and eventually die.[204]

Calcium and Magnesium   1,000 to 1,500 milligrams of calcium plus 500 to 750 milligrams of magnesium daily. Calcium eases breathing by relaxing the muscles surrounding the bronchial tubes. Taking one or two calcium tablets each hour during an asthmatic episode often decreases its severity. Magnesium, essential for calcium assimilation, is commonly deficient in COPD patients.[17]

Manganese European doctors have had good results with asthma patients when 5 milligrams were taken twice each week for 10 weeks.[57]

Tissue Salts One 6X tablet of Kali. Mur. and/or one 6X tablet of Kali. Phos. dissolved under the tongue each 20 minutes during an attack, then once every 3 hours for the remainder of the day.

Folk Remedies

Eating minced raw garlic or a spoonful of garlic cooked with vinegar and sugar before breakfast each morning was an 1880's cure for asthma. Other suggestions from folk healers follow.

Daily Preventive Maintenance Spread honey over thin slices of onion on a plate, cover overnight, then take a teaspoonful of the liquid four times a day. Or take 5 drops of anise oil mixed with a teaspoon of honey before each meal. Or take 1 tablespoon of lightly crushed mustard seed mixed with molasses or water each morning and evening. Or take 2 teaspoons of bee pollen granules (or the equivalent in tablets) every day.

For Wheezing and Shortness of Breath Pour boiling water over sliced apples, let cool, then strain and sip a cupful for 30 minutes (1 tablespoon of apple cider vinegar or 2 teaspoons of cooked, mashed cranberries stirred into a glass of water can be substituted for the apple liquid). Or combine 1 tablespoon *each* honey, lemon juice, and whiskey and take during attacks. If neither ACTH nor cortisone have been prescribed, take ½ teaspoon *each* salt and baking soda dissolved in a little water, then drink a glass of orange juice or milk. Apply a poultice of honey and bee pollen around the throat or a pack of castor oil-saturated cloth around the lung and kidney areas, cover to keep warm, and leave in place for 2 or 3 hours.

Exercise

Improbable as it may seem to someone struggling for breath, exercise is essential for everyone with respiratory problems.

Breathing Exercises Shallow breathing, which draws air into and out of the upper portion of the lungs, leaves carbon monoxide and mucus trapped in the bronchial tubes. Deep breathing, which expands the stomach on inhalation and retracts it on exhalation, expels all the air and strengthens the muscles to build up resistance to future attacks. Breathing out twice as long as breathing in, then pretending to blow out a candle for three puffs dislodges stale air; so does blowing up balloons.

Passive Exercise Gravity can help get rid of trapped mucus when the upper body is draped face-down across a bed with the head resting on the hands on the floor.

Posture Slumping compresses the diaphragm and reduces the amount of available air. The rigidity of military cadets is no longer advised, but erect posture pays dividends in breathing capability. Standing against a wall with shoulders, hips, and heels flush, then holding that pose while walking away from the wall establishes the correct posture. Imagination can help keep shoulders relaxed, head erect, back straight, and steps light. If pretending to be a puppet on a string or having a weight-supporting balloon attached to the top of your skull lacks appeal, *Men's Health* (October 1991) suggests imagining that a huge bird is clutching your hair and hovering overhead to support your weight.

Aerobic Exercise Walking, the ideal exercise for persons with COPD, strengthens muscles so they require less oxygen and conditions bronchial tubes so they become less reactive. When the air is cold, breathing through the nose or wearing a gauze mask helps warm the air before it reaches the lungs. If the outdoor air is frightfully cold, shopping malls or home exercycles, ski machines, and treadmills offer safe options for exercising.

Nerve Pressure and Massage

To relieve shortness of breath:

- Using a tongue depressor or the handle of a tablespoon, press down on the floor of the mouth at the root of the tongue, then on top of the tongue as far back as possible without causing gagging. See the Introduction for optional timing.

- Use the index finger to press and massage inward and downward in the hollow of the throat between the collarbones.

- Lean the back against a doorframe and press to massage the area from just below the shoulders to the base of the rib cage, 3 inches on each side of the spinal column.

○ Massage the tops and bottoms of hands and feet about 1 inch below the second and third fingers or toes.

Sources (see Bibliography)

1, 2, 3, 5, 6, 14, 17, 26, 29, 42, 47, 50, 57, 58, 59, 60, 63, 75, 87, 89, 98, 112, 123, 144, 164, 168, 171, 173, 176, 177, 190, 202, 203, 204, 205, 239, 244, 255, 256, 257, 281, 283, 293, 302, 304, 305, 316, 321

Athlete's Foot

Technically termed tinea pedis, athlete's foot is neither limited to athletes nor confined to feet. An infection caused by a fungus commonly found in gyms or on swimming pool decks, it usually makes its first appearance as itchy redness between the toes. The condition is highly contagious because the dead skin that flakes off houses fungi eager for a new host or for a new location—toenails, fingernails, scalp, and the moist folds of armpits or groin are particularly susceptible.

Well-ventilated shoes allowed to air dry for a day between wearings and absorbent socks changed when they become damp from perspiration help keep feet dry and undesirable to fungus. To avoid reinfection, spray disinfectant inside shoes (or wipe them with white vinegar) as soon as they are removed, take showers instead of tub baths, use cotton towels only once, and wear cotton socks that can be laundered in extra hot water with bleach. After the flaking-off stage is past, switch to spun acrylic socks (which draw moisture away from the feet) and rinse them in a strong vinegar solution.

Treatment begins with daily washing, thorough drying, and a dusting of powder. David M. discovered that he could eliminate cleanup chores by blow-drying his toes with a hair dryer, then placing his feet in a large paper bag before sprinkling them with talc. (According to the June 1991 issue of *Prevention*, cornstarch should not be used as a powder for athlete's foot—it actually feeds the growing fungus.)

Nutritionists suggest helping the body fight the infection by supplementing the daily diet for 1 month with yogurt or acidophilus capsules, 25,000 IU beta carotene, a B-complex tablet, 500 to 3,000 milligrams vitamin C in divided doses, 400 IU *each* vitamins D and E, and 15 to 50 milligrams of zinc (see note on page xii). Acupressurists recommend using the eraser on a pencil to press the top of the foot at the base of the little toe where it joins the fourth toe. Press for 10 seconds, release for 10 seconds, and repeat for a total of 30 seconds of pressure each morning and evening.

Folk Remedies

The old-fashioned practice of soaking infected feet in salt water has been vindicated by science—a 5- to 10-minute foot bath in a warm saline solution (1 teaspoon salt per cup of water) discourages the fungus and reduces perspiration.[293] For added benefits, apply a paste of baking soda and water as soon as the feet are dry, then rinse it off after a minute or so. Other remedies, old and new, include

○ Twice daily, coat with aloe vera gel, onion juice, or vitamin E oil. Or with an ointment made from ¼ cup lanolin, 2 tablespoons cod liver oil, and 1 tablespoon *each* garlic powder and honey. Or with an antifungal lotion prepared by combining ½ cup 100-proof vodka with twenty minced garlic cloves, and 1 tablespoon *each* ground cinnamon and cloves in a dark glass bottle. Cover tightly and let stand in a cupboard for 2 weeks, shaking the bottle every other day.

○ Twice daily, dust the feet with garlic powder and, for a few days, wear minced fresh garlic in closed-toe shoes. Garlic is believed to be more effective than nonprescription antifungal drugs.[17]

○ Once a day, soak feet in an herb tea foot bath of goldenseal, thyme, or a half-and-half mixture of thyme and camomile teas. Other soaking options are a strong solution of apple cider vinegar, or cinnamon water prepared by simmering a dozen broken cinnamon sticks in 6 cups of water for 5 minutes and steeping until lukewarm.

○ Once a day, splash feet with apple cider vinegar or diluted rubbing alcohol or garlic juice. Let dry for 30 minutes, then rinse with clear water.

○ At bedtime, cover the affected areas with raw honey or plain yogurt, or with a water-based paste of baking soda, powdered vitamin C, or dry red clover tea. Sleep in cotton socks, then wash the feet in the morning.

Sources (see Bibliography)

2, 6, 16, 17, 41, 42, 53, 57, 87, 98, 109, 111, 112, 148, 150, 166, 186, 190, 202, 205, 226, 234, 246, 278, 282, 283, 293, 300, 306, 311, 312, 313

Backache and Sciatica

A back attack usually appears suddenly from strain (an abused muscle) or sprain (a partially torn ligament) and is accompanied by painful muscle spasms that immobilize back muscles to protect them and the spinal nerves. The cause can be as obvious as bending over to lift a heavy object instead of keeping the back straight and utilizing leg and arm muscles or as subtle as sitting in the same position for several hours. Muscle tension from emotional stress can trigger a spasm or a nagging backache; either of which may be alleviated by the relaxation methods described in the Introduction. Pain in the lower back, sometimes termed lumbago, may be caused or aggravated by poor posture, high-heeled shoes, lack of exercise, dietary deficiencies, too-soft beds, genetic predisposition, or excess weight, which can engender the same type of back pain as pregnancy does—physicists calculate that back muscles must exert a force of 50 pounds to counterbalance a 10-pound paunch in front of the spine.[177] Sciatica (pain along the sciatic nerve from buttock to ankle) may occur independently of or in conjunction with other back pain. Pressure from a herniated disk may be responsible for sciatica, but more commonly the sciatic nerve is pinched by tightened muscles attached to the hip—sciatica has been instigated by sitting on a bulging wallet.[300] As explained in *Berkeley Wellness Letter* (January 1993), the mechanical vibrations of long hours behind the wheel of a car or truck, or work that requires repetitive lifting may be responsible for sciatic attacks.

A 10- to 20-minute application of ice at the onset of a back attack deadens pain, relieves spasms, and minimizes swelling. Alternating the chilling with 15 to 30 minutes of heat widens arteries and veins to speed blood flow to and from the constricted muscles. Lying in bed with a pillow under the knees is the usual choice for the few days of mandatory inactivity. Lying on the floor with a thin pillow under the neck and head, and the lower legs resting on the seat of an upholstered chair may be more comfortable for sciatica sufferers. Assuming this position within 10 minutes of the first warning twinge of an incipient back attack may abort it or at least make it milder.

Acute back pain that continues unabated after 2 days of complete bed rest or that is accompanied by fever or vomiting should be evaluated by a physician.

Diet and Supplements (see note on page xii)

Good nutrition helps prevent and correct many back problems. Drinking a glass of fresh, raw potato juice (mixed with beet, carrot, or celery juice for additional enzymes and palatability) daily has brought relief to some lumbago and sciatica sufferers. Protein and vitamin C are necessary for strong supportive tissue. The entire B complex is essential for the health of nerve tissue. Calcium and other minerals help to avoid or relieve backaches brought on by gradual demineralization of the bones.

Mike H. had been examined by his doctor and manipulated by an osteopath, but his back continued to spasm and freeze every few months, and the two-day recovery layovers were jeopardizing his truck-driving job. So when his mother-in-law presented him with a gift-wrapped package of vitamin pills and a jug of cranberry juice, Mike agreed to give the supplements a try. With each morning's glass of juice he dutifully gulped down a multivitamin-mineral, a B-complex tablet, 1,000 milligrams of time-release vitamin C with bioflavonoids, and 400 IU of vitamin E. The combination worked. Mike still drives his 18-wheeler and has almost forgotten that he ever had a bad back—but he doesn't forget to take his vitamins.

Sciatic pain has responded to a month of therapy with the same vitamins and minerals that Mike took, plus 50 milligrams of zinc and 1,000 to 2,000 micrograms of sublingual B_{12}. Mag. Phos., a tissue salt, is recommended for acute back pain with spasms. One teaspoon of the tablets may be taken each 3 hours for 12 hours, then three tablets dissolved under the tongue three times each day.

One folk remedy for a back attack triggered by an emotional crisis is uva ursi tea, bed rest, and one or two mild alcoholic drinks. Herbalists advise white willow bark, either in capsules or steeped for a beverage, because it is a natural salicylate with the same anti-inflammatory power as aspirin.[293] Other herbs for back pain are burdock, comfrey, juniper, oat straw, slippery elm, and valerian.

Posture

Sitting, standing, and walking correctly are both prevention and treatment for chronic backache. Slouching, slumping, or leaning forward puts added pressure on the spinal disks. Proper posture, with head and chest high, stomach and buttocks tucked in, keeps the spine aligned. Keeping the knees slightly flexed while standing and frequently shifting weight from one foot to the other or propping one foot on a chair rung or low shelf reduces back strain. Rocking chairs or 30-second "standing breaks" relieve the spinal strain of protracted sitting. When relaxing in an upholstered chair, select a recliner or use a footstool to elevate the knees above the hips.

Exercise

Anyone with a serious back problem should see an orthopedist before undertaking any exercise program and then follow the individualized regimen advised for strengthening back and abdominal muscles. Gentle stretches often prevent or alleviate chronic backache. These unobtrusive exercises can be practiced during the day.

- ○ Sit on a straight-backed chair with both feet on the floor. Gradually allow the body to droop forward until the head is between the knees with hands dangling on the floor, then tighten the abdominal muscles and slowly pull back up. Alternate with an elbow stretch: Bend both elbows, then move one elbow down behind the back and raise the other to the head. Reverse and repeat.

- ○ Lean back against a wall with the feet 12 inches away from the baseboard. Tip head, shoulders, and pelvis forward to press the beltline against the wall.

Low-impact aerobics like swimming, stationary cycling, and walking are good for the back. Jogging or sports involving jumping or twisting can be damaging to bones and muscles. Floor exercises should be performed slowly, and daily repetitions gradually increased to no more than 10—gain without pain is the goal.

- ○ To improve muscle flexibility and strength, and have a back massage at the same time: (1) Lie on the back with arms at the sides, knees bent, and feet flat on the floor. Tilt the pelvis and lift buttocks so the small of the back presses against the floor, hold for 5 seconds, then relax. (2) Extend hands between the thighs and slowly curl head and shoulders up off the floor. Hold for 3 seconds and roll back down, then relax. (3) Bring the knees up to the chest with arms hugging them, hold for 5 seconds, then return to the bent-knee position.

○ To strengthen thigh muscles and prevent or relieve sciatica, lie on the left side with left knee bent. Extend the right leg and raise the right foot toward the ceiling three times. Turn over and repeat with the left leg.

Nerve Pressure and Massage

○ With the thumbs, press inward and upward under the arch of each eyebrow. Maintain pressure for 10 seconds, release for 10 seconds, and repeat three times each day.

○ Press and massage the spot on the back of each hand where the long bones of the fourth finger and the little finger meet.

○ Every other day, massage the bottom of each foot for a minute or two. On alternate days, massage both hands—especially the pad at the base of the thumb, the center of the palm, and the pad between thumb and first finger.

○ For pain in the center of the back, massage the top of the foot at the center of the inner rim of the arch and/or the top of the hand between the wrist and the web of the thumb. For lower back pain, massage the inside rim of the foot from the arch to the heel and/or massage the top of the hand at the base of the thumb.

Sources (see Bibliography)

2, 3, 6, 17, 26, 29, 41, 57, 59, 60, 72, 82, 87, 98, 111, 112, 115, 135, 159, 160, 166, 175, 177, 186, 207, 218, 233, 250, 255, 256, 257, 265, 291, 293, 300, 316

Bad Breath (Halitosis)

When not due to the consumption of garlic, onions, or exotic spices, halitosis is most often caused by mouth-dwelling bacteria that produce offensive gases from food fragments and oral debris sequestered between the teeth and in the rough texture of the tongue. If brushing teeth and tongue after every meal is not feasible, bad-breath microorganisms may be controlled by a before-bed brushing to quell the bacterial activity responsible for "morning breath" and by brushing and flossing after breakfast rather than immediately upon arising. Swishing and spitting (or swallowing) a mouthful of water after each meal or snack helps dispense with potentially malodorous bits of food between brushings.

If good oral hygiene and home remedies do not resolve the problem, health care professionals should be consulted. Chronic halitosis can stem from a multitude of sources—digestive disturbances, intestinal sluggishness, periodontal disease, and sinus or throat infections—or may signify more serious conditions such as diabetes, duodenal ulcers, hypoglycemia, kidney or liver malfunction, and respiratory disorders.

Diet

Foods like garlic, onions, and curry contain aromatic compounds that enter the bloodstream, circulate through the lungs, and are exhaled as offensive breath for up to 24 hours. Other notorious breath destroyers include blue, Camembert, and Roquefort cheeses; fish, especially canned tuna and the anchovies on pizza; and spicy deli meats. In lieu of sucking breath mints, eating fresh parsley (which follows the same metabolic path as garlic to release pleasant aromas through the lungs) or chewing a few anise, cardamom, dill, or fennel seeds will help mask offending odors.

A high-fiber diet emphasizing whole grains and an abundance of fresh fruits and vegetables is essential for optimum digestive performance and the prevention or correction of bad breath. Apples and crunchy, mouth-scrubbing foods like raw celery and carrots are recommended snacks. Many cases of chronic halitosis can be attributed to malodorous gases that rise back up through the digestive tract from undigested food fermenting in the intestines and slowing elimination. Chewing foods thoroughly and eating in a relaxed atmosphere assists digestion. Nervous tension restricts the flow of digestive juices, and as explained in *Natural Health* (October 1992), overeating can overwhelm the stomach's digestive enzymes and send partially digested food into the small intestine.

Eating yogurt may be helpful because the *Lactobacillus* culture it contains reinforces beneficial bacteria that battle odor-producing intestinal microorganisms. Taking two acidophilus capsules before each meal dispensed with Virgil D.'s bad breath and got rid of the terrible taste he had in his mouth for 6 months following treatment with antibiotics—apparently, the antibiotics had decimated the friendly flora while curing his infection.

Drinking generous amounts of nonalcoholic beverages between meals improves digestion and helps prevent unpleasant "desert breath" from a dry mouth. Saliva is a natural bacteria-suppressing cleanser. Anything that dries the mouth (alcohol, antianxiety drugs, medications such as decongestants and diuretics, smoking, stress) allows bad-breath microorganisms to flourish.

Supplements (see note on page xii)

A deficiency of B vitamins can be responsible for bad breath. Some cases of halitosis have been cleared by taking 50 milligrams of niacinamide with each meal, plus a high-potency B complex tablet and 50 milligrams of B$_6$ once a day.[98] Halitosis caused by a lack of zinc may be corrected by taking 30 to 60 milligrams of the mineral every day.[6, 293] Divided daily doses of 1,000 to 6,000 milligrams of vitamin C with bioflavonoids help rid the body of excess mucus and toxins that can instigate offensive breath.[17]

Folk Remedies

Chewing two sprigs of parsley dipped in vinegar or sucking a lemon wedge sprinkled with salt is said to fend off garlic or onion breath. Dissolving a pea-sized piece of myrrh in the mouth at bedtime or sucking a small chunk of cinnamon bark during the day is believed to freshen breath. To prevent or correct halitosis, folk practitioners advise brushing the teeth and tongue twice a day with baking soda or with a paste of baking soda and hydrogen peroxide, then rinsing thoroughly. Or, every morning, brush the tongue and gums with a little powdered cloves or powdered myrrh. Drinking a cup of peppermint tea every day may also be helpful—peppermint enters the bloodstream and is exhaled through the lungs in the same manner as parsley.

Mouthwash

Tests conducted by *Consumer Reports* (September 1992) show that rinsing with mouthwash can cover even garlic breath for 10 to 20 minutes. Medicinal mouthwashes can protect against bacterial buildup for as long as 3 hours,[186] but the frequent use of products containing more than 25 percent alcohol has been linked to an increased incidence of oral cancer.[254] For a nonalcoholic, bacteria-inhibiting mouth rinse, swish with a half-and-half mixture of hydrogen peroxide and water for 30 seconds.

Double-strength teas brewed from antiseptic herbs are time-honored mouth rinses for temporary control of halitosis. If desired, 1 or 2 tablespoons of brandy or vodka may be added to each cup to enhance the germicidal qualities of allspice, anise seed, cinnamon, clove, echinacea, eucalyptus, fenugreek, horsetail, goldenseal, myrrh, peppermint, rosemary, sage, sandalwood, thyme, or winter savory. Combinations can be prepared by steeping the following herbs in 2 cups of boiling water for 10 minutes and straining before using:

○ One teaspoon *each* dried mint, rosemary, and crushed fennel seeds.

○ Two sprigs chopped raw parsley, three whole cloves, and ¼ teaspoon *each* powdered goldenseal and myrrh. If desired, ¼ teaspoon crushed anise or caraway seeds, or ⅛ teaspoon ground cinnamon may be included.

Sources (see Bibliography)

6, 17, 29, 42, 43, 50, 53, 87, 98, 108, 109, 149, 165, 173, 176, 179, 186, 202, 254, 256, 293, 300, 301, 312, 313

Bedsores

Also known as decubitus ulcers or pressure sores, bedsores bedevil the bedfast. They begin as reddened, tender areas over thinly padded bony prominences such as elbows, hip bones, heels, the base of the spine, and even ears and the back of the head. If ignored, dangerously deep, slow-to-heal ulcers can develop. Prevention is easier than cure. When prolonged bed rest is a necessity, medical-supply houses offer spot-relieving foam doughnuts for hips or heels, and bed-sized sheepskins, multi-contoured foam mattresses, or plastic pressure pads that ripple air in and out of narrow tubes.

Removing the pressure at the first signs of redness usually aborts the sores. Bedridden 82-year-old Cora J., ensconced in her electronically adjustable bed on a fluffy fleece with cushions to protect pressure points, was confident that she needn't worry about bedsores. Rather than vegetate in sloth, however, Cora became a one-person calling committee for her church and social groups. With her handset containing an on/off button as well as a dial, she could tuck the phone against the pillow and chat for hours without having to hold it in her hand. When one ear wearied of the pressure, she simply switched sides. Then her daughter noticed Cora's red ears. She immediately attached sticky-backed foam around the telephone's earpiece and twisted nylon stockings into an ear-sized doughnut for additional pressure relief. Within a few weeks, the tenderness disappeared and Cora's ears regained their normal hue.

Besides utilizing protective padding, body position should be changed every 2 hours if the physical condition allows. Daily baths with mild soap, thorough rinsing and drying (moist skin, particularly from incontinence, encourages pressure sores), and gentle massage with petroleum jelly over the pressured points help strengthen skin and stimulate circulation.

43

Diet and Supplements (see note on page xii)

Even with proper care, the development, severity, and healing time of bedsores can hinge on nutritional factors because the body's reserves are depleted by the physical stress of illness. A diet replete with fruits, vegetables, and whole grains, plus ample protein and fluids, replenishes the reserves and hastens healing, as does reinforcing other remedies with dietary supplements.

Vitamin A At least one-half beta carotene, 10,000 to 35,000 IU daily. This healing vitamin is partially responsible for the strength of new tissue formed at the site of the sore.

B Complex One or two high-potency tablets daily. All the B vitamins are needed to combat the stress of illness.

Vitamin C and Bioflavonoids 1,000 to 4,000 milligrams of vitamin C in divided doses daily, preferably with 100 to 400 milligrams of bioflavonoids—both guard against the capillary fragility that allows bedsores to form. If ulcers have formed, the combination can reduce healing time from months to weeks. Misting the sores with a 3 percent solution of vitamin C crystals and water further speeds healing.

Vitamin E 100 to 1,200 IU daily. Vitamin E improves circulation to help avoid bedsores and to heal existing ones more rapidly.

Minerals One daily multi-mineral (containing 2 milligrams of copper) plus 30 to 60 milligrams of zinc. Among the numerous minerals necessary for the synthesization of new proteins for wound healing, the key mineral is zinc. Copper supplementation is suggested because the therapeutic amounts of zinc can reduce the absorption of copper, which is essential for connective tissue replacement.[248]

Folk Remedies

Sprinkling a thick layer of granulated sugar over an open bedsore and covering it with an airtight dressing is a time-tested remedy—adding a bit of powdered vitamin C may increase the benefits. Spreading raw honey on a gauze pad and placing it over the sore is another ancient but viable curative that has produced healing within two weeks.[42] Adding a crushed zinc tablet to the honey may make the application even more beneficial.

Other folk treatments include

- ○ Sponging with hydrogen peroxide or the juice of fresh, ripe cucumbers; or with a mixture of one tablespoon powdered alum (available in pharmacies) and ¾ cup water.
- ○ Dusting the sores with cornstarch.
- ○ Applying aloe vera gel; an egg white beaten with 2 tablespoons of wine; or a coating of castor oil, cod liver oil, or liquid lecithin (available in health food stores). Or a poultice of freshly grated garlic combined with vegetable oil.

Sources (see Bibliography)

2, 17, 41, 42, 75, 84, 87, 92, 109, 122, 135, 144, 150, 159, 203, 233, 248, 268, 283, 294, 315

Bedwetting (Enuresis)

In adults, enuresis is labeled incontinence. Women may become incontinent after a hysterectomy or as a result of weakened pelvic muscles from numerous pregnancies. An enlarged prostate gland is often responsible for the problem in men. Most childhood bedwetting is due to a combination of genetic inheritance, delayed development of the nervous system controlling elimination, insufficient bladder capacity, and the susceptibility of bladder controls to the influence of stress from excitement or anxiety. Other factors are bladder hypersensitivity or exceptionally deep sleep created by allergic reactions to foods, and low blood sugar, which can be initiated by stress as well as sugar and can leave the nervous system without sufficient energy to transmit a message from a full bladder up to the brain. Nocturnal enuresis is not of medical concern until after the age of 6 unless there is obvious neurological disease—10 percent of 5-year-olds still wet the bed; many of them continue to do so until the age of 8 or 9.[75] If a child also has difficulty with daytime bladder control, however, professional diagnosis is warranted to rule out infection or structural abnormality of the urinary tract, diabetes, or spinal-cord damage.

Patience and positive reinforcement have proven more effective than scolding or threats, which increase anxiety and exacerbate the problem. Toddlers can be roused and taken to the bathroom once or twice during the night, then rewarded with gold stars on a "dry tonight" chart. Older children can either respond to an alarm clock or to an alarm system that signals the first few drops of moisture, then, if necessary, accept responsibility by covering the wet spot with a cloth-topped waterproof pad and donning dry pajamas.

A half-hour's relaxation in bed before the final bathroom visit often pays dividends, especially when combined with parental tenderness. Coping with the divorce and having to move back home with her 6-year-old had been such a nightmare that Judy K. hoped Benjy's "Mom, my bed's wet" was merely part of a bad dream. It wasn't. The next morning, as Judy was apologetically explaining that this was Benjy's first nighttime accident in over a year, her mother offered a suggestion. "Why don't you try giving him a back rub after he's tucked in bed, then have him go to the bathroom. You never had a bedwetting problem but that's how I helped your older brother solve his after we moved here from the farm. Little ones react to stress, too, you know." The nightly reassurance was just what Benjy needed; there were no more embarrassing mishaps.

Diet and Supplements (see note on page xii)

The kidneys are active for only a short period after a drink is taken, so liquids need be restricted for only an hour or so before bedtime. Herbalists suggest a cup of cornsilk tea 1 hour before bed. The tea is prepared by steeping fresh cornsilk in boiling water, straining, then stirring in a spoonful of honey. When children are able to voluntarily postpone urination as long as possible, bladder capacity may be improved by drinking extra fluids during the day. Cranberry juice is beneficial to the bladder and is credited with stopping some cases of enuresis. A cup of fennel-seed tea daily, chilled and sweetened with honey if desired, is advised by folk healers. Incontinent adults may benefit from a cup or two capsules of buchu or uva ursi tea. Caffeine-containing beverages, carrots, and grapefruit juice are mild diuretics that may need to be avoided after lunchtime.

Including cabbage, cantaloupe, fish, and leafy green vegetables in a diet containing ample protein is recommended. Nutritional deficiencies or a hereditary need for exceptionally high amounts of certain vitamins and minerals may be responsible for bedwetting at any age. Taking a multivitamin-mineral tablet containing at least 10 milligrams of iron has been beneficial in some instances, and additional supplements may be helpful for brief trial periods.

> **Magnesium** 200 to 600 milligrams, plus 25 to 100 milligrams of B6, depending on body weight, daily. Bedwetting may be due to a deficiency of magnesium. Vitamin B6 helps correct muscle weakness and improves bladder control but increases the need for magnesium.[98]
>
> **Vitamin C and Niacin** 500 to 1,000 milligrams of vitamin C plus up to 150 milligrams of niacin have proven beneficial when taken in divided doses each day.

Vitamin E   100 IU for children 6 to 12; 600 IU for adults. Vitamin E collaborates with vitamin A to normalize bladder function.[17]

Tissue Salts   One tablet *each* 3X Ferr. Phos, Kali. Phos., and Nat. Phos. dissolved under the tongue three times each day has corrected some cases of enuresis.

Folk Remedies

Cinnamon   Chewing stick cinnamon just before retiring is thought to have an astringent effect on the urinary system.

Epsom Salts   ½ teaspoon stirred in liquid and taken after supper was an old-fashioned remedy that has been scientifically justified—epsom salts equals magnesium sulfate—but it has a laxative effect, and it should not be used by anyone with kidney disease.

Honey   For those who are neither diabetic nor hypoglycemic, 1 teaspoon to 1 tablespoon raw honey taken just before retiring is believed to act as a mild sedative and to attract and hold body fluid to spare the kidneys.

Nerve Pressure and Massage

Once each day, press and massage the hollow on each side of the back of the neck between the spine and the bottom of the ears, the joint crease closest to the tip of the little finger; and/or the second crease closer to the hand, the hollow behind and slightly below each anklebone, and the web of skin where the big toe and the next toe meet.

Sources (see Bibliography)

41, 42, 57, 63, 64, 75, 80, 86, 87, 98, 144, 159, 162, 172, 176, 186, 203, 204, 226, 234, 255, 261, 281, 282, 283, 284, 293, 312, 313, 317

Bites

Most bites are merely unpleasant incidents, but even nonvenomous nibbles—animal or insect—may be potentially hazardous because of allergic reactions, secondary infections, and transmitted diseases. To augment specific remedies and any necessary medical treatment, orthomolecular physicians suggest these therapeutic supplements (see Note on page xii).

B vitamins 50 milligrams of B₆ plus 100 milligrams of pantothenic acid immediately after the bite to help detoxify poisons and prevent allergic reactions. Then, one high-potency B-complex tablet daily to promote antibody production.

Vitamin C 1,000 to 2,000 milligrams immediately; 4,000 to 10,000 milligrams in divided doses during the first day; then 3,000 milligrams daily. Accompanying the vitamin C with bioflavonoids enhances the detoxifying, antiallergy action.

Calcium Gluconate Up to 1,500 milligrams daily to reduce pain and lessen the likelihood of stomach irritation from vitamin C.

Animal Bites

First-Aid Tip Clean the wound with soap and running water for 5 minutes to remove contaminating agents; splash with hydrogen peroxide or other antiseptic, if desired; then apply a sterile dressing. An ice pack may be placed over the bandage to alleviate pain.

If the wound is superficial, the animal is a healthy pet, and the human has had a tetanus shot within five years, no further treatment should be required unless there is subsequent swelling, redness, or drainage. Deep gashes or a bite from a stray or wild animal warrants medical attention and a rabies alert. Herbalists recommend teas or capsules of echinacea, golden-seal, or red clover. Holistic doctors advise a 2-week regimen of taking two odorless garlic capsules with each meal (garlic is a natural antibiotic) and 500 milligrams daily of the detoxifying amino acids L-cysteine and L-methionine.[17]

Mosquitoes and Flying Pests

Horseflies produce a painful bite. Gnats are a menace if they attack in a swarm. Mosquitoes are the most prevalent flying annoyances. The itchy red bites are allergic responses to substances in the insect's saliva or feces, which are deposited at the site and can cause secondary infections. Typically, mosquitoes prefer men to women, dirty to clean, and are attracted to the color blue; but individual body aroma also plays a role. Mosquitoes were spoiling Cynthia F.'s vacation at the lake. Before the first itchy bites cleared up, she acquired new ones. Then a bite-free friend shared her secret: bleach baths. Cynthia followed instructions, swishing 4 tablespoons of chlorine laundry bleach in her bath water and soaking for 15 minutes before dressing for the evening cookout. To her delight, the mosquitoes zoomed right past her in search of more appealing targets.

Wearing body-covering garments is another form of protection. For some people, the daily consumption of brewer's yeast or fresh garlic acts as an insect repellent. For others, taking 60 milligrams of zinc every day for a month, or taking 100 milligrams of B_1 or niacin immediately before and every 3 or 4 hours during exposure is effective.

Bite treatment depends on the availability of remedies and the intensity of the itch. To avoid contamination with disease or infection: wash the bite area with soap and water, then dab with disinfectant. To relieve itching or pain, moisten the site and rub with an aspirin tablet, or apply a paste of water plus baking soda, crushed charcoal tablets, meat tenderizer, or table salt. Other options include covering the bite with aloe vera gel, ammonia, epsom salts dissolved in warm water, eucalyptus oil, lemon juice or vinegar, or with this prepare-ahead folk remedy: 1 teaspoon *each* cinnamon, cloves, ginger, lemon peel, orange peel, and sassafras combined with 1 cup vinegar and allowed to stand in a covered glass container. Shake once daily for 10 days, then strain and bottle.

Ticks

Although its bite is usually harmless and relatively painless, a tick can inject disease-causing bacteria while drawing blood. Precautionary measures include wearing a long-sleeved shirt and tucking pants into socks or boots. Slippery materials such as nylon make it difficult for ticks to grab a foothold, and donning a hat will deter them from settling on the scalp. A daily body inspection and clothing check is wise—ticks often crawl around for a long time before selecting a bite site.

A tick's mouth has a sharp probe with backward pointing barbs. After tapping into a blood source, it injects bacteria as it feeds, so the sooner the tick is removed, the less likely the chance of infectious organisms being transferred. A drop of oil or alcohol may be applied to partially immobilize the tick, but folk remedies for making it back out by aggravating it with a hot match or suffocating it with petroleum jelly or nail polish may instigate the secretion of more bacteria so are being forsaken in favor of fast removal.[300]

○ Use tweezers or tissue-covered fingers to grip the tick as close to the skin as possible and gently pull straight up without jerking, twisting, or squeezing the body—any of its fluids could cause an infection.

○ Cleanse the area with soap and water, disinfect with alcohol or hydrogen peroxide, then apply a small bandage if needed.

○ Save the tick in a bottle labeled with the date, geographical location, and body site of the bite. Incorporating a piece of damp paper towel will preserve the tick for up to 6 weeks in case suspicious symptoms develop and medical evaluation is necessary. Rocky Mountain spotted fever (which actually is most prevalent in the South and East) usually makes its presence known within a week by fever and a rash of reddish black spots on wrists and ankles.[281, 300] Lyme disease (which has been reported in 43 states) starts with a red rash around the bite in 60 to 80 percent of cases.[186] Joint and muscle pains, fever, swollen glands, and dizziness are other Lyme-disease symptoms that may occur from 3 days to a month after the bite.

Chiggers

Unlike ticks, in that they neither embed their heads nor suck blood, chiggers attach themselves to humans with claws, feed for about 3 days by secreting enzymes that liquefy skin cells, and then drop off. Long-sleeved shirts, long pants, socks, and shoes provide some protection from these parasites, which lurk in lawns and other areas covered with vegetation.

Chiggers are so small (approximately $1/20$ of an inch) that they are seldom noticed until tiny red welts and severe itching results several hours after their enzymes make initial contact. To dislodge the insects, lather with soap, scrub with a brush, then rinse thoroughly. An ice pack helps control swelling. To relieve itching, apply a paste of baking powder and ammonia or use any of the remedies suggested for mosquito bites. If the itchiness is widespread, a lukewarm bath with cornstarch sprinkled in it may bring relief.

See also **Snakebite and Spider Bite**

Sources (see Bibliography)

2, 6, 17, 20, 41, 42, 46, 50, 57, 64, 69, 72, 75, 87, 92, 98, 104, 109, 111, 135, 144, 148, 151, 159, 169, 173, 176, 186, 196, 202, 203, 207, 216, 264, 281, 282, 284, 285, 293, 300, 301, 311, 313, 322

Black Eyes

W hether called a shiner or a subcutaneous extravasation, a black eye provides a living-color experience. A blow to the cheekbone or eyebrow area damages tiny blood vessels beneath the skin, allowing blood and other fluids to leak into soft surrounding tissue to cause swelling and discoloration. Blood looks blue below skin level; when deprived of the oxygen in the bloodstream, red blood turns purple and makes the skin appear black, especially the thin, translucent skin around the eyes. After blood seepage ceases, the body's healing forces begin the resorbing process, which produces multicolor changes from purple to blue to green to yellow before finally returning to normalcy in about a week. If a painkiller is needed, acetaminophen is advised; aspirin is an anticoagulant that slows clotting, increasing the potential for further oozing from ruptured blood vessels. Professional evaluation is warranted for any injury that might have damaged the bone of the eye socket or that results in vision disturbances.

Treatment

First-Aid Tip Immediate chilling, without pressure on the eye, slows the internal bleeding to minimize swelling and discoloration. An ice pack is the first choice, but anything cold suffices. Raw meat is no longer believed to be more effective than a can of soda or a package of frozen peas. For Brett B., a popsicle furnished the chill, and his two almost-black eyes turned out to be a blessing in disguise. Moving to a new school just before the end of the term had left him feeling friendless, but "making" the Little League team was some compensation, and he was determined to make a good impression at the first game. Next up, wearing a batter's helmet and standing in front of the players' bench, Brett was glancing toward his mother in the snack bar when a batted ball struck him in the unprotected center of his forehead. Too groggy from the blow to be embarrassed by being carried to the car by the coach while his mother ran beside them, holding a popsicle to his forehead, he was grateful for the pain-relieving coldness enroute to the emergency room. X-rays revealed no bone damage; the quick chilling averted most of the eye discoloration, leaving only raccoon like black rings around his eyes, plus the bonus of a bump that was a perfect replica of the baseball—complete with the imprint of stitches from the seam. The visual effect was so fascinating that Brett was surrounded by avid viewers who quickly became new friends.

Immediately applying a cotton pad saturated with witch hazel may be beneficial. Grated raw potato encased in cheesecloth is another option. Leeches were once employed to suck the blood from black eyes. More appealing is the modern method of continuing to apply an ice pack for 10 minutes at a time (a longer period could cause frostbite) to control discoloration, pain, and swelling. To make an eye-sized ice pack, place crushed ice in a plastic sandwich bag and tuck it in a stretchy sweat band. If the eye is still tender after a day or so, warm, moist compresses may speed healing and the absorption of discoloring fluids.

Supplements (see note on page xii)

Taking 2,000 milligrams of vitamin C in divided daily doses encourages the disappearance of discoloration. All of the other antioxidants (see Introduction) act as scavengers of the free radicals produced when blood vessels are damaged.[98] The tissue salts Ferr. Phos. and Kali. Mur, taken in the 3X potency at 10-minute intervals during the first hour, then reduced to two or three times a day, may help reduce both discoloration and swelling.

Folk Remedies

Herbs have long been utilized as a treatment for black eyes. Any of the following may be brewed into tea for drinking or for saturating cloths to be used as warm compresses, or they may simply be moistened and sandwiched between pieces of cloth as a poultice for the eye: comfrey, dandelion, fenugreek, hyssop, lobelia, mullein, parsley, pekoe, rose hip, slippery elm, thyme, turmeric, yarrow.

Sources (see Bibliography)

6, 41, 42, 53, 57, 64, 69, 75, 92, 98, 111, 135, 148, 168, 186, 187, 202, 264, 284, 293, 294, 299, 313, 322

Body Odor

Perspiration is an essential regulator of body temperature. When the body accumulates too much heat from external warmth or from physical or mental stress, the output from over two million sweat glands increases to cool the body by evaporation of the liquid on the skin's surface. Most perspiration is an odorless fluid composed of water, salt, and trace elements secreted by the eccrine sweat glands distributed over the entire body. After puberty, the chemical composition of perspiration produced by apocrine sweat glands, concentrated in the armpits and genital areas, carries a faint scent and is rich in organic material ideal for bacterial reproduction. Within a few hours, bacteria normally present on the skin multiply and decompose in these secretions to cause the body odor considered so offensive in twentieth-century America. In earlier cultures there was no such taboo. Male virility and female attractiveness were judged by the potency of perspiration odor, and philters filled with sweat were worn as aphrodisiacs. Other civilizations, however, attempted to overpower natural odors with sweet fragrances. Egyptians concocted perfumes in 2000 B.C.; ancient Romans applied aromatics to all parts of their bodies and to their pet animals; Elizabethan and colonial gentlemen as well as ladies, who seldom bathed more often than once a month, flaunted lacy handkerchiefs drenched with eau de cologne to camouflage natural aromas.

Excessive sweating without apparent cause (hyperhidrosis) usually begins during the early teens, then self-adjusts by the age of 30. Episodes of severe sweating accompany fevers, may relate to low blood sugar or metabolic dysfunctions, and frequently occur during menopause. Emotional stress (anger, fear, excitement) triggers localized sweating on the forehead, palms, and soles of the feet as well as under the arms.[258] Deodorants mask odor; some temporarily reduce bacterial action. Antiperspirants, which need be only 20 percent effective to be so labeled, reduce the output of perspiration. There is no firm evidence linking the aluminum compounds in commercial products with the high aluminum levels of

Alzheimer's patients, but for those who wish to avoid possible problems from the assortment of chemicals they contain, there are many alternatives.

Baths

Daily bathing is essential for odor control. People who perspire heavily may need to shower morning and evening as well as after strenuous activity. Removing underarm hair once a week eliminates that haven for malodorous bacteria. Scrubbing armpits with a soapy washcloth removes residual secretions and bacteria more effectively than does hand-lathering. To banish serious body odor, nurses and therapists have their patients soak for 15 minutes in a tub of water containing 3 cups of tomato juice.[109]

Deodorant soaps, especially those containing antibacterial agents, cut down on the number of bacteria on the skin. Individual reactions may necessitate experimentation with different brands. Earl T.'s experience is an extreme example: He washed with a bar of clean-smelling deodorant soap provided by his hotel and emerged from the shower smelling as if he had been doused with spoiled milk. The odor became so obvious during breakfast that Earl had to shop for a bar of his regular soap, then shower again before approaching the clients on his morning schedule. If all bath soaps prove unacceptable, antibacterial surgical scrubs are sold without prescription in most pharmacies.[293]

Clothing

Loosely fitting garments fashioned from porous fabrics allow perspiration to evaporate before it becomes a breeding medium for bacteria. But unless regularly changed, clothing collects odors that can negate the benefits of daily bodily cleansing.

Diet and Supplements (see note on page xii)

Caffeine and other stimulants in beverages and medications can trigger excess perspiration due to nervous tension. Garlic and spices such as cumin and curry may be responsible for offensive body odor, as the pungent essence is excreted through the sweat glands. Some cases, such as Sybil R.'s, result from other flavorful foods. Sybil lusted after chip dip—the real thing, made from sour cream and dried onion soup mix. Calorie and cholesterol consciousness kept her passion bridled until she discovered nonfat sour cream. With a variety of fresh vegetables for dunking, she nibbled all weekend and polished off the last of a big bowl of onion dip for a Sunday-night snack. On Monday morning, savoring the remembered flavor and basking in the afterglow of guilt-free indulgence, Sybil was astonished when a coworker asked who brought the onion dip. By the time the third person wanted to know where she had stashed the chip dip, Sybil was embarrassed. Mouthwash and breath mints did not improve the situation; but the lingering aroma dissipated by late afternoon and indulging in more prosaic portions of her fabulous fat-free dip occasioned no odor problems.

Dietary supplements often reduce both perspiration and odor. One high-potency B-complex tablet plus 500 milligrams of magnesium daily help quell the secretions of bacteria-encouraging liquid. Clinical studies indicate that 30 to 50 milligrams of zinc each day dramatically reduce body odor in some cases.[165] Some individuals have reduced perspiration odor by taking two chlorophyll tablets with each meal. The biochemic remedy for offensive odor is to dissolve three 6X tablets of the tissue salt Silicea under the tongue each morning and evening.

Folk Remedies

Herbalists suggest drinking 1 cup of sage tea every day to reduce sweat-gland activity. A handful of fresh sage leaves blended with a cup of tomato juice has been found even more effective.[36] Natural deodorant-antiperspirants utilized for generations include:

○ Sponge bathing with 1 tablespoon of ammonia or cologne in 1 quart of water.

○ Dabbing the armpits with alcohol, white vinegar, witch hazel, or a mixture of white willow bark tea and borax.

○ Rubbing the armpits with a spoonful of deodorizing liquid made by crushing and squeezing leaf lettuce or chrysanthemum leaves or by grating raw turnip and squeezing the juice through cheesecloth.

○ Powdering clean, dry armpits with baking soda or cornstarch, or a mixture of the two; or a blend of baby powder and baking soda; or with rice powder or talc.

See also **Foot Odor**

Sources (see Bibliography)

36, 42, 49, 52, 53, 65, 75, 87, 98, 109, 135, 165, 186, 202, 216, 252, 256, 258, 281, 283, 284, 293, 300, 313

Boils, Sties, Carbuncles, and Felons

Sometimes called a furuncle, a boil is a painful, raised area of skin surrounded by swollen, inflamed tissue, usually instigated by a staphylococcus infection at the root of a hair follicle. As white blood cells battle the infection, dead cells and bacteria accumulate as pus in the abscess until the boil bursts and the skin begins to heal. A sty is a little boil amid the eyelashes, with inflammation of one or more of the sebaceous glands of the eyelids. Carbuncles also are staph abscesses, often appearing as a cluster of small boils, but are more severe because the infection penetrates deeper into underlying layers of skin and muscle. A felon, or whitlow, is an abscess at the terminal joint of a finger or toe. It may be superficial (triggered by an injury to the base or side of the nail) or deep seated, involving the bone. The infection may be caused by a bacterium that enters the body through a cut or by the herpes simplex virus responsible for cold sores. Felons require professional treatment if they do not heal after 2 or 3 weeks of self-help. Most boils respond to home care, but medical intervention should be sought if a red streak appears near the boil or if the boil is close to the nose or is accompanied by a fever.

An incipient sty or other boil may be aborted by holding an ice chip against the spot. To bring a developing boil to a head, apply warm, moist compresses for 20 to 30 minutes three or four times a day. To open a sty that has come to a head, pull the eyelash out of its infected follicle and carefully wash the drainage away from the eye. Other boils that appear ready to burst can be opened by pricking with a sterilized needle, then gently squeezing to help release the waste material. After cleansing and disinfecting the area, warm compresses should be continued for several days to assure complete drainage. To avoid possible spread of the infection, showers instead of tub baths are recommended, sterile techniques should be used when dressing the boil, and hands should be thoroughly scrubbed before touching food—staph bacteria can cause food poisoning.[293]

Diet and Supplements (see note on page xii)

Improving nutrition and including supplements may shorten the duration of the infection and strengthen the body's defense against a recurrence. Apricots, bananas, citrus fruits, onions, and tomatoes are considered especially beneficial. Eating several cloves of garlic every day (or taking two garlic capsules with each meal) provides natural antibiotic action. One or two glasses daily of any combination of the juices from beets, carrots, cucumbers, lettuce, and spinach has been found helpful. Drinking at least eight glasses of water a day and incorporating high-fiber foods plus a tablespoon of miller's bran in the diet will help avoid the constipation that may be associated with an outbreak of boils.

Vitamin A 25,000 IU in the form of beta carotene plus 100 to 600 IU vitamin E. Some authorities advise 50,000 to 75,000 IU of vitamin A each day during the infection.[17] The combination of A and E speeds healing and is necessary for proper immune system function.

B Complex One comprehensive tablet daily to help combat the stress of infection and to aid the body's production of antibodies.

Vitamin C 500 to 1,000 milligrams every 2 hours for several days, then 1,000 to 8,000 milligrams in divided doses daily. Vitamin C has antibacterial, anti-inflammatory properties that stimulate the immune system.

Zinc 15 to 50 milligrams per day promotes healing and may prevent the formation of boils.[98]

Tissue salts 3X-potency tablets, as directed:

○ During an attack of boils, take alternate doses of 2 tablets of Ferr. Phos. and Kali. Mur. at hourly intervals, plus 2 tablets of Silicea three times a day.

○ When the boil is ready to drain, take three tablets of Silicea every 2 hours. For a sty, alternate the same amount of Ferr. Phos with the Silicea. If the boil continues to drain without healing, change the remedies to Calc. Sulph. and Nat. Sulph., two tablets of each at 2-hour intervals.

❍ For carbuncles, add four tablets daily of Calc. Fluor. to the dosages recommended for boils.

❍ For external compresses, in ½ cup hot water, dissolve three doses of whatever tissue salts are being taken internally.

Folk Remedies

Folk medicine dealt with boils for thousands of years before the advent of antibiotics. While some of the old remedies such as puncturing a sty with a cat's whisker or rubbing it with a gold wedding ring are no longer advised, many of their suggested ingredients are acknowledged as healing agents.

Bread Stale bread soaked in hot milk, applied and reapplied as a continuous hot poultice, is said to bring a boil to a head by the time a mixture of 4 slices of bread and 1 cup of milk is exhausted. Poultices prepared from breadcrumbs and honey are preferred by some folk healers.

Egg The skin of a raw egg can be used to draw a boil to a head. A poultice of mashed, hard-cooked egg white is also considered helpful.

Flour A poultice of warm milk and flour (with 1 tablespoon salt added to each cup of flour if desired) was a basic remedy. During the early 1800s, a paste of flour and ground ginger or dry mustard was used to draw abscesses that were not near an eye.

Fruit Placing raw figs over boils was advised by Hezekiah (*Isaiah 38:21*); over 2,400 years later, folk healers are still using the same treatment. Eating one dozen oranges or grapefruit daily was an early specific for furuncles and carbuncles. To relieve the pain of a felon, a hole can be cut in a lemon and the finger or toe can be inserted. For body boils, thick slices of lemon, the inside of ripe banana peel, or poultices of crushed raw cranberries can be applied under a bandage.

Herbs Burdock root, cayenne, comfrey, dandelion, echinacea, goldenseal, oatstraw, red clover, sarsaparilla, and slippery elm teas are recommended as internal remedies for boils. Aloe vera gel can be applied to a sty several times a day. For external compresses or poultices, the selection includes alfalfa seeds, bayberry root bark, black pekoe tea, chickweed, comfrey, ground fenugreek, sage leaves, or a combination of triple-strength sassafras and slippery elm teas thickened with cornmeal.

Honey Use plain or blend half-and-half with cod liver oil, apply directly to the boil, cover with a sterile dressing, and replace three times a day.

Salt For boils other than sties, apply a compress squeezed out of a solution of 1 tablespoon epsom salts or table salt in 1 cup of hot water; for felons, soak in the mixture.

Vegetables Warm poultices of the following vegetables (mixed with castor oil, if desired) have been effective when renewed every few hours: ground cabbage or lightly steamed cabbage leaves; grated raw or cooked carrots; cooked, minced garlic; green blades of leeks, finely chopped; grated raw or cooked white potato; or thin slices of raw pumpkin or tomato. Cooked onion was 12-year-old Steven F.'s magic potion. Determined not to be a bother during the long-awaited summer with his grandparents, embarrassed by the location of his problem, and fearing he had a fatal disease, Steven postponed mentioning the sore on his buttock until the pain became unbearable. Finally, he asked his grandfather's advice. "What you've got is a boil on your behind, and it's about ready to pop," was the reassuring diagnosis. "Help me concoct this magic potion and we'll make it disappear." They chopped half an onion, cooked it with a little water, stirred in a tablespoon of sugar, and bandaged the mixture over the boil. Three such treatments were all it took. The boil burst, drained with the help of warm-water compresses, and the remainder of the visit was so great that Steven remembers it as his "magic vacation."

Sources (see Bibliography)

6, 17, 20, 21, 57, 64, 65, 75, 87, 92, 98, 111, 117, 124, 135, 143, 144, 148, 150, 151, 159, 166, 168, 173, 176, 186, 202, 203, 205, 213, 218, 226, 228, 241, 281, 282, 283, 285, 293, 304, 312, 313, 316

Bronchitis

A cute bronchitis, usually a viral infection accompanying or resulting from a cold or the flu, is a temporary inflammation of the upper respiratory tract. The incessant cough may be expected to linger for a month, but if even a mild fever persists longer than 5 days a physician should be consulted to preclude the presence of bacterial infection or to abolish it with antibiotics. Chronic bronchitis develops insidiously from the irritation of repeated bouts of acute bronchitis and/or smoking and lasts longer with each recurrence. Eventually, the airways narrow and partially clog with a profusion of thick mucus that must be coughed up. Untended chronic bronchitis can progress into emphysema.

During a bout of bronchitis, staying indoors and using a humidifier or vaporizer may relieve congestion, especially if apple cider vinegar or eucalyptus leaves are added to the steamer. Cigarettes should be avoided—tobacco smoke can paralyze the hairlike bronchial-tube filters (cilia) so that they are unable to help propel mucus along its normal expulsion route. Cough expectorants rather than cough suppressants should be used. Postural drainage—lying face-down with the head lower than the chest for a few minutes—expedites clearance of the sputum.

Unusual sleeping positions may be necessary. George C. had coughed until he was exhausted, but he could not relax and fall asleep. Lying down made breathing even more difficult. Propping himself up on pillows in the bed or leaning back in the recliner didn't help. He ran hot water in the shower and inhaled the mist while imagining breathing deeply in a wooded glade, but he was still too uncomfortable to sleep. In desperation, he sat on the floor to watch television, faced the recliner, and leaned forward against a pillow to rest his head on the elevated foot rest. Awakened several hours later by the beeping sound of the television station's sign-off, George realized he had found a solution for getting some sleep during a bronchitis attack.

Diet

Hot, spicy foods have been used throughout antiquity to treat pulmonary problems—capsaicin, from hot red pepper, is chemically similar to an ingredient in most modern cough and cold medications. The heat that makes tongues tingle and eyes water from hot pepper, curry, horseradish, and mustard also stimulates bronchial glands to release a flood of "internal tears" that thin mucus, relieve bronchoconstriction, and wash away irritants. Onions induce the same watery secretions—which may account for the folk remedy of eating several slices of onion with tomato and minced garlic every day. Garlic is an antioxidant, a mucus regulator, and an anticongestant when combined with vitamin C. Polish physicians have used garlic extract to cure children afflicted with chronic bronchitis, and garlicky chicken soup (fifteen garlic cloves per quart of broth) sparked with black pepper and/or curry powder has been a bronchitis remedy since it was prescribed by British doctors in the 1880s.[56] Eating one well-spiced meal every day, or drinking a glass of water or tomato juice sprinkled with 10 to 20 drops of hot pepper sauce, is the dietary prescription. If fiery foods cannot be tolerated by the stomach, gargling with the pepper water may increase expectoration and help clear air passages.

All kinds of fruits and vegetables and their juices (especially apricots, beets, carrots, celery, citrus, cucumber, green pepper, papaya, pineapple, and tomatoes) are beneficial if no allergic reactions occur. Drinking at least 2 quarts of liquid a day favorably affects the viscosity of phlegm so it can be expelled. Alcoholic or caffeine-containing beverages are not recommended—their diuretic propensities result in the loss of body fluid. Strong, regular coffee or tea may be an exception in times of emergency because the bronchodilating effect is similar to that of the time-honored medication, theophylline.[29] To flush mucus out of the body, herbalists suggest drinking 1 cup of fenugreek seed tea each hour during the first day, then 4 cups a day. Other teas believed beneficial are camomile, cayenne, chicory, comfrey, dandelion, echinacea, eucalyptus, ginger, licorice, mullein, parsley, peppermint, rose hip, rosemary, saffron, sage, savory, slippery elm, and yarrow.

Supplements (see note on page xii)

Vitamin A 25,000 IU in the form of beta carotene twice daily for 1 month, then 25,000 IU daily to help heal and protect lung tissue.

B Complex One comprehensive tablet daily to activate enzymes needed for healing.

Vitamin C and Bioflavonoids 3,000 to 5,000 milligrams of vitamin C and 200 to 600 milligrams of bioflavonoids, in divided daily doses to fight infection and promote healing.

Vitamin E 100 to 400 IU twice daily, to protect against damage by free radicals, prevent internal oxidation of vitamin A, and improve breathing.

Zinc 50 milligrams daily to accelerate healing.

Bee Pollen 1,000 milligrams or 1 teaspoon of granules daily.

Tissue Salts One 12X tablet *each* Ferr. Phos. and Nat. Mur. twice daily during bouts of bronchitis, plus these specifics: For fever, take one 6X Ferr. Phos. tablet every half hour until temperature is normal. For soreness in the chest or larynx, take three tablets of 6X Ferr. Phos. each 4 hours, and three tablets of 6X Calc. Sulph. between those doses.

Folk Remedies

Beverages Liquefy a can of asparagus in an electric blender and refrigerate. Each morning and evening, mix ¼ cup of the asparagus with water for a hot or cold drink.[2] Or boil fresh cranberries in water for 10 minutes, then whir in a blender with an equal amount of pear juice; drink several glasses daily. Or boil four chopped figs in 2 cups of water for 6 minutes, cover until cool, then refrigerate and sip half a cup of the liquid each morning and night. Or stir 1 or 2 tablespoons of raw honey into a cup of scalded milk and sip to relieve bronchial distress.

Ointments and Poultices Warm a tablespoon of petroleum jelly with four minced garlic cloves; massage into the chest while still warm. Or blend 2 tablespoons of warm castor oil with 1 tablespoon of turpentine, rub on the chest at bedtime, and cover with flannel—in severe cases, apply the mixture several times a day. Or use boiled bay leaves or chopped onions fried in lard as a before-bed poultice.

Nerve Pressure and Massage

For short-term relief from bronchial distress, press or massage each point (intermittently or steadily) for 30 seconds to 2 minutes.

○ Press the bridge of the nose with fingers and thumb, then press in and up under the bony shelf on the cheekbones above the nostrils.

○ With the thumb and fingers, pinch up and down the back of the neck.

○ Press against each side of the breastbone, between the collarbone and the first rib; then press and massage the center of the chest.

○ Extend the left arm, palm up. Press and massage a point 1 inch toward the hand from the inner hollow of the elbow 1 inch toward the outside of the forearm on the same side as the thumb; repeat with the right arm. Then squeeze both sides of the thumbnail on each hand with the thumb and index finger of the opposite hand.

○ Press a point the width of 1 hand directly above the navel.

○ Hold the right foot with the left hand and use the right hand to rub the area directly beneath the toe pads. Start under the big toe, and if there is any tenderness, massage it out with a circular, rolling motion. Repeat with the left foot.

Sources (see Bibliography)

2, 6, 17, 26, 29, 42, 50, 56, 57, 59, 60, 64, 89, 98, 135, 144, 148, 150, 153, 159, 164, 166, 173, 176, 179, 186, 202, 203, 204, 205, 218, 228, 233, 247, 256, 264, 281, 282, 285, 293, 302, 304, 306, 312, 313

Bruises

Black-and-blue marks usually appear from bumps or blows that, without breaking the skin to cause external bleeding, injure small blood vessels so that blood seeps into surrounding tissue to create discoloration and possible swelling. Deprived of the bloodstream's oxygen, the leaked red blood darkens to purple, then the bruise gradually changes color from blue to green to brownish yellow as the body conducts its complex healing maneuver called hemostasis. First, platelets (tiny blood-clotting cells) form a temporary plug in the damaged blood vessels. Then, while the seeped blood is being resorbed, proteins called clotting factors permanently repair the ruptures to prevent further blood loss. Any disturbance of the elements required for this natural process can result in additional bleeding or bruising and can delay the normal recovery time of about 1 week.

Treatment

Cold The immediate application of ice or any chilled substance slows the seepage from injured blood vessels to limit the size of the lump and the intensity of its color. To avoid the possibility of frostbite, use ice intermittently and remove it for a few minutes each time the area feels numb. If the bruise is on an arm or leg, elevating the injured part will decrease local blood flow.

Heat Immediately plunging a bruised fingernail or toenail into very hot water may relieve the agony by softening the nail so that it yields to accommodate the swelling beneath it.[202] For other bruises, hot compresses can be used after the first 24 hours to stimulate circulation and hasten the resorption of discoloring fluid in the tissues.

Supplements (See note on page xii) Taking 2,000 milligrams of vitamin C immediately, then supplementing the diet with vitamins A, B complex, C, and E, plus selenium and zinc, assists blood vessel repair and speeds healing. Taking one tablet *each* of the 3X tissue salts Ferr. Phos. and

Kali. Mur. each 10 minutes for 1 hour after the bruising occurs, then two or three times a day, may reduce both swelling and discoloration. For topical application: the same two tissue salts can be dissolved in water and sponged over flesh bruises; for bruises on shins or other bones, use dissolved Calc. Fluor., then cover with a moisture-retaining bandage.

Easy Bruising

Internal conditions are responsible for the appearance of black-and-blue marks with little or no apparent reason. In some instances, a slight bump or constrictive clothing results in a bruise; in others, called spontaneous bruising or purpura, no external pressure need be exerted.

○ Allergic reactions to drugs, foods, or bacteria can cause an inflammation of blood vessels beneath the skin resulting in spontaneous hemorrhaging and bruising called allergic purpura.

○ Common purpura, sometimes termed senile purpura because it frequently occurs in the middle-aged or elderly, may appear as wine-colored spots that fade away in 2 or 3 weeks without turning blue. Dietary deficiencies or anti-inflammatory medications that destroy vitamin C can weaken the collagen fibers (synthesized from protein and vitamin C) supporting blood vessel walls, leaving fragile blood vessels that rupture at the slightest provocation. Taking divided doses of 500 to 5,000 milligrams of vitamin C plus 100 to 1,000 milligrams of bioflavonoids daily may correct the problem.[17, 272]

○ Blood-clotting platelets are essential for the prevention of easy bruising. This blood-clotting function can be curtailed by aspirin or aspirin-like drugs, large amounts of alcohol or cayenne pepper, and by high doses of fish-oil supplements.[151, 177] Deficiencies of B_{12} and folic acid can decrease the body's production of platelets; daily supplementation with a B-complex tablet and additional folic acid may be beneficial.

Easy bruising or purpura that continues or is excessive warrants medical evaluation. The problem may be a side-effect of prescribed medications, and/or might be accompanied by internal hemorrhages or could be an indication of bone-marrow disorders or other diseases.

Folk Remedies

The 1835 edition of *The American Frugal Housewife*[69] advises a poultice of wet brown paper dipped in blackstrap molasses for healing a bruise. The inside of a ripe banana peel; bread soaked in vinegar, kerosene, or turpentine; or 30 minutes of hot fomentations were alternatives when ice was not available. Immediately rubbing the area with damp fingers dipped in sugar is said to prevent a black-and-blue mark from developing. The more intrepid steeped a handful of tobacco in warm water for several hours, applied the tobacco to the bruise, and drank several spoonfuls of the liquid. Soaking the bruised part for 15 minutes several times a day in a quart of hot water containing ¼ cup of apple cider vinegar is a solution for swelling.

Herb Teas The following can be used for hot compresses: alfalfa, comfrey root, fenugreek, hyssop, lobelia, mullein, oregano, parsley, pekoe, rose hip, thyme, turmeric, and yarrow.

Poultices When bandaged over a bruise, these are said to hasten healing: bread blended with water or milk; a paste of arrowroot and water or cornstarch and castor oil, boiled slippery elm bark or soapwort roots; heated salt; minced raw ham or minced parsley mixed with butter; grated raw cabbage, potato, or turnip; or chopped boiled onion, plain or mixed with an equal amount of raw salt pork.

Saturating a cotton ball with witch hazel and binding it over bruised spots may help prevent discoloration. Aloe vera gel is another bruise healer. Five-year-old Dewain H. was so excited about spending a whole week at his grandparents' lakeside cabin that he dashed toward the front porch the moment they arrived, tripped over a rock, and banged his head on a flowerpot. Dewain's grandfather snatched a half-frozen package of hamburger out of the ice chest and pressed it against the reddening streak at the corner of Dewain's eye above the cheekbone until the pain was deadened. Then his grandmother smoothed aloe vera gel over the area, and when her finger slipped, over half the skin between his eye and eyebrow. For most of the next week, Dewain looked as if he had been experimenting with eye makeup. The aloe-treated areas changed directly from red to yellow without bothering with blue, then returned to normal before the three-quarters of a black eye progressed through the usual purples and greens.

By the time Dewain got home, the evidence had disappeared, but his grandparents corroborated his tale of terrible injury and its colorful aftermath.

Sources (see Bibliography)

6, 17, 42, 45, 50, 53, 57, 64, 69, 75, 87, 98, 112, 144, 146, 148, 150, 151, 168, 176, 177, 179, 187, 202, 205, 224, 256, 264, 272, 276, 281, 283, 284, 299, 304, 312, 313, 317, 322

Bruxism (Tooth Grinding)

Tooth grinding occurs during sleep or as an unconscious habit during the day. The underlying cause may be unresolved stress (teeth clenching is an instinctive reaction to anger or emotional tension), jaw muscles attempting to grind away unevenness such as the high point of a crown or filling when the teeth are brought together, hypoglycemia (related to low adrenal function), or dietary deficiencies. Continued bruxism can wear away tooth enamel; increase teeth's sensitivity to heat and cold; loosen teeth and contribute to periodontal disease; cause morning headaches, sore jaw muscles, and painful chewing; and can eventually lead to TMJ (temporomandibular joint syndrome) by forcing the jaw joint out of balance.

Sleeping on the back avoids unnatural pressure on the jaws and teeth. When sleeping on one side, placing a contoured foam pillow under the face and another under the free arm helps reduce strain on the neck and jaw muscles. A soft mouth guard (sold in sporting goods stores) may be used temporarily to protect the teeth from nocturnal damage,[293] but if home remedies do not alleviate the problem, a dentist should be consulted to make sure the teeth fit together properly and, if necessary, to design a plastic bite plate.

Diet and Supplements (see note on page xii)

Nutritionists advise cutting back on caffeine and refined carbohydrates such as candy and white-flour products. Many doctors believe that bruxism is a nutritional problem that can be corrected with supplements in addition to a daily multivitamin-mineral.[98]

Taking a B-complex tablet once or twice a day, 3,000 to 5,000 milligrams of vitamin C in divided daily doses, and 50 milligrams of zinc often helps compensate for and reduce stress reactions.

Deficiencies of calcium and pantothenic acid have been linked to tooth grinding. Taking 1,200 to 1,500 milligrams of calcium (to help regulate involuntary muscle movement), 500 to 750 milligrams of magnesium (to assist calcium assimilation), and 100 to 1,000 milligrams of pantothenic acid (in divided daily doses for muscle coordination) has helped many cases of bruxism.[17, 301] Sometimes, calcium, magnesium, and a little extra protein are all that is needed. Five-year-old Jason A.'s nighttime tooth grinding lessened after his mother started giving him chewable calcium wafers as after-dinner and before-bed treats. When she mixed a pulverized magnesium tablet with peanut butter for a half-sandwich bedtime snack, Jason's tooth-grinding stopped completely.

Exercise

Teeth need to touch only when chewing or swallowing. The passive exercise of positioning the tongue against the roof of the mouth behind the front teeth helps keep teeth slightly separated while the lips remain together.

○ To relieve the neck and shoulder tension often experienced by people with bruxism, several times a day, shrug each shoulder and hold for a few seconds, then shrug both shoulders at the same time; gently roll the head clockwise, then counterclockwise several times; conclude by holding the chin up and slowly turning the head to look over each shoulder ten times.

○ Daytime stretching of jaw muscles may relieve facial tension and soreness from nighttime gnashing. With the mouth wide open, slowly shift the jaw from left to right, then drop the lower jaw. Repeat three times.

○ Overactive mouth muscles may be calmed by the exercise of munching on raw apple, cauliflower, or carrot just before retiring.

Stress Management

The problems of bruxism are often related to today's pressure-packed lifestyles. When changing jobs, spouses, or children is impractical, taking three deep breaths and practicing any relaxation technique (see Introduction) may help overcome teeth grinding. Including an affirmation such as,

"My mouth muscles are relaxed. I will sleep soundly, and soundlessly, all night," may be helpful.

Sources (see Bibliography)

17, 41, 42, 47, 49, 75, 80, 98, 108, 111, 186, 207, 234, 281, 283, 293, 301, 312

Burns

A first-degree burn causes pain, redness and mild swelling but no blisters. Second-degree burns extend below the skin and are characterized by blisters as well as pain, redness, and swelling. A third-degree burn evidences a white or charred appearance from deep tissue damage and may be temporarily painless due to the destruction of nerve endings. Third-degree burns should be cooled with cold water, then receive immediate medical attention. Flood a chemical burn of the eye with water or milk for 5 to 10 minutes, then get professional assistance.

First-Aid Tip for First- and Second-Degree Burns If the burn is under clothing, dousing the area before removing the garment may prevent the hot cloth from causing a deeper burn. Cool the burned skin for 20 to 30 minutes or until pain diminishes by running cold tap water over the area, immersing it in cold water, or applying cold compresses. If discomfort persists, cold compresses or an ice pack may be applied at intervals throughout the first 24 hours. To reduce skin sensitivity, a topical ointment may be used between cold applications and covered with a light, nonadherent dressing. Blisters are nature's protective bandage so should be left intact. If blisters break, wash the area twice daily with soap and water, then cover with a sterile dressing. Widespread second-degree burns, or those on the face, hands, genitals, or feet, should receive medical care.

Diet and Supplements (see note on page xii)

For victims of severe burns, nutritional consultants advise drinking at least eight glasses of water daily, eating ample protein, consuming high-potassium foods (apricots, bananas, leafy greens, baked potatoes with skin) and edibles that increase the ratio of sulfur in the diet (cabbage, corn, garlic, kale, kohlrabi, soybeans, watercress);[149] and including dietary supplements.

Vitamin A In the form of beta carotene, up to 100,000 IU daily for 1 week, then 25,000 IU a day for maintenance to fight infection and promote healing.

B Complex One comprehensive tablet twice a day to compensate for the stress of serious burns. Taking an additional 200 milligrams of PABA with each meal during the painful period may ease the discomfort.

Vitamin C 1,000 milligrams per day, up to 1,000 milligrams per hour for the first few days. When taken immediately, vitamin C helps prevent shock. It also helps prevent infection, aids healing, and when taken with bioflavonoids, improves the tensile strength of connective tissue.

Calcium and Magnesium 1,500 milligrams of calcium plus 750 milligrams of magnesium to help structure proteins for healing and to compensate for loss of body fluids.[17]

Vitamin D 400 to 1,000 IU daily for 1 month to assist with the assimilation of vitamin A and calcium.

Vitamin E 100 to 1,000 IU daily to speed healing and help prevent scarring.[266, 267]

Selenium 200 micrograms daily until healing is complete, to help prevent infection and to increase tissue elasticity.

Tissue Salts Immediately following the accident, take one 3X tablet *each* Ferr. Phos. and Kali. Mur. at 10-minute intervals for 1 hour. For serious burns, Kali. Phos. can be included.

Zinc—50 to 100 milligrams daily for 2 to 4 weeks to stimulate healing.

Folk Remedies

To help prevent shock from a severe burn, folk practitioners advise sipping one of these beverages: ½ cup cold water mixed with 1 teaspoon salt and ½ teaspoon baking soda; cool cayenne tea (two capsules may be substituted); or cooled, strong tea made from 1 tablespoon skullcap, 2 teaspoons valerian, and 1 teaspoon hops.

For immediately cooling of minor burns, milk or apple cider vinegar is believed more effective than water. For rapid pain relief, equal parts of apple cider vinegar, brandy, and water can be combined and applied constantly until the pain is gone, then the burn can be covered with a vinegar-soaked bandage. For pain relief and speedy healing after the initial cooling, a coating of cod liver oil, garlic oil, or sesame oil can be applied; or one of the other folk remedies may be utilized.

Aloe Vera Gel One of the oldest, best-known, and most effective treatments for burns, aloe vera gel is not only a soothing, healing agent but has also been found to reduce peeling and may help prevent infection.[254] Erna V., cafeteria manager for an elementary school, decorates the kitchen windowsills with potted aloes she calls "burn plants." With students standing in line for lunch, neither she nor the other cafeteria workers have time for lengthy cooling of the minor burns they frequently encounter. After a chilling swipe with an ice cube, they cover the burned spots with aloe vera gel squeezed directly from the end of a broken-off segment of one of the decorative plants.

Baking Soda Sprinkle the soda over the burn and bind with a soft cloth, or cover with a paste of baking soda (combined with flour, if desired) blended with water or egg white. A mixture of baking soda and olive oil can be used to help heal a severe burn and reduce scarring.[149]

Cornmeal and Charcoal Apply a poultice made with two parts cornmeal and one part powdered activated charcoal, moistened with milk.

Eggs Cover the burned skin with a beaten raw egg then drench with alcohol to "cook" it into a protective film. Or beat the egg with 2 tablespoons castor oil or olive oil, spread the mixture on soft cloth, and apply over blistered burns.

○ Beat the white of an egg (with or without 1 tablespoon of lard), apply to the burn, and let remain for 1 hour.

○ If the throat is burned from hot liquid, beat an egg white with water and sip slowly.

Flour Cover a superficial burn with flour (over a coating of lard or molasses, if desired) and wrap with clean cloth to exclude the air.

Fruits and Vegetables To relieve minor burns, apply apple butter or grated apple mixed with olive oil; the inner surface of a ripe banana peel; mashed cabbage leaves; grated or juiced carrots; slices of raw onion; or ground raw pumpkin, radishes, or turnip. Replace every 15 minutes or when the poultice dries. For more severe burns, sliced, grated, or ground raw white potato bandaged over the burn is said to encourage healing from the inside without leaving a scar.

Herbs Folk healers recommend cool compresses of tannic-acid-containing teas such as beriberi leaves, blackberry leaves, pekoe, sassafras, sumac leaves, sweet gum, or white oak bark. Modern herbalists suggest making a paste of boiling water and any of these herbs: burdock, chickweed, comfrey, fenugreek, goldenseal, hyssop, marshmallow, pennyroyal, plantain, or slippery elm, then sandwiching the mixture between two pieces of cloth before applying the poultice over a coating of vitamin E oil.

Honey Probably the most ancient remedy for burns, raw honey has been found to have antibacterial properties and is used in some hospitals. It can be applied directly to the skin to counteract pain. Adding bee pollen granules to the honey or combining equal parts of honey and wheat germ oil blended with comfrey leaves to make a paste is believed to speed healing. If desired, the honey mixtures may be covered with a dry bandage.

Oatmeal Apply a poultice of oatmeal and cold water.

Sugar To hasten pain relief, sugar can be added to the water used for the initial cooling. When sprinkled on the surface of oozing burns, granulated sugar is believed to encourage healing by pulling out the excess moisture. To ease the pain of a burned tongue, sprinkle it with sugar or with a few drops of vanilla extract.

Yogurt Plain yogurt, reapplied as it dries, often provides swift relief from painful burns and is reported to speed healing.

Nerve Pressure

To activate natural healing, press inward and upward below each eyebrow an inch out from the nose. Apply pressure for 10 seconds, release for 10 seconds, and repeat for 30 seconds of pressure once each day.

Sources (see Bibliography)

2, 6, 17, 21, 42, 61, 64, 66, 69, 75, 84, 87, 92, 98, 111, 117, 135, 142, 143, 144, 149, 150, 151, 159, 164, 166, 171, 176, 180, 186, 202, 203, 205, 228, 254, 256, 257, 266, 267, 281, 284, 293, 294, 299, 300, 304, 312, 313, 316, 322

Bursitis

The body's joints are surrounded by tiny, fluid-filled sacs (bursae) to ensure frictionless movement. Bursitis occurs when 1 of the 156 bursae becomes painfully inflamed from an injury, from overuse of the joint, or from the irritation of calcium deposits on a bursa wall. Stress, which prevents proper assimilation of nutrients, can be a contributing factor. Shoulders, elbows, hips, and knees are its most common locations. Bunions, which may be either genetically inherited or caused by ill-fitting shoes, are a form of bursitis that may require surgical correction.

During the acute phase of bursitis, the afflicted joint should be allowed to rest without being totally immobilized. Anti-inflammatory painkillers such as aspirin or ibuprofen are recommended.[111] If the joint is hot to the touch, applying ice packs on a schedule of 10 minutes on/10 minutes off helps relieve the pain. (For homemade, joint-conforming ice packs, see "First-Aid Supplies" in the Introduction.) If the joint does not feel hot, warm compresses may bring relief. If pain remains after a few days, medical attention may be necessary for treatment of an underlying infection or for surgical removal of calcium deposits. As soon as the pain subsides, gentle exercise helps prevent the formation of fibrous bands of tissue (adhesions) that can permanently limit movement of the joint.

Diet and Supplements (see note on page xii)

Some nutritionally oriented doctors recommend increasing protein consumption, reducing purines (see "Gout"), eating six small meals daily, and accompanying each meal with acidophilus yogurt or capsules. Including generous amounts of carrots, citrus fruits, tomatoes, green vegetables, and calcium-containing foods, and taking a daily multivitamin-mineral plus additional supplements may also be of help.

Vitamin A In the form of beta carotene, up to 60,000 IU daily for 1 month; 50,000 IU for 2 weeks; then 25,000 IU each day to speed healing and bolster the immune system to help prevent recurrence.

B Complex One high-potency tablet daily, plus 1,000 micrograms of sublingual B_{12} for 10 days, then the same amount every other day for 3 weeks to relieve pain, aid tissue repair, and improve nutrient absorption. Accompanying the B_{12} with a 50-milligram tablet of B_1 often improves its effectiveness.

Vitamin C with Bioflavonoids 1,000 milligrams every hour or 2 during the first few days, then 2,000 to 5,000 milligrams in divided doses each day for several weeks to help relieve inflammation and potentiate the immune system.

Calcium and Magnesium 1,500 milligrams of calcium plus 750 milligrams of magnesium in divided daily doses. Calcium requires magnesium for utilization by the body, and deposits can form in the tissues from calcium that has been pulled from the bones to compensate for a deficiency of the mineral.[86, 317]

Vitamin D 400 to 600 IU daily during the acute period to assist in the absorption of calcium.

Vitamin E 400 to 1,000 IU daily as an anti-inflammatory agent during the painful phase, then 100 to 400 IU each day to help prevent the formation of calcium deposits or scar tissue in the affected joint.

Tissue Salts During the acute stage, three tablets 3X-potency Nat. Mur. can be taken three times each day with 1 teaspoon apple cider vinegar stirred into a glass of water. To help disperse fluid in the joint, alternate doses of Nat. Sulph. may be taken. For slow-to-heal bursitis, dissolve three tablets of 3X Silicea under the tongue three times a day.

Exercise

The following are two easy exercises for bursitis of the shoulder. (1) Stand in a corner and "walk" the fingers up the wall as high as possible without overstretching. (2) While standing, lean forward and let the arm swing back and forth like a pendulum, gradually increasing the arc. Bertha A. was bedfast with another ailment and couldn't perform either of those exercises. To prevent her bursitis from becoming a frozen shoulder, her son attached a T-shaped pillar of hollow pipe to the head of her bed with comfortable handgrips anchored to a rope threaded through the crossbar. By grasping the grips, Bertha used her good arm to gradually elevate the bad one and improve her range of movement.

Folk Remedies

To hasten recovery, folk healers advise keeping the afflicted joint extra warm at night by wrapping flannel around a knee or by sleeping in a sweater.

Apple Cider Vinegar and Honey Stirring 2 teaspoons *each* apple cider vinegar and raw honey into a glass of water to accompany each meal is believed to correct the calcium precipitation that may instigate bursitis.

Herbs For bursitis sufferers, a cup or two daily of any of these teas is suggested: alfalfa, burdock, camomile, chaparral, fenugreek, lobelia, oat straw, white willow, yarrow, or yucca. For external relief, boil 1 tablespoon cayenne pepper in 2 cups apple cider vinegar for 10 minutes and use the liquid for a warm compress. Poultices provide additional options: Moisten comfrey, crushed flaxseed, or mullein with boiling water, stir in a spoonful of vegetable oil, then spread the paste between pieces of gauze and apply to the painful area after coating it with olive oil to protect the skin.

Oils Smooth castor oil over the afflicted joint, cover with flannel, and keep warm with hot towels or a heating pad. After the pain is no longer acute, massage the joint with warmed olive oil once a day to relieve soreness and help prevent a return of bursitis.

Potato Juice Slice a scrubbed potato very thin, cover with water in a large glass, and let stand for 8 to 12 hours. Strain and drink the liquid on an empty stomach. If preferred, potato juice may be made in an electric juicer and diluted half-and-half with water.

Sea Water Taking 2 or 3 teaspoons of bottled sea water daily for 6 to 9 months has cleared some cases of chronic bursitis.[128]

Nerve Pressure and Massage

For Bursitis in Any Joint Press and massage the palm of each hand or the sole of each foot from the ball of the foot to the beginning of the heel pad.

For Bursitis in the Shoulders or Arms Press and massage 3 inches across the center of the upper edge of the collar bone on both sides and just below the ends of the collarbones where they meet the shoulders. Then press or massage each palm just below the pad of the little finger or the sole of each foot below the pad of the little toe.

For Bursitis in the Hip or Leg Massage a 2-inch area on the back of each hand on the outside just above the wrist or on the outer edge of the top of the foot between the anklebone and the beginning of the heel pad.

Sources (see Bibliography)

2, 6, 17, 27, 42, 63, 65, 75, 80, 82, 86, 87, 98, 111, 128, 144, 148, 159, 164, 171, 172, 176, 186, 200, 201, 206, 244, 256, 262, 264, 281, 283, 293, 301, 317

Canker Sores

Medically identified as aphthous ulcers, canker sores have annoyed humanity since ancient times—Hippocrates coined the other medical term for them, aphthous stomatitis, in the fourth century B.C. Although hereditary predisposition may play a role in the frequency of their appearance, the official cause of these painful craters inside the mouth is considered to be a temporary malfunction of the immune system[254] that can be triggered by minor injuries inside the mouth, fatigue, psychological stress, illness with fever, menstrual cycles, nutritional deficiencies, or sensitivity to certain foods. The cankers, with their open white centers and red borders, can occur singly or in clusters, can be as small as a pinhead or as large as a quarter and usually last from 4 to 20 days. Sores that do not heal in 3 weeks should receive medical attention to preclude bacterial infection. Home remedies may alleviate pain, hasten the healing process, and reduce the possibility of recurrence.

Diet and Supplements (see note on page xii)

Highest on the list of foods that trigger cankers are cherries, chocolate and other sweets, citrus fruits, nuts, pineapple, plums, and tomato products. Eliminating all suspects for a month, then reincorporating them one at a time every 3 or 4 weeks, may identify the dietary culprit. During an outbreak, a bland diet with no acidic fruits, nuts, or salty, spicy, or sugary foods avoids irritating the cankers. Swishing a swallow of milk over the sores before and several times during a meal lessens the discomfort of eating.

Eating plain yogurt is especially helpful for canker sores. Taking two to five capsules of *Lactobacillus acidophilus* with each meal as a preventive measure is effective for some individuals. Lilly E. prefers chewable acidophilus tablets. Frequently plagued by painful mouth ulcers, she avoided her known instigators—pineapple and raw tomatoes—and took acidophilus capsules or ate yogurt to treat the cankers that appeared at random intervals. After experimenting with the 500-milligram tablets, Lilly found that taking two of them each morning and evening prevents the outbreaks of unknown origin. And by dissolving two extra tablets in her mouth before a meal, she can enjoy both tomatoes and pineapple without an adverse reaction.

A nutritious, well-balanced diet can be an important factor in canker control. Studies show that 15 percent of the people with canker sores are deficient in iron and B vitamins.[50] Taking individual supplements in addition to a daily multivitamin-mineral often shortens the duration of the sores and helps prevent their reappearance.

Vitamin A   In the form of beta carotene, 50,000 IU daily for 1 week, then 25,000 IU a day for 2 weeks to spur healing.

B Complex   One to four high-potency tablets daily have reduced the active time of canker sores to as little as 48 hours when the B vitamins were accompanied by a calcium-magnesium supplement.[301] Taking 25 to 100 milligrams of niacin or niacinamide with each meal often corrects and prevents these sores.[87, 313] Several studies report excellent results when 2,000 micrograms of sublingual B12 and folic acid are taken twice daily on an empty stomach.[17]

Vitamin C with Bioflavonoids   500 to 1,000 milligrams at the first sign of a canker sore and each hour for the first day, then 1,500 to 5,000 milligrams in divided daily doses until healing is complete.[186]

Vitamin E   When a canker first appears, coat it with vitamin E from a pierced capsule and repeat at frequent intervals.

Tissue Salts   Three or four times a day, dissolve alternating doses of four tablets *each* 6X Kali. Mur. and Kali. Phos. under the tongue.

Zinc   30 to 60 milligrams daily, or one zinc lozenge dissolved in the mouth every 3 hours for 2 days to speed healing and enhance immune function.

Folk Remedies

Contemporary folk remedies call for holding a moist teabag over the sores, dissolving an antacid tablet in the mouth, or protectively coating the tender craters with a swish of milk of magnesia to relieve pain. Older treatments include eating an apple after every meal, dabbing the cankers with aloe vera gel, or diluting the gel with water for a mouth rinse several times a day. An assortment of other options follows.

Baking Soda or Table Salt To temporarily relieve pain and to encourage healing, use a strong solution of either soda or salt and water as a mouth rinse.

Blackstrap Molasses Several times each day, keep a glob of this healing substance next to the sore.

Herbs Applying just a touch of tincture of myrrh (a 2,000-year-old remedy available in most pharmacies) to the center of a canker, or holding a pinch of dry mustard or myrrh against the sore for five minutes, is temporarily painful but is said to heal the sore within 2 days.[149, 312] A solution made from 1 tablespoon of dried, grated pomegranate rind boiled in 1 cup water until reduced by half is believed equally effective.[144] The basic folk medicine canker cure is a frequent mouth rinse with any of these teas brewed triple-strength: burdock, camomile, goldenseal, red raspberry, sage, or strawberry.

Hydrogen Peroxide Place a drop of 3 percent peroxide on each canker, or dilute the peroxide with water and swish it in the mouth before spitting it out.

Sources (see Bibliography)

6, 17, 42, 49, 50, 65, 75, 87, 98, 109, 112, 135, 144, 148, 149, 165, 166, 176, 202, 207, 254, 256, 281, 283, 293, 300, 301, 312, 313

Cataracts

Centuries ago, the name "cataract" was coined from the conception that misty vision and white pupils were caused by a kind of waterfall descending from the brain. Babies can be born with cataracts as the result of an inherited disease; eye injuries or steroid drugs can trigger them at any age; diabetes or exposure to X-rays contribute to their formation. Senile cataracts, however, are the most common form. To some degree, they affect most people over the age of 65, but in many cases the opacity is confined to the edge of the lens, where it does not impair vision.[75]

Once accepted as a normal tribulation of aging, cataracts are now considered a degenerative condition only in that the thickening and clouding of the eye's transparent lens often results from accumulated cell damage due to years of exposure to sunlight's ultraviolet rays. Wearing sunglasses designated Z80.3 or prescription glasses with a UV-protective film lessens the risk of cataracts and slows their growth.[186] Tanning booths intensify the risk because they utilize penetrating UVA radiation in preference to the UVB rays that are more likely to produce a sunburn.[300] When visual impairment warrants, advances in modern medicine have reduced surgical removal to an outpatient procedure, but postponement, retardation, or regression is a preferable option.

Diet and Supplements (see note on page xii)

Although no single nutrient is effective in delaying eye aging and defeating cataracts, favorable responses have been achieved when all dietary essentials are supplied. Dr. Rinse's "breakfast formula" (devised by a chemist as a cure for atherosclerotic complications and publicized during the 1970s) has proven beneficial for preventing and correcting some cataracts.[222] For a simplified version of the formula, combine 1 tablespoon *each* brewer's yeast, lecithin granules, and raw wheat germ with 1 teaspoon powdered calcium and a small amount of milk. Stir in hot or cold cereal and/or yogurt, add fruit and sweeten to taste with brown sugar or honey, then accompany it with a multivitamin-mineral, 500 milligrams of vitamin C, and 100 IU of vitamin E. Nutritional experts of that decade advised drinking two glasses of vegetable juices daily—8 ounces of carrot juice mixed with any combination of beet, celery, cucumber, parsley, and spinach—and including cantaloupe, citrus fruits, red-orange and leafy-green vegetables, unsaturated oils, and whole grains in the diet.[173, 218, 226]

By 1985, holistic ophthalmologists were not only preventing and retarding cataracts but were reversing some of them with a low-fat diet stressing fish, fowl, and fresh produce supplemented by a multivitamin-mineral, a B-complex tablet, 500 milligrams vitamin C, 400 IU vitamin E, and 20 milligrams *each* manganese and zinc.[43, 177] In 1988, Gary Price Todd, M.D., stated in *Eye Talk* that by taking nutritional supplements, 50 percent of his cataract patients had their vision restored without surgery.[17]

Recent studies validate these earlier successes. The B vitamins, especially B$_2$, have been found protective of the crystalline lens of the eye.[151] A study reported in *American Journal of Clinical Nutrition* (January 1991) shows that people who eat less than 4 daily servings of fruits and vegetables are almost six times more likely to develop cataracts than those who consume generous quantities of foods rich in vitamin C and carotenoids such as beta carotene and vitamin E. Another study, reported in *Archives of Ophthalmology* (February 1991), revealed that adults taking multivitamins are 37 percent less likely to have cataracts than people who do not use supplements and that high intakes of vitamins B$_1$, B$_2$, niacin, C, and E, plus beta carotene and iron reduce the risk of cataracts.

The January 1993 issue of *Berkeley Wellness Letter* explains that all of those vitamins, along with selenium, are antioxidants that combat the tissue-damaging, lens-clouding free radicals created by exposure to ultraviolet light, cigarette smoke and other environmental hazards, and by the body itself. Many ophthalmologists prescribe over-the-counter "eye vitamins" containing these antioxidants plus zinc for their cataract patients.[124] Thelma O. had endured complications following the removal of a cataract from one eye and dreaded having the next surgery so soon after moving from the Midwest to Boston. When her new doctor suggested that she take a comprehensive multiple plus 1,000 milligrams of vitamin C, 400 IU of vitamin E, and an over-the-counter eye vitamin formula every day for 6 weeks before the operation and for a month afterward, Thelma was willing to experiment. She was delighted with the outcome. No problems this time, and such rapid healing that she was soon reading comfortably with contact lenses.

With medical approval, and in addition to a comprehensive multiple, nutritionists and naturopathic doctors recommend the following daily supplements.

Vitamin A in the form of Beta Carotene   100,000 to 200,000 IU for 1 month, then 50,000 to 75,000 IU.

B Complex   One comprehensive tablet, plus 50 milligrams *each* B_1, B_2, and B_6; and 100 to 500 milligrams pantothenic acid.

Vitamin C with Bioflavonoids   500 to 6,000 milligrams in divided doses.

Vitamin E   100 to 600 IU.

Calcium and Magnesium   1,000 milligrams of calcium plus 500 milligrams magnesium.

Selenium   50 to 200 micrograms.

Zinc   30 to 50 milligrams.

Tissue Salts   Four tablets of 6X Calc. Fluor. plus two of 6X Silicea.

Folk Remedies

The ancient practice of smearing the eyelids with a mixture of honey and ox dung to correct cataracts has been forsaken, but honey is still utilized by folk healers. Placing a drop of raw honey in the corner of the eye each night is said to instigate improvement within 2 months, and sipping a blend of 2 teaspoons *each* honey and apple cider vinegar in a glass of water at each meal is believed to retard or reverse cataract growth. Other reportedly successful home remedies follow.

Cod Liver Oil or Linseed Oil   Place two drops of cod liver oil in the afflicted eye each night for 1 month. If no improvement is evident, substitute one drop of linseed oil (from a pharmacy).

Epsom Salts   Dissolve in warm water and use a mild solution as an eye wash.

Herbs   Aloe vera juice may be used as an eye drop. Herbalists advise filtered camomile or eyebright tea (not a tincture) for twice-a-day eye washing. Taking four or five capsules of eyebright each morning and evening is said to enhance the benefits.[176, 312] Drinking a cup of cayenne tea daily is believed to delay the development of cataracts. Other herbs considered beneficial are bayberry, chervil, goldenseal, and red raspberry.

Potato   Spread peeled, grated raw potato between pieces of gauze and place over the eyelid for an hour or more each day.

Sea water   Place 2 drops of bottled sea water in the eye each morning and night, then swallow a spoonful of the water.

Nerve Pressure and Massage

❍ Once or twice each day, press each point for 30 seconds: Press up under the eyebrows on each side of the bridge of the nose; press the small notch in the bone surrounding the eye, about ¼ inch toward the nose from the lower outside corner of the eye; then use the index fingers to press under each ear at the back of the jawbone and pull forward.

❍ Once a day, on the side on which the cataract is located, massage the area at the bottom of the second toe and the one next to it, as well as the base of the index and middle fingers. Then press and massage the sole of each foot between the ball of the foot and the beginning of the arch.

Sources (see Bibliography)

2, 6, 17, 26, 43, 45, 46, 47, 49, 59, 60, 64, 72, 75, 82, 86, 87, 89, 98, 112, 124, 146, 150, 151, 164, 172, 173, 176, 177, 186, 190, 213, 218, 222, 226, 256, 262, 281, 283, 294, 300, 303, 312, 316

Chapped, Sore Lips

Thin skinned and devoid of oil glands, lips can chap from exposure to dry air, sunshine, or cold temperatures unless covered with a protective barrier. Doctors and cosmetologists advise wearing sunscreen-containing lip balm or lipstick with an SPF rating of at least 15 to guard against skin-damaging ultraviolet light, and an air-excluding coating indoors and overnight. Humidifying dry indoor air may also help counteract dry lips.

Lip licking can instigate lip chapping because the externally applied saliva draws internal moisture with it when it evaporates. Lip-licker's dermatitis (red, irritated skin surrounding the lips) can develop from continuing to moisten chapped lips with the tongue.[293] Chronically sore lips may be due to allergic reactions to foods or to ingredients in chewing gum, cosmetic products, mouthwash, or toothpaste. Experimenting with the elimination of suspect foods or different brands of gum, cosmetics, and mouthwash, or brushing the teeth with baking soda may correct the problem.

Diet and Supplements (see note on page xii)

Drinking at least eight glasses of water every day helps moisturize lips from the inside. Adding a tablespoon of polyunsaturated oil to an otherwise low-fat diet may rectify lip dryness and scaling. Dietary deficiencies of B vitamins often result in lip problems. Since the entire B complex functions synergistically, taking a comprehensive, high-potency tablet twice a day can offset any increased demands created by therapeutic daily supplementation with individual B vitamins.

○ Fifty milligrams each of B_2 and B_6. A lack of B_2 makes lips crinkle, flake, and feel chapped; can cause cracks at the corners of the mouth (cheilosis); and eventually may shrink the upper lip until it practically disappears. Clinical studies also show that a deficiency of B$_6$ produces sore lips.[86]

○ Folic acid (400 micrograms) and pantothenic acid (100 milligrams) taken in addition to the other B vitamins, often prevent and correct lip ulcers and other sore-lip problems.

Topical applications of vitamin E from a snipped capsule help heal sore lips, and for some individuals, oral vitamin E supplementation is successful. Craig S. was a large man with a small aggravation—a split lip. Before he began taking 400 IU of vitamin E twice a day, his lower lip would chap and crack after the first cold spell. Salves and ointments had no effect; the painfully cracked lip persisted until spring. After one winter with the supplement and without lip discomfort, Craig experimented by cutting his vitamin-E intake in half—and developed a sore lip that recovered only after 3 weeks of daily supplementation with 800 IU of vitamin E.

Homeopathic practitioners suggest taking three tablets of the 3X tissue salt Calc. Fluor. three times a day for chapped lips and sores at the corners of the mouth.

Folk Remedies

Rubbing beeswax or unwaxed cucumber skin over dry lips may help lubricate the surface. The folk remedy favorite, petroleum jelly, proved to be the most effective therapy for chapped lips when tested by *Consumer Reports* in February 1991; other old-fashioned treatments may be equally beneficial. To heal severely chapped lips, apply petroleum jelly or one of the following lip soothers every half hour for a few days, then gradually reduce the frequency as healing progresses.

○ Cod liver oil, honey, borax dissolved in honey or glycerin, glycerin mixed half-and-half with lemon juice, or a blend of 4 teaspoons glycerin and 1 teaspoon tincture of benzoin can be smoothed on; or triple-strength white oak bark tea may be sponged over the lips.

○ Protective pomades: In a heat-proof dish in a pan of boiling water, stir 3 tablespoons olive oil into 1 tablespoon melted beeswax or paraffin—if desired, add 2 teaspoons of honey. Or stir 4 tablespoons petroleum jelly into 2 tablespoons melted beeswax or paraffin. Pour the lip salve into small containers with snug-fitting lids. If either mixture becomes too hard, reheat over hot water and stir in a few drops of olive oil.

Sources (see Bibliography)

6, 32, 42, 45, 46, 53, 65, 66, 75, 86, 87, 92, 93, 98, 129, 135, 150, 186, 202, 207, 218, 250, 276, 281, 283, 293, 300

Colds and Flu

The common cold can be caused by any of 200 viruses, usually a rhinovirus.[300] Influenza is instigated by different viruses classified in groups as type A, B, or C. Type A is responsible for over 90 percent of flu cases and for major epidemics. The less severe type B occurs in localized outbreaks; type C evidences even milder, coldlike symptoms. Stomach flu results from bacteria or gastrointestinal viruses unrelated to influenza.

Colds announce their arrival with a stuffy nose, scratchy throat, mild malaise, and sometimes chilliness and a low grade fever. The onset of the flu is more dramatic: fever up to 103 degrees, headache, and pronounced bodily discomfort. Both are "caught" by inhaling microscopic droplets of the exhaled virus (a sneeze can throw droplets 6 feet through the air at a speed of 100 miles per hour),[112] or by touching a virus-contaminated object (hand, stair rail, telephone) and then touching the eyes, nose, or mouth. These viruses are contagious shortly after initial exposure and for several days thereafter as the body develops antibodies with which to counteract them. Flu and cold symptoms are indications of the body's efforts to eradicate the viruses. A runny nose guards against further invasion. Fever and inflammation of the nasal passages help contain the spread of the infection—the viruses are sensitive to any elevation of body temperature. Annual flu shots, formulated for each year's variation of type A, are recommended for the elderly, the chronically ill, and for other high-risk individuals such as health care workers.

Flu and colds usually are self-limiting miseries that spontaneously disappear in less than 2 weeks; severity and duration are related to the competence of the body's immune system. Antibiotics are of no avail against viruses, but if complications appear or if a fever over 101 degrees persists longer than 4 days, medical evaluation should be obtained. Bacterial infections, which do respond to antibiotics, may coexist with or may follow a severe cold or bout of flu. Aspirin, acetaminophen, or ibuprofen can be used to relieve muscle pain and headache for adults; children with viral infections should not be given aspirin because of its association with Reye's syndrome. Natural therapies can ameliorate discomforts and reinforce the immune system to help prevent an extended siege or a relapse.

Diet

Eating small amounts of "light" natural foods at frequent intervals and drinking at least ½ cup of liquid each hour while awake are recommended for the first few days. Fruit and vegetable juices—apple, apricot, beet, carrot, citrus, grape, tomato—are especially beneficial. Hot beverages, broths, and soups help relieve sinus and chest congestion. A nutrient-laden broth can be made by cutting the outside half-inch off of two well-scrubbed potatoes and boiling these peelings for 30 minutes with a sliced carrot in 2 cups of chicken broth, then straining before sipping. Onion soup, liberally laced with garlic and cayenne pepper, is considered even more effective than the proverbial chicken soup. Garlic contains allicin, which wards off bacterial complications and, along with fiery foods (curry, horseradish, hot mustard, red pepper, Tabasco sauce), acts as a decongestant by loosening secretions. A recent study showed that dairy products are not mucus makers to be shunned during a cold,[51] so low-fat milk, cottage cheese, and yogurt can be ingested to provide calcium and protein as well as some of the dietary iron essential for the production of antibodies.[98]

Supplements (see note on page xii)

Under the stress of infection, the body consumes key nutrients more rapidly than they can be replenished by most diets, and an insufficiency of any nutrient can diminish immune defenses. If dairy products are being avoided, 1,000 milligrams of calcium plus 500 milligrams of magnesium are advised, and in addition to a daily multivitamin-mineral, nutritional consultants and holistic doctors recommend supplementation as follows.

Vitamin A In the form of beta carotene, 25,000 to 75,000 IU until recovered, then 10,000 to 25,000 IU for at least 1 month to prevent recurrence.

B Complex One comprehensive tablet each morning and evening, to combat the stress of illness, to speed healing, and to encourage the production of antibodies.

Vitamin C with Bioflavonoids 250 to 1,000 milligrams daily to help prevent colds and flu; 1,000 to 24,000 milligrams in divided doses to hasten recovery. Vitamin C has been a topic of controversy since the 1970s, when Linus Pauling publicized his success with megadoses.[223] Clinical studies have produced conflicting results, but there is an abundance of positive anecdotal evidence. Countless colds reportedly have been aborted by taking from 250 to 1,000 milligrams of vitamin C at the onset and repeating the dosage at intervals of from 1 to 3 hours. In some cases, vitamin C has been effective when taken in the midst of an already severe infection. Signa S. is one example. Even though her flu was being complicated by a bacterial infection, 90-year-old Signa insisted on staying at home in Minnesota. Her daughter Ingrid engaged a part-time nurse, arranged for the town's only physician to stop in twice a day, and tried to convince her sister on the West Coast that everything possible was being done for their mother. But Signa's condition worsened despite antibiotics and oxygen, and when the doctor prescribed an hourly dose of 1,000 milligrams of vitamin C taken with half a glass of water and a soda cracker, Ingrid's sister threatened legal recourse if Signa was not moved to a city hospital. Three days of the vitamin C regimen resolved the cross-country debate. Signa was standing in the kitchen brewing a pot of tea when the next California call came through, and she answered the phone herself!

Tissue Salts At the first sign of a cold, take one 6X Ferr. Phos. every 15 minutes for 1 hour, then three tablets every 2 hours. For chilling and aching, take 3X Nat. Sulph. at 30-minute intervals. For a runny nose or watery eyes, take one 3X Ferr. Phos. every 2 hours, plus one 3X Nat. Mur. each hour. When there is stuffiness, take three doses daily of Kali. Mur. in the 6X potency—if accompanied by thick mucus, take one 12X Kali. Sulph. three times a day. For convalescent aches and weariness, take 12X Kali. Mur. and Kali. Sulph. alternately twice each day, plus one 12X Kali. Phos. at bedtime.

Zinc One zinc gluconate lozenge dissolved in the mouth every 2 or 3 hours for 3 days, then one every 4 hours for 1 week, to shorten the duration of symptoms.[293]

Exercise

Bed rest is important while fever is present. When the temperature is normal, however, and bodily malaise permits, walking a mile or two every day can make breathing easier by constricting nasal blood vessels and opening the air passages. According to an article in *The Physician and Sports Medicine* (June 1990), people who exercise regularly may continue with their program during a cold if all symptoms are above the neck; but strenuous workouts should not be attempted if there are symptoms below the neck, fever, or a bad cough.

Folk Remedies

Folk medicine utilizes the nutritional and medicinal properties of foods, herbs, and flowers. "Conserve of roses," prescribed for colds in 1669, contained vitamin C—half a pound of rose petals was simmered with dark sugar before being eaten plain, stirred into milk, or spread on toast.[275] Hot lemonade sweetened and spiced with honey, cinnamon, and cloves is as comforting today as it was when flu was called "the grippe."

Alcohol The possibility of alcohol-dilated blood vessels increasing nasal congestion is of little concern to folk practitioners. They suggest eating a steak and drinking a glass of apricot or blackberry brandy at the first sign of a cold, lacing a glass of lemonade with bourbon or rum, adding 3 tablespoons of brandy to a cup of honey-sweetened pekoe tea sprinkled with nutmeg; or mixing whiskey half-and-half with honey and taking a tablespoonful every hour. Dark beer, heated with a teaspoon of sugar, is an old German curative for the flu. The "silk hat cure," popular during the 1800s, consisted of placing a tall silk hat on the right-hand bedpost, then lying quietly and sipping brandy until there appeared to be silk hats on both bedposts.

○ For the physical discomforts accompanying a cold, *Mother's Book of Daily Duties*, published in 1850, advises bottling three-cents-worth of garlic with 1 cup of rye whiskey and taking a tablespoon of the mixture several times a day; other experts of the era suggested brandy or vodka as the steeping liquid.

○ Nighttime cold remedies called for stirring ½ cup *each* sherry and hot milk with 1 tablespoon sugar and seasoning it with cinnamon and nutmeg; or combining the juice of a lemon with ¼ cup *each* maple syrup and hot water, then adding 2 tablespoons of brandy.

Baking Soda Sipping soda water at the onset is a time-honored method of aborting a cold. Suggested strength ranges from ¼ teaspoon to 1 tablespoon of soda per glass of water. Taking an aspirin or its equivalent with the liquid increases the benefits. During the first day of a cold, a glass of "lemon soda" can be sipped every 2 or 3 hours. To prepare, stir 1 teaspoon soda in ½ cup boiling water. Stir the juice from half a lemon into ½ cup cold water. Combine the mixtures by pouring one into the other, then into a glass.

Baths Attempting to "sweat out" a cold or the flu by soaking in a tub of hot water can weaken the body and leave it more susceptible to secondary infections.[148] A 20-minute hot foot bath, however, may squelch chilliness at the onset and may relieve existing headache and nasal congestion.

Garlic In addition to its antibiotic and decongestant capabilities, garlic may be a cold stopper when two to four garlic cloves are minced and swallowed at the onset or when a garlic clove is held between teeth and cheek, lightly scored with the teeth but neither chewed nor swallowed.

Herbal Teas One or two cups (or the equivalent in capsules) daily of camomile, dandelion, echinacea, elder, fenugreek, goldenseal, horchound, lemon grass, licorice root, mullein, peppermint, rose hip, rosemary, saffron, sage, sarsaparilla, savory, skullcap, slippery elm, or yarrow may be helpful. For added benefit, add fresh lemon juice or a teaspoon of dried, grated grapefruit peel to each cup of tea. Herbal decongestants include weak catnip, cayenne, ephedra (ma huang), or ginger tea; a combination of equal amounts of boneset and hyssop offers pain relief as well.

○ A combination said to cure a cold in 24 hours when taken freely is prepared by steeping 1 teaspoon *each* bay leaf, cinnamon, and sage in 1 cup boiling water.

○ For colds or flu with headache and nausea, simmer 1 teaspoon each coriander seeds and minced garlic with ½ teaspoon ground ginger and 1 tablespoon honey in 2 cups of water until reduced to 1 cup. Strain and sip throughout the day.

Honey Samuel Pepys' cold remedy, recorded in his diary for 1660, was to go to bed and take a spoonful of honey mixed with a grated nutmeg. For chest congestion, 1 tablespoon horseradish mixed with enough honey to be palatable is recommended. A Vermont remedy calls for stirring 2 tablespoons *each* honey and apple cider vinegar in a glass of hot or cold water and drinking three glasses during the day, plus another at bedtime.

Ice The Eskimo remedy for a drippy nose is to immerse it in snow or ice water. Oriental folk healers secure a piece of ice on the bottom of the big toe three times a day to activate a cold-curing acupuncture point.

Milk At the first sign of a cold or the flu, scald a cup of milk, stir in a tablespoon of butter, sprinkle the surface with ground black pepper, and drink while hot. Alternatives to stir into the scalded milk include ½ teaspoon ground cinnamon or ginger plus honey to taste; or 1 tablespoon honey, 1 teaspoon butter, and ½ teaspoon garlic powder. Other options call for simmering six chopped figs in 1 quart of milk for 1 hour, then drinking a cup of the liquid three times a day; or combining 1 cup *each* molasses and hot milk, then letting it stand for 10 minutes before straining and drinking.

Nose Drops and Inhalants A 1650's remedy for snuffiness (a sniffly cold) was to apply rubbed sage leaves to the nostrils. During the reign of Queen Victoria, orange rinds, thinly pared and rolled inside out were thrust into the nostrils to relieve cold symptoms. Contemporary folk medicine suggests clearing nasal passages with a drop or two of plain saline solution (¼ teaspoon salt in ½ cup warm water) or a mixture of ¼ teaspoon *each* salt, garlic oil, and powdered vitamin C with the water.

Plasters and Poultices A mustard plaster is the folk remedy favorite for chest congestion, but neither it nor the poultices should be applied to irritated skin. To prepare a plaster, mix equal parts of dry mustard and flour to a paste with warm water, or blend the mustard with egg white. Spread the paste between layers of gauze and coat the chest with olive oil before applying the plaster. Cooked, mashed onions can be substituted for either mustard mixture, or a piece of flannel can be dipped in boiling water, sprinkled with turpentine, and placed over the chest as hot as can be borne. An alternative is to blend 2 tablespoons lard with 1 tablespoon turpentine, rub the mixture on chest and throat, then cover with woolen cloth.

Steam Inhaling steam for 10 minutes twice a day not only mois-turizes and helps clear air passages, it also makes the nose untenably hot for cold and flu viruses, which flourish in normal nasal temperatures.[118] Cover the head with a towel and, with eyes closed, breathe in the vapors from a container of boiling water. To enhance the effect, inhale the steam from steeping teas of eucalyptus, juniper, pine, rose geranium, or rosemary, singly or in combination.

Nerve Pressure and Massage

To Relieve Cold or Flu Symptoms Press and massage from the top of the head down to the hollow at the base of the skull; massage across both eyebrows for 1 minute; press the center of the breastbone and a point 3 inches directly below the navel; press and massage 1 inch below the hollow of each elbow, and the hollows on the underside of the knees; or massage the big toes and the pads beneath them and the middle toes.

For a Head Cold Press the end of the jawbone just below the earlobe, then the center of the lower jawbone directly beneath the outer corners of the mouth.

For a Runny Nose Begin at the bridge of the nose and massage down to the base of the nostrils. Or squeeze the point where the eyebrows would meet above the nose.

For Sneezing Press the same point above the nose, or press directly under the center of the nose.

To Stimulate the Immune System Use the index and middle fingers to massage the back of each wrist and the top of each foot where it meets the ankle.

Stress Management

Medical research has established a definite link between emotions and infections. Studies reported in the *New England Journal of Medicine* (August 1991) show that a high level of psychological stress lowers resistance to viral infections and nearly doubles the chances of catching a cold. Mounting evidence indicates that practicing relaxation techniques and positive imagery (see Introduction) can shorten the duration of a viral infection and begin to lessen its impact in as short a time as an hour or two by mobilizing the healing forces of the immune system.[118, 186]

Sources (see Bibliography)

2, 6, 14, 17, 20, 22, 26, 32, 42, 49, 51, 57, 59, 60, 63, 64, 65, 69, 75, 87, 98, 111, 112, 116, 118, 135, 144, 148, 150, 153, 159, 164, 168, 171, 186, 202, 203, 211, 223, 224, 244, 254, 281, 284, 285, 293, 294, 299, 300, 301, 304, 312

Cold Sores (Fever Blisters)

Whether called cold sores or fever blisters, these uncomfortable eruptions around the mouth are caused by the herpes simplex type-1 virus (HSV-1). Most people are infected with this virus during childhood by a "kissing cousin" or other doting admirer. The initial exposure may pass unnoticed or may produce a flulike illness with lesions on the lips. Subsequently, the virus lies dormant in facial nerves until the body's defenses are weakened by illness, stress, or sunburn; then fever, sunshine, or environmental factors such as cold wind or ultraviolet light reflected from snowy ski slopes, sandy beaches, or shimmering water can trigger an outbreak. Cold sores signal their arrival with a tingly sensation several hours before the first blister appears. Glands in the neck may become tender, and within a few days the painful blisters burst and become encrusted, then heal in 1 to 3 weeks. Medical assistance should be sought if the lesions linger longer or if they develop near the eyes.

HSV-1 is so eager to proliferate that care must be taken during all stages of an outbreak. Besides no kissing, there should be no sharing of eating or drinking utensils, or towels or washcloths; and, for self-protection, three new toothbrushes should be purchased—a toothbrush can harbor, and spread, the herpes virus for 7 days.[186] The first new brush should be used during the tingly phase, the second when a blister appears, and the third after all scabs have disappeared.

Wearing a lip sunscreen with a sun protection factor of at least 15 (SPF 15) guards against environmental triggering of the herpes virus. Studies have shown a definite link between stress and reactivation of the herpes simplex virus.[98] Practicing the relaxation techniques described in the Introduction and utilizing home remedies may help speed healing and prevent future flareups.

Diet and Supplements (see note on page xii)

Strengthening the immune system with a nutritious diet plus a daily multivitamin-mineral provides a defense against reactivation of the herpes virus. During an attack, eating an abundance of alkaline foods (bananas, raw vegetables, skim milk); limiting arginine-rich comestibles such as beer, chocolate, coconut, cola beverages, corn, gelatin, grain cereals, nuts, and peas (arginine is an amino acid on which the herpes virus thrives); and avoiding citrus fruits and high-fat or sugary foods may reduce the number of cold sores and the length of time they are active.[109, 186] Eating unflavored yogurt once a day, or taking acidophilus capsules with each meal, inhibits HSV-1. In one survey, 69 percent of cold-sore victims reported success with this treatment.[49] Since *Lactobacillus acidophilus* inactivates but does not destroy the virus, a maintenance dosage of two to six capsules daily may be helpful for people who are subject to frequent outbreaks. Other supplements also have been found to have a direct effect on the herpes virus.

B Complex One or two high-potency tablets daily, plus optional B vitamins. Taking 500 milligrams of pantothenic acid at the first sign of a sore and every hour or 2 for a full day may abort its formation—or at least shorten its duration.[301] Some cold sores respond to a combination of the pantothenic acid plus 50 milligrams of B_6 and 500 milligrams of vitamin C; others clear in a day or two when 50 to 350 micrograms of B_{12} are taken twice daily.

Vitamin C 150 to 1,000 milligrams every hour when a cold sore warns of its approach, then 2,000 to 6,000 milligrams in divided doses each day until healing is complete. Accompanying the C with a calcium tablet or taking it with milk helps prevent stomach irritation.

Vitamin E 400 IU daily, plus topical applications of vitamin E squeezed from a snipped capsule. Covering the E oil with powdered vitamin C may prove even more effective.

Lysine 50 to 3,000 milligrams at the first tingle, then the same amount taken twice a day with water or juice between meals. With medical consent, people who have more than three cold sores a year may be able to prevent future outbreaks by taking a maintenance dosage of

100 to 3,000 milligrams of this amino acid.[293] Greta C. had been beset by cold sores since childhood but had not experimented with lysine until a tingly lip threatened disastrous embarrassment just a few days before she was to speak at an important conference. Greta held ice chips on the lip while her secretary dashed to a health food store for lysine. She took 2,000 milligrams immediately, another 2,000 before bed, and the same amount twice daily for the next 2 days. The incipient blister did not develop. With her physician's approval, Greta is successfully fending off future flareups by taking 400 milligrams of lysine three times a day.

Tissue Salts   Three 6X tablets of Silicea every 3 hours each day during the blister stage.

Zinc   20 to 60 milligrams daily in tablet form, or a zinc lozenge dissolved in the mouth every 3 hours for 2 days, then two lozenges daily. To hasten healing, pulverize a zinc supplement and apply to the blister with a moist cotton swab.

Folk Remedies

Consuming liberal quantities of unsalted baked potato and rubbing the blister with sliced garlic are Russian remedies. A French favorite is dabbing the sore with the residue from red wine evaporated on a saucer or freeze dried in a small container. American practitioners advise frequent applications of aloe vera gel; or aborting an incipient blister by covering the tingling spot for 3 hours with a cloth saturated in a solution of hot water and as much salt as can be dissolved (renewed as soon as it cools), then sponging the area with brandy every hour or so. Other self-help treatments follow.

Drying Liquids   Drink buttermilk with each meal and dab some on the blister, or swab the sore with rubbing alcohol or witch hazel.

Herbal Remedies   Drinking one to three cups daily of red clover tea may speed healing. An equal quantity of strong sage tea, with 1 teaspoon powdered ginger stirred into each cup, is said to work miracles when a bit of the beverage is sponged over the sores three times a day. Triple-strength burdock, goldenseal, marjoram, or raspberry tea may be swabbed over the sores. Tea tree oil (used by Australian Aborigines and World War II soldiers as oil of melaleuca) is now available in health food stores, as is tincture of myrrh, which has been used since biblical times to stop pain and encourage healing.

Soothing, Healing Coatings The sores can be covered with chilled heavy cream or commercial cold cream, a dab of the individual's own earwax, petroleum jelly, or with a combination of 1 tablespoon raw honey and 1 teaspoon apple cider vinegar.

Sources (see Bibliography)

2, 3, 6, 17, 42, 49, 53, 56, 57, 61, 65, 75, 87, 98, 109, 135, 141, 148, 150, 151, 159, 165, 176, 186, 201, 205, 207, 254, 281, 283, 293, 301, 312, 313

Colitis and Inflammatory Bowel Disease

All types of inflammatory bowel disease (IBD) produce abdominal pain and cramping, a frequent urge to defecate, and bouts of diarrhea. Precise identification requires medical evaluation, which should be obtained if the symptoms persist for more than 5 days. By definition, *colitis* is inflammation of the colon (large intestine); *enteritis* is inflammation of the small intestine or of the entire intestinal tract; *ileitis* is inflammation of the lower half of the small intestine; *ulcerative colitis* is continuous inflammation with bleeding sores on the lining of the colon all the way to the anus; and *Crohn's disease* is identified by inflamed sections of the colon above the rectum.

Colitis instigated by infections, antibiotic treatment, or nutritional deficiencies usually responds to home remedies.[75] Ulcerative colitis or Crohn's disease generally attacks in early adulthood and recurs at intervals varying from a few months to a few years. Symptoms can include blood and pus in watery stools, fever, and weight loss and warrant immediate medical attention plus frequent monitoring. A family history of colitis appears to correlate with Crohn's disease or ulcerative colitis, but dietary inadequacies play a role, and smoking increases the risk of IBD. Although the link between stress and IBD is not fully understood, it has been established that anxiety and emotional stress can precipitate an attack and that the degree of stress influences the severity of colitis by causing the brain to generate a substance that attacks intestinal cells and activates defensive inflammation and pain.[204] Besides practicing some of the relaxation techniques described in the Introduction, establishing a program of regular exercise may help offset the effects of stress.

Diet

Eating small, low-fat, high-protein meals at frequent intervals and thoroughly masticating all foods helps avoid bowel irritation caused by improperly digested food being shunted on to the colon. IBD sufferers may be sensitive only to certain foods such as yeast, wheat, or dairy products (lactase supplements may prevent aggravation from the undigested lactose in milk). Fat-rich or fried foods exacerbate diarrhea; highly spiced foods, nuts, and seeds can irritate an inflamed colon. A disturbance in carbohydrate metabolism can lead to colitis. In some cases, simply avoiding all forms of sugar clears the condition.[42, 162]

For the first day of a diarrhetic attack, a diet of broth, gelatin, diluted fruit juices, and caffeine-free soft drinks may be beneficial (see "Diarrhea"). Although some physicians still prescribe a bland, low-residue diet for patients with chronic colitis, most gastroenterologists advise gradually increasing the amounts of soluble fiber (gums, pectin, and some hemicellulose) to help move material through the small intestine without taxing the colon.[186] Good sources are apples, barley, brown rice, brussels sprouts, carrots, legumes, oat bran, and sweet potatoes. Granulated, quick-cooking tapioca can be combined with unflavored gelatin and maple syrup then fluffed with stiffly beaten egg whites for a pudding said to have a healing effect on the intestinal tract if eaten regularly.[150] Pectin, which is also available as a supplement, offers bonus benefits: It soothes inflamed membranes and speeds healing by nourishing cells in the lining of the colon.[45] If unprocessed wheat bran can be tolerated, gradually incorporating from 2 teaspoons to ½ cup of this insoluble fiber with daily meals helps regulate bowel activity by absorbing approximately eight times its own weight in water.

To perform its function, fiber must be accompanied by six to eight glasses of liquid each day. Nutritional consultants recommend apple, beet, broccoli, cabbage, cantaloupe, carrot, papaya, and strawberry juice, as well as the juice of leafy greens because the enzymes in fresh fruit and vegetable juices are quickly absorbed to help rebuild the collagen sheath on the intestinal tract. Herbal teas of alfalfa, camomile, comfrey, dandelion, feverfew, papaya, red clover, and slippery elm have proven beneficial; as has the folk remedy of 2 teaspoons *each* apple cider vinegar and honey stirred into a glass of water and taken before meals.

By reinforcing beneficial flora (which can be destroyed by antibiotics) and inhibiting inflammation-instigating bacteria in the intestines, acidophilus (from capsules or yogurt) can be invaluable for colitis sufferers. Sheldon A. and a series of doctors had unsuccessfully battled his ulcerative colitis for years. When the cramps and bloody diarrhea returned just a few months after he had had a section of his colon removed, Sheldon opted for nutritional therapy instead of another round of prescription drugs. Eating acidophilus yogurt daily provided *Lactobacillus* bacteria to protect his intestines, and taking supplemental apple pectin, glucomannan, and psyllium apparently cured Sheldon's IBD—at least he remains symptom-free.

Dietary Supplements (see note on page xii)

Colitis forces nutrients through the intestinal tract before they can be properly absorbed. A daily multivitamin-mineral, a mineral supplement containing calcium, magnesium, and zinc, plus separate vitamin supplements may help prevent nutritional deficiencies and encourage healing. To hasten recovery, holistic doctors suggest taking alfalfa tablets (for chlorophyll and vitamin K) and garlic capsules (for antibiotic action) with every meal.[17]

Vitamin A In the form of beta carotene, 25,000 IU to help prevent infection and to aid tissue repair.

B Complex One comprehensive tablet. During flareups, an additional 50 milligrams *each* B_6 and pantothenic acid, plus 1 to 5 milligrams of folic acid. Crohn's disease may necessitate B_{12} supplementation as well.

Vitamin C with Bioflavonoids 1,000 to 5,000 milligrams of a non-acidic form such as calcium ascorbate in divided doses to strengthen tissues and help combat toxins that irritate an inflamed intestinal tract.

Vitamin E and Unsaturated Fatty Acids (UFA) Cold-pressed vegetable oils or capsules of primrose oil plus 100 to 400 IU of vitamin E provide essential UFAs for cell formation and tissue repair.

Nerve Pressure and Massage

○ Press and massage the top of the cheekbones next to the ears.

○ Beginning beneath the pad of the little finger, use the opposite thumb to massage across the palm of each hand, paying particular attention to any tender spots.

○ Massage the shins of both legs from just below the knees to midcalf.

○ Massage just below each outside ankle bone, then massage both soles from the heel pads to the outside of the feet.

Sources (see Bibliography)

6, 10, 17, 42, 44, 45, 50, 58, 59, 60, 75, 87, 98, 101, 112, 150, 162, 164, 176, 186, 190, 201, 204, 207, 244, 255, 256, 279, 281, 283, 296, 300, 305

Conjunctivitis and Blepharitis

Conjunctivitis is the clinical term for inflammation or infection of the thin membrane (conjunctiva) covering the whites of the eyes and lining the eyelids. It is also known as pinkeye or bloodshot eyes. When the conjunctiva becomes irritated, the tiny blood vessels that run through it to provide nourishment dilate to carry away toxic substances and bring protective antibodies to the surface of the eye, making the eye appear pink or red. Temporarily bloodshot eyes can be caused by dust, tobacco smoke, or other environmental pollutants, or by lack of sleep, overexposure to sun or wind, overindulgence in alcohol, or swimming in chlorinated water. Chronically red or irritated eyes may be due to nutritional deficiencies or may be an allergic response of the conjunctiva. Among hayfever sufferers, allergic conjunctivitis (itchy, watery, red eyes) is usually seasonal. Other cases may be provoked by cosmetics, contact lens cleaning solutions, or redness-relief eyedrops.

Conjunctival infections may be bacterial (spread by hand-to-eye contact from anything that has been in contact with infectious matter from the eyes), or from viruses associated with colds, herpes simplex (fever blisters), or illnesses such as measles. Pinkeye is a painful, highly contagious form of conjunctivitis. Blepharitis (inflammation or infection of the oil-producing glands in the eyelids) causes the exudation of a sticky discharge that can glue the eyes shut overnight, create crusty eye margins, and irritate the eyes. It can result from seborrhea, excessive rubbing of the eyes, or from any of the conjunctivitis instigators.[124]

Meticulous personal hygiene helps prevent recontamination or transmission of eye infections. Hands should be washed before and after touch-

108

ing the eyes, linens should be laundered separately, and eye makeup should not be shared. According to the _Johns Hopkins Medical Letter_ (November 1990), an eyepatch should not be worn unless advised by a doctor because it could foster proliferation of the infectious organisms. Most cases of conjunctivitis clear up by themselves within 2 weeks and can be alleviated with home remedies. But if the condition gets worse instead of better after 5 days, or if there is a greenish-yellowish discharge, a physician should be consulted—medical analysis is essential to determine the correct treatment and avoid potentially serious eye damage.

Cold and Heat

Cold compresses shrink engorged blood vessels to relieve bloodshot eyes and the puffy, itchy miseries of allergic conjunctivitis. Warm compresses soothe irritated eyes. Alternating cold with heat for 5 minutes each is often effective. Hot compresses may be helpful in treating blepharitis. After Lyle J.'s crusty eyes were diagnosed as chronic, noninfectious blepharitis, he resigned himself to the daily chore of carefully removing the scaly residue with a cotton-tipped swab dipped in a tablespoon of water mixed with a drop of baby shampoo. Then a friend with the same problem suggested he try "draining out the glunk" before it had a chance to clump around his lashes. Each night at bedtime, Lyle held a hot, wet washcloth over his eyes for 5 minutes; then for another 5 minutes, he gently stroked downward on his upper lids, upward on the lower lids. There was some improvement every morning, and within 2 weeks there were no crusts to be cleaned off. Forewarned that the treatment was not a cure, Lyle gradually extended the time between draining sessions to a maintenance level of twice a week.

Supplements (see note on page xii)

To help maintain healthy eyes, many eye care experts recommend a daily eye formula tablet containing vitamins A, C, and E, and the minerals copper, selenium, and zinc. For treating conjunctivitis, therapeutic dosages of the following supplements may be beneficial.

Vitamin A In the form of beta carotene, 10,000 IU three times a day for 1 week (under medical supervision, 100,000 IU in emulsion form for up to 1 month), then 25,000 IU daily. Itching, burning eyes and conjunctivitis symptoms may be caused by a lack of vitamin A. An infection fighter, this vitamin is especially important during viral conjunctivitis.[17, 109]

B Complex One comprehensive tablet daily. Constantly bloodshot eyes due to a deficiency of vitamin B_2 have been cleared by taking an additional 15 milligrams of B_2 plus a tablespoon of brewer's yeast every day.[313] Insufficient B_2 may also be responsible for inflamed, itchy eyelids, sticky accumulations at the base of the lashes, and cracks at the corners of the eyes.

Vitamin C with Bioflavonoids 1,000 to 5,000 milligrams in divided daily doses to promote healing, strengthen capillary walls, and protect the eye from further damage.

Tissue Salts Three 6X tablets dissolved under the tongue three or four times a day: Ferr. Phos. for inflammation without purulent discharge, Kali. Mur. for "sandy" eyelids or inflammation with a whitish discharge, Nat. Phos. if there is a yellowish discharge and the eyelids stick together in the morning.

Zinc 25 to 50 milligrams daily unless included in an eye formula supplement.

Folk Remedies

For inflamed, irritated eyes and pinkeye, folk healers suggest drinking the juice of a lemon stirred into a cup of hot water each morning before breakfast, downing a minced raw onion mixed with a glass of beer each evening, eating a portion of goat's milk yogurt and applying a poultice of the yogurt daily, placing slices of raw cucumber or potato over the eyelids, or immersing the face and blinking the eyes twice a day in a basin of water to which a tablespoon of salt has been added.

Compresses and Poultices Applying a cloth-wrapped poultice of warm, cooked apples is the advice given in *Consult Me*, a medical reference published in 1872. Grated raw cucumbers or potatoes, or beaten egg white are other options. Herbalists suggest compresses of moistened tea bags or cloths squeezed out of strong teas made from camomile, catnip, eyebright, fennel, horsetail, pekoe, red raspberry leaf, or slippery elm. Gauze pads saturated with witch hazel and placed over the closed eyes for 15 minutes may help relieve irritation.

Eyedrops and Eyewashes For a soothing eyewash, stir ¼ teaspoon baking soda or honey in ½ cup water. When using drops, pressing the corner of the eye next to the nose reduces the amount of the medication passing into the body through the lacrimal (tear) duct.[116] With conjunctivitis, no eye medication should be used without a doctor's approval. Antihistamine drops may relieve allergy-related discomfort but can have an irritating effect of their own and can adversely affect viral conjunctivitis; get-the-red-out drops sometimes create redness; even artificial tears contain preservatives that can instigate allergic reactions. An eye care specialist should be consulted before using commercial eyedrops more than four times a day for 2 consecutive weeks.[293, 300]

Herbal eyewashes or drops of regular-strength teas (which should be filtered or finely strained) include bayberry, catnip, fennel, goldenseal, and red raspberry leaf. Unless susceptible to hay fever, borage, camomile, or elderflower can be used. A half-and-half blend of chervil and parsley acts as a soothing disinfectant. A combination of ⅛ teaspoon *each* powdered camomile, comfrey, and goldenseal steeped in a cup of boiling water for 15 minutes has also proven effective.[150] To relieve irritation, add a teaspoon of warm pekoe tea to ¼ cup water.

Nerve Pressure and Massage

❍ To relieve watery eyes, press and massage the webs between the second and third fingers of both hands. For inflammation and granulated lids, squeeze the joints of the first and second fingers of the hand corresponding to the irritated eye.

❍ For eye infection, press the underside of the cheekbone, 1½ inches in from the ear, for 10 seconds, release for 10 seconds, and repeat three times once each day.

Sources (see Bibliography)

2, 6, 17, 26, 29, 47, 53, 64, 65, 75, 76, 92, 98, 108, 109, 111, 124, 135, 143, 150, 151, 164, 176, 186, 202, 213, 234, 255, 256, 281, 293, 294, 300, 306, 312, 313

Constipation

Defined as the infrequent, difficult passage of stool, constipation is often self-perceived or self-inflicted—normal bowel emptying can vary from three times a day to twice a week. Misconceptions regarding the necessity of "daily regularity" can develop laxative dependency. Stimulant laxatives irritate the delicate lining of the intestinal tract, reduce nutrient absorption, and often remove not only the waste matter that should be expelled but also the still-liquid material in the tract above. This prevents a normal bowel movement for the next day or so and creates the impression of further constipation. Laxatives become an addiction when their regular use weakens the normal reflexes and produces an inert colon that requires constant cathartic fixes. Aside from an occasional 8-ounce enema of tap water, enemas are utilized mainly for colon cleansing prior to certain medical procedures and should be given at home only on the advice of a physician.

Physical activity speeds the movement of food through the digestive tract and stimulates peristaltic action. A brisk walk each morning may help correct chronic constipation. Setting aside a few minutes for undisturbed visits to the toilet at the same time each day helps establish regular bowel habits. As explained in *Harvard Health Letter* (February 1991), deliberately delaying the response to nature's signal produces hard, dry stools and trains the bowel to malfunction.

Any persistent change in usual frequency, or failure to defecate for longer than 1 week, warrants investigation by a physician to rule out the possibility of an underlying disorder or the need for alternative medications. Certain antacids, antidepressants, diuretics, and drugs for control of cholesterol or blood pressure can be responsible for constipation. Emotional stress, with its accompanying muscular tension, can cause it. So can lack of exercise or changes in eating habits due to travel or other circumstances.

Diet

Increasing the daily intake of fiber and fluids usually prevents or corrects chronic constipation. The soluble and insoluble fibers of fruits, vegetables, dried legumes, nuts, and whole grains increase fecal bulk for bowel regularity. Bananas and other fibrous foods are rich in potassium, which is essential for muscle contraction. Prunes and prune juice stimulate contraction of the intestinal wall with a cathartic action. Foods like apples, cabbage, and carrots have ¼ the constipation-relieving effect of wheat bran (miller's bran), which is considered nature's best laxative; the insoluble fibers of rice bran and corn bran are more effective than oat bran.[186] A study of three-hundred chronically constipated, laxative-dependent patients showed that adding ½ tablespoonful of bran to the morning oatmeal resolved the problem for 60 percent of the cases. For the remainder, ½ cup of prune juice a day was added, and within a year, 90 percent were off laxatives.[56]

At least 2 quarts of water or other liquids are needed daily to augment a high-fiber diet—fiber's stool-bulking, stool-softening action is achieved through expansion as it absorbs many times its own weight in water. A glass daily of the juice from fresh apples, cabbage, carrots, cucumber, papaya, or spinach—in any combination—is believed especially helpful.[218] Alcoholic or caffeine-containing beverages are mildly diuretic, which offsets their liquid assets. For persons unaccustomed to caffeine, however, a cup of strong coffee may induce a bowel movement very quickly.[308] Herbalists suggest a cup of herbal tea daily: barberry, buckthorn, cascara sagrada, flaxseed, or senna leaf.

Supplements (see note on page xii)

A daily multivitamin-mineral plus optional supplements offsets possible deficiencies resulting from nutrient malabsorption due to constipation.

Vitamin A In the form of beta carotene, 25,000 IU daily to maintain the health of the lining of the intestinal tract and to help prevent infection from retained fecal material.

Acidophilus Two capsules with each meal, or a daily serving of acidophilus yogurt to help replenish the "friendly," B-vitamin-producing bacteria forced out of the gastrointestinal tract by laxatives.

B Complex One comprehensive tablet daily to assist the digestive process and, along with deliberate relaxation (see Introduction), help counteract constipation induced by emotional stress. Additional B$_1$,

B_6, and niacinamide have been helpful in some cases; taking from 100 to 500 milligrams of pantothenic acid has restored regularity for other people.

Vitamin C   One teaspoon of the powdered form can serve as a quick-acting laxative. Marlene K.'s limited experience with laxatives had involved so much abdominal cramping and so many dashes to the bathroom that she dared not take one in the middle of a week-long convention; yet she was so miserably constipated she had to have relief. Marlene's roommate resolved the dilemma. She handed Marlene a bottle of vitamin C crystals and a 6-ounce of fruit juice. "I never travel without this emergency laxative," she said. "Stir a teaspoon of the C into the juice and drink it down. You'll have results in about an hour." The combination was as efficient as promised, allowing Marlene to relax and enjoy the full schedule of convention activities.

Psyllium   Although it is the principal ingredient of some over-the-counter bulk laxatives, psyllium is a dietary supplement that can be taken for years without ill effects (*Harvard Health Letter*, March 1991). One teaspoon of powdered psyllium in a glass of water expands eight to ten times and has a soothing effect on the entire gastrointestinal system as it bulks stools and eases their expulsion.[111]

Tissue Salts   6X potency unless otherwise directed.

○ If there is discomfort in the bowel, take Ferr. Phos. every half hour until relieved. If there is no movement and the tongue is white, take Kali. Mur. at bedtime and early in the morning for several days. If the tongue is yellow, substitute Kali. Sulph.

○ If there is difficulty in expelling the stools: take Calc. Fluor. and Silicea, one dose of each at bedtime and in the morning. If the bowel movement is dry, substitute Nat. Mur. and Nat. Sulph. for a few days. If there is no desire to defecate, take one dose each 12X Calc. Fluor. and Kali. Phos. at bedtime and again in the morning for several days. If all efforts at stool fail, use Nat. Phos. at half-hourly intervals until a bowel movement results.

Folk Remedies

An Egyptian papyrus inscribed in 1550 B.C. prescribes castor oil for constipation, but this once-universal laxative is no longer recommended because it irritates the lining of the colon. Eating an apple or two every day or an avocado mashed with a little apple cider vinegar or lemon juice, or experimenting with other home remedies, are healthier options for keeping constipation away.

Before-Breakfast Beverages Drink fresh cabbage juice. Or half-fill a blender container with shredded cabbage, sprinkle with salt and let stand overnight, then liquefy with a cup of water. Or boil raw escarole and drink the warm liquid. Stir 1 teaspoon pulverized flaxseed or 2 teaspoons cornmeal in a glass of cool water. Or steep six whole cloves in ½ cup boiling water overnight and strain before drinking. Add 1 tablespoon fresh lemon juice to a cup of hot water. Or stir 2 teaspoons apple cider vinegar into a glass of water and add 2 teaspoons of honey, if desired.

Figs Cook figs in milk; drink the liquid and eat the figs. Or stew the figs in olive oil until tender, then add a little honey and lemon juice and simmer until thickened. Or mix ½ pound *each* ground figs, prunes, and raisins with ½ cup unprocessed bran and press into a shallow pan. Cut into 1-inch squares, store in the refrigerator, and eat one piece daily.

Honey Eating several tablespoons of raw honey every day is an old remedy believed to be even more effective when 1 teaspoon of bee pollen granules is added and the mixture spread on whole-grain bread. German peasants preferred their honey stirred into a cup of hot, dark beer.

Olive Oil and Lemon Juice Combine 1 teaspoon of each and take before breakfast every morning.

Onions Eat roasted onions at bedtime. Or cover a minced onion with fresh vegetable juice, let stand overnight, strain, then take 2 teaspoons of the liquid in a glass of water twice daily before meals. Or try the 3,500-year-old Egyptian remedy of cooking onions in beer and drinking a glass of the liquid every day for 3 days.

Nerve Pressure and Massage

❍ Press and massage a spot on both cheekbones parallel with the nostrils, 1½ inches toward the ears. Massage the base of both nostrils, then the cleft of the chin.

❍ Simultaneously press the center of the back of the neck and the navel; then press or massage points 3 inches directly above, below, and 2 inches to the left of the navel.

○ Massage the center of the palm of each hand.

○ Place the palm of one hand on the abdomen and rub clockwise; then massage the back of each calf midway between the hollow of the knee and the top of the ankle.

○ On the right foot, press just below the inside of the nail on the big toe, and under the pad of the little toe. Then massage the bottom of each foot from the base of the middle toe to the heel pad.

Sources (see Bibliography)

6, 10, 17, 21, 40, 51, 52, 56, 57, 59, 60, 64, 65, 66, 72, 75, 76, 86, 87, 89, 98, 101, 111, 112, 117, 135, 144, 147, 150, 151, 152, 164, 166, 171, 176, 186, 201, 202, 203, 218, 240, 254, 256, 265, 280, 293, 294, 300, 302, 304, 305, 306, 308, 312, 313

Corns and Calluses

Resulting from persistent friction and pressure, corns occur either on top of the toes or between them; calluses of thickened skin develop on soles and heels to protect the flesh over bony prominences. Plantar's warts have a hard surface similar to a callus but contain blood vessels and nerve endings, so may require professional removal. Paring down corns or calluses with a razor blade is too hazardous to attempt; podiatrists caution that over-the-counter corn medications contain acid that can cause potentially dangerous ulcerations in healthy tissue. Wearing comfortable shoes and applying moleskin pads around corns or calluses provide temporary relief. Natural remedies offer permanent removal.

Diet and Supplements (see note on page xii)

Eating an abundance of potassium-rich foods such as bananas and leafy greens, and supplementing the diet with 25,000 IU of beta carotene and 100 to 600 IU of vitamin E provide prevention as well as treatment. Drinking a glass daily of apple or cranberry juice, or a blend of water and 2 teaspoons *each* apple cider vinegar and raw honey; or taking two 3X tablets of the tissue salts Kali. Mur. and Silicea three times a day may be beneficial.

Folk Remedies

Massaging calluses and corns twice daily with aloe vera gel, oil squeezed from capsules of vitamin A or E, castor oil, a paste of baking soda and water, or a salve prepared from equal parts of soft soap and roasted onions are old-fashioned sure-cures.

Foot Baths Soapy or plain warm water relieves pain and softens corns or calluses. For more pronounced effect, use the water in which oatmeal has been cooked, or add one of these substances to the water: baking soda, camomile tea, dry mustard, epsom salts, or table salt.

Callus Removal Pumice stone, a callus file, a nail brush, a coarse towel, or a handful of moistened salt can be rubbed over calluses after a foot-bath soaking. (To ease the departure of dead skin, apply a coating of glycerin before using pumice or a callus file.) After rinsing and drying, smooth on hand cream, petroleum jelly, white vegetable shortening, or a blend of 2 teaspoons vegetable oil and 1 teaspoon cider vinegar.

To hasten the disappearance of calluses, rub them with a mixture of 2 teaspoons lemon juice, 1 teaspoon camomile, and a crushed garlic clove. Cover with a plastic bag for 5 minutes, then rinse in warm water and remove the layer of dead skin with a pumice stone.

Callused Toes Calluses on toes may call for special treatment. Vanity plus discomfort instigated Valerie D.'s callus-removing home remedy. Wearing high-heeled sandals had created calluses on the bottoms of her big toes. The calluses remained painful even when she wore more sensible shoes. To depose the calluses, Valerie mixed two crushed aspirin tablets with ½ teaspoon *each* lemon juice and water, patted the paste over the callused spots, covered her toes with plastic sandwich bags and pulled on a pair of ankle-high nylons to hold them in place, then tucked her feet under a heating pad set on *low*. After 10 minutes, she gently removed the dead skin with a nail brush, washed her feet, and rubbed the contents of a vitamin E capsule into her now-smooth toes.

Callused, Cracked Heels Restore to normalcy with a before-bed routine of scrubbing with a nail brush after soaking, rubbing vitamin E oil into the crevices, adding a coating of petroleum jelly, and sleeping in cotton socks.

Soft Corns Between the Toes Dislodge by dabbing them with castor oil, petroleum jelly, or rubbing alcohol, then wrapping the adjoining toes with plain or turpentine-saturated wool yarn or strips of castor oil-soaked cloth.

Protuberant Corns These have perturbed humans ever since Egyptians contrived the first shoes from woven reeds 4,000 years ago. In

1829, the *American Frugal Housewife*[69] stated that securing the cut side of half a raw cranberry over a corn each night would draw it out in less than a week; the 1886 edition of *Dr. Chase's Recipes: Information for Everybody*[66] recommends binding cotton over the corn, then saturating it three times daily with turpentine.

Other on-the-spot treatments include bandaging the corn overnight with a paste of breadcrumbs and apple cider vinegar, brewer's yeast, and lemon juice, or powdered white chalk and water; a half-and-half mixture of baking soda and petroleum jelly; a piece of raw garlic, vinegar-soaked onion, or fresh papaya or pineapple; or the pulp side of a slender wedge of lemon.

More complex methods call for soaking feet in warmed castor oil or a foot bath of dry mustard and water, then either saturating the corn with apple cider vinegar or surrounding it with petroleum jelly and applying a touch of iodine to the top of the corn.

Sources (see Bibliography)

2, 46, 53, 64, 66, 69, 85, 92, 98, 109, 111, 135, 144, 150, 159, 166, 172, 179, 186, 202, 203, 206, 207, 234, 256, 284, 293, 304, 306, 312, 313, 317

Coughs

Coughing is the body's method of expelling harmful material (a bit of food swallowed the "wrong way," dust, excess mucus) from the respiratory tract. A productive cough should be encouraged with an expectorant. A nonproductive, barking cough that appears toward the end of a cold should be subdued with an antitussive (cough suppressant), as should all dry, hacking coughs. They serve only to irritate the airways and lead to more coughing. An occasional cough, which can release a burst of air at a speed of 500 feet per second, is normal. A cough that lasts longer than a month should be medically evaluated to rule out the possibility of an underlying physical disorder. A tickling cough without throat soreness may be due to nervousness or cigarette smoking, may be an indication of allergy, or may simply be the result of a lack of moisture.

Lubricating the throat with extra liquids and inhaling warm, moist air not only benefits a dry cough but also helps loosen any secretions that should be expelled. When using a vaporizer, adding a few drops of peppermint or spearmint oil produces a chemical that liquefies phlegm.[186] Draping a towel over the head and breathing the vapors from a bowl of steaming water containing 1 teaspoon tincture of benzoin per pint may be equally efficient. Benzoin is available from pharmacies and is also used as an antiseptic.

Folk Remedies

For instant relief from a dry, irritating cough, folk healers suggest sipping ¼ cup of water containing ¼ teaspoon apple cider vinegar, gargling with salt water, or, for the intrepid, smoking equal quantities of ground coffee and pine sawdust in a clean pipe and swallowing some of the smoke. Eating eight dried juniper berries before breakfast each morning is said to clear a persistent cough. Taking a spoonful of cod liver oil, vegetable oil, or honey before retiring may calm nighttime coughs. Cough-relieving syrups to be taken by the teaspoonful can be made from equal parts of honey, glycerin or olive oil, and lemon juice or apple cider vinegar. Okra, cut very fine, can be substituted for honey or sugar to thicken any cooked cough syrup.

Alcohol Alcohol is used in many cough preparations. To stop a coughing spasm, take 1 teaspoon sugar dissolved in 1 teaspoon whiskey, or add 1 tablespoon butter and 3 tablespoons whiskey to 1 cup boiling water and drink as hot as possible. Cough syrups to bottle and take by the spoonful include: four sticks of horehound candy dissolved in a pint of whiskey; equal amounts of honey, lemon juice, and gin, or of honey, olive oil, and rum; or ¾ cup gin and ½ cup sugar mixed with the strained liquid from ½ cup sunflower seeds boiled in 5 cups water until reduced to 2 cups.

Herbal Cough Syrup Prepare by simmering 4 tablespoons dry raspberry tea in 1 cup water until reduced by half, then mixing the strained liquid with 2 tablespoons honey and 1 tablespoon lemon juice. Or by blending 1 tablespoon *each* slippery elm powder and boiling water, then stirring the mixture into ½ cup of honey.

Herb Tea Anise, eucalyptus, or peppermint tea is believed to suppress the brain's cough center.[118]

Juice Utilize to stop an irritating cough. For a syrup, fresh carrot or cherry juice can be mixed half-and-half with honey. Or ⅔ cup lemon juice can be simmered with ½ pound brown sugar and a tablespoon of almond oil. Sipping hot grapefruit juice sweetened with honey is an alternative cough queller.

Milk-Based Beverages These may mollify a cough. Stir 1 teaspoon *each* honey and sesame oil into 1 cup hot milk. Or simmer three chopped black mission figs in 1 cup milk, let stand for an hour, strain, and reheat before drinking. To ease coughing spasms, sip the strained liquid from equal amounts of barley, oats, and rye cooked in milk.

Onions A time-honored cough cure. Slices of raw onion layered in a dish with honey or sugar, and covered and allowed to stand for 8 to

12 hours produce a liquid to be taken by the teaspoonful each 2 hours. For a bottled syrup, cook minced onions or leeks in wine vinegar, strain, then combine the liquid with an equal amount of honey.

Expectorants

Hot soup, especially chicken or onion, eases the expectoration of harmful secretions. Fresh lemon juice, mixed with a little honey, if desired, acts as an expectorant when taken by the spoonful. Fiery condiments (black pepper, garlic, horseradish, hot mustard, red pepper) ingested with food in quantities sufficient to cause a tingly mouth and watery eyes are even more effective. Eating a clove of garlic every 3 hours is believed beneficial. Taking ½ teaspoon horseradish with 2 teaspoons of honey often relieves coughing spasms, as does a spoonful of syrup made by steeping peeled garlic cloves in honey. Herbalists recommend sipping tea made from fenugreek, gumweed, mullein, thyme, or wild cherry bark. Licorice tea is considered an excellent expectorant that also relieves smoker's cough.

Expectorant Cough Syrups Taken by the teaspoonful as needed, these soothe raspy throats, help clear congestion associated with colds or the flu, and are helpful for persons with asthma or bronchitis.

○ Simmer 1 teaspoon *each* anise seeds and dried thyme in 2 cups of water for 10 minutes. (If desired, 1 teaspoon *each* horehound and licorice root may be included.) Strain, then stir 1 cup brown sugar or honey into the hot liquid.

○ Stir ½ teaspoon cayenne pepper and 2 tablespoons honey into a mixture of ¼ cup *each* apple cider vinegar and water.

○ Steep 1 tablespoon *each* horseradish and crushed mustard seeds in 1 cup boiling water for 20 minutes. Strain and stir in enough honey to make a syrup.

Tissue Salts For an expectorant, dissolve three 6X tablets of Kali. Mur. under the tongue every two hours. If fever is present, substitute Kali. Sulph. Taking three 6X tablets of Ferr. Phos. every two hours is advised for a hard, dry cough.

Nerve Pressure and Massage

○ Stimulate each point for 30 seconds: With the index fingers, press inward and upward against the underside of the cheekbones just above the nostrils; press in and pull down on the top of the breastbone at the hollow of the throat; massage the hollows beneath the collarbones on both sides; then press the center of the breastbone.

○ To stop a fit of coughing, squeeze the joint nearest the tip of the middle finger with the fingers of the opposite hand; or press both sides of the right thumbnail; or press and massage the lower joint of the right index finger; or press upward on the roof of the mouth.

○ To stop a nervous cough, press the upper lip beneath the nose.

Sources (see Bibliography)

17, 20, 21, 32, 51, 57, 58, 64, 65, 69, 75, 84, 85, 92, 110, 111, 116, 117, 118, 135, 144, 148, 150, 159, 164, 171, 172, 186, 202, 203, 224, 254, 255, 264, 265, 281, 293, 294, 300, 312, 313

Dandruff

Although no one has ever perished from terminal dandruff, snowy shoulders and "that little itch" are social embarrassments. Causes include allergic reactions, dietary deficiencies, emotional stress, hairspray or shampoo residue, hormonal fluctuations, illness, infrequent shampooing, a too-dry or too-oily scalp, or a sunburned head. Severe dandruff that does not respond to home remedies and relaxation techniques (see Introduction) warrants a visit to a dermatologist and possible treatment for seborrheic dermatitis, a scaly, itchy rash that may also appear on the face, chest, and back.

Diet and Supplements (see note on page xii)

The complex carbohydrates in fruits, vegetables, and whole grains supply nutrients essential for scalp health. Studies show that many cases of dandruff are related to diets high in saturated fat, sugar, and refined carbohydrates.[98] Taking a daily multivitamin-mineral plus optional supplements often clears dandruff problems.

Vitamin A In the form of beta carotene, 25,000 to 35,000 IU daily for 1 month to prevent dry scalp and the dead-cell accumulation of dandruff.

B Complex One comprehensive tablet once or twice daily. An additional 100 to 300 milligrams of PABA has cleared intractable dandruff that had spread to the eyebrows and sides of the nose.[301]

Vitamin E and Vegetable Oil Taking 20 to 400 IU of vitamin E plus a tablespoon of canola or olive oil with the daily diet may correct dry, flaky dandruff.

125

Lecithin   One tablespoon of granules daily or two capsules with each meal protects and strengthens cell membranes of the scalp.[17]

Selenium   50 to 100 micrograms daily enhances the action of vitamin E and helps prevent the hardening of tissues that can result in scaly dandruff.

Tissue Salts   Two daily doses of both Kali. Sulph. and Nat. Mur. in the 12X potency for 2 or 3 weeks.

Zinc   30 to 50 milligrams, or the equivalent in zinc lozenges dissolved in the mouth at intervals, daily for 1 week. In some instances, zinc supplementation has halted the itching and scaling of dandruff within 7 days.[42]

Preshampoo Treatments

Although an overly oily scalp can instigate dandruff, an occasional oil treatment helps loosen and soften the scales. Massage warmed castor oil, corn oil, olive oil, or petroleum jelly into the scalp and cover with a hot, moist towel for 30 minutes before shampooing. To ease the itching and scabbing of severe dandruff, apply vitamin E oil to the scalp twice a week before going to bed, then shampoo the following morning.

○ Fifteen minutes before shampooing, massage the scalp with any of these dandruff destroyers: a half-and-half mixture of vinegar and water (for increased benefits, add 1 tablespoon bee pollen granules per cup); equal parts of triple-strength rosemary and sage tea; an infusion of 1 tablespoon dried mint simmered with ½ cup water and ¼ cup vinegar, strained after cooling. Or massage the scalp with warmed peanut oil, then with fresh lemon juice; or use just the lemon juice.

○ At bedtime, rub aloe vera gel on the scalp. Or squeeze grated ginger root through cheesecloth and combine the liquid with an equal amount of sesame oil before massaging it into the scalp. Cover either treatment with a towel or sleep cap and shampoo out the next morning. Repeat two or three times a week until the dandruff disappears.

Apple Cider Vinegar Pouring warm vinegar over the hair and wrapping with a towel for 1 hour before shampooing has cleared some cases of intractable dandruff when repeated twice a week for a month.[42]

Salt Combine ½ cup salt with enough water to make a paste. Rub into the scalp, wait 5 minutes, then rinse out. Whitney B. liked to wear dark sweaters to accentuate her fair skin and light blond hair, but she did not like the white flakes that drifted onto her shoulders. An old folk remedy solved the problem. Twice each week she stirred a tablespoon of salt into a raw egg, rubbed the mixture into her scalp, and let it remain for 5 minutes before rinsing with lukewarm water and shampooing as usual. Now free of dandruff, Whitney continues to use the salty egg treatment once a week to prevent a recurrence— and because she delights in the body and radiance it gives her hair.

Shampoos and Rinses

Shampooing daily with a mild shampoo diluted half-and-half with water has proven more satisfactory for many people than using harsh, medicated products. If conditioners or cream rinses are used, they should be applied only to the hair, not to the scalp. Dandruff may result from an overly alkaline condition that can be corrected by adding a tablespoon of lemon juice or vinegar to the final rinse, or by using one of these folk remedy rinses.

○ Before the final rinse, massage the scalp with a combination of ¼ cup apple cider vinegar, 1 tablespoon witch hazel and two crushed aspirins; or with a mixture of 1 tablespoon *each* witch hazel and water plus 1 teaspoon lemon juice.

○ For a final rinse, use double-strength tea brewed from camomile, catnip, celery seed, chaparral, chive, nettle, rosemary and mint, sage, thyme, or wintergreen. Adding a spoonful of vinegar may increase the benefits.

Tonics

To combat between-shampoo flakiness, dab the scalp with a cotton ball moistened with one of these mixtures: 1 teaspoon apple cider vinegar stirred into 1 cup water; glycerin and rosewater (available in pharmacies); a half-and-half blend of double-strength rosemary and sage teas (if desired, a teaspoon of borax can be dissolved in each cup); a blend of equal parts of witch hazel and any commercial mouthwash; or a solution of 1 tablespoon witch hazel or lemon juice in ¼ cup water.

Sources (see Bibliography)

6, 17, 32, 41, 42, 53, 64, 74, 75, 82, 87, 89, 98, 135, 144, 150, 159, 176, 177, 186, 196, 203, 205, 207, 219, 225, 256, 262, 293, 300, 301, 304, 305, 312, 313

Dermatitis, Eczema, and Prickly Heat

Dermatitis (from Latin words for inflamed skin) and eczema (meaning "to boil out" in ancient Greek) are often used interchangeably as terms for noninfectious, itchy, blistery rashes. Skin may redden and swell, the small blisters may weep and crust, and in some cases fissures or flaking may occur. Whatever the type of rash, dermatologists agree that scratching creates a vicious cycle resulting in more itching and more rash, as well as possible infection. Over-the-counter antihistamines may reduce itching by preventing histamines from reaching sensitive skin cells. Topical steroid preparations can control the itch but should not be used for long periods. Besides being absorbed through the skin to cause possibly adverse reactions, the relief provided by steroids may mask a more serious skin problem.[201] Any rash that does not respond to a week or two of home treatment should be diagnosed by a dermatologist. There are two basic types of this skin disorder, with many variations and myriad causes.

1. **Atopic dermatitis or eczema,** generally begins in the skin folds at elbows and knees but may cover any part of the body. Usually affecting allergy-prone individuals, the rash may appear almost immediately or develop days after being triggered by environmental, internal, or psychological factors such as emotional stress, extreme heat or cold, dust or pollens, or food allergies.

2. **Contact dermatitis** is induced by either an allergen or an irritant touching the skin. The patches of rash develop within 2 to 48 hours and correspond to the area of contact. Skin-care products produce 28 percent of contact dermatitis.[112] Other causative substances in-

clude detergent residue or dry-cleaning chemicals left in clothing; the formaldehyde in nail polish, some plastics, and all permanent-press fabrics; metal alloys (especially nickel) in jewelry, watchbands, and clothing fasteners; plants (see "Poison Ivy"); rubber (in bathing caps, condoms, elastic, gloves, and shoes); and soaps and shampoos.

Subclassifications offer clues to identification and future avoidance of the instigators.

Actinic Dermatitis/Photodermatitis Caused by a reaction to sunlight or other sources of ultraviolet radiation, this reaction usually appears within 2 hours after exposure.

Asteatosis Eczema/Winter Itch Dry cold air and indoor heat can dry sensitive skin, making it more susceptible to itchy irritations that may blister and peel (see "Dry Skin" for moisturizing remedies).

Hand Dermatitis/Housewives' Eczema This usually results from contact with substances such as dust, or chemicals in detergents and household cleansers. Itchy blisters may develop on the fingers or palms, or the hands may become covered with scales and painful cracks. Wearing rubber or plastic gloves over thin white cotton gloves when in contact with any irritant speeds healing and helps prevent recurrence.

Infantile Eczema An intensely itchy rash with tiny red pimples that weep when scratched, it usually begins on the inner creases of knees and elbows but may occur on the diaper area. This type of atopic dermatitis, common in babies under the age of 18 months, often is precipitated by allergies to foods such as eggs, milk, and orange juice. Home remedies call for coating the rash with petroleum jelly; dressing the baby in lightweight, all-cotton clothing to avoid overheating or skin irritation; and, with the pediatrician's approval, experimenting with a food-elimination diet.

Seborrheic Dermatitis Also called inflammatory dandruff of the skin, this appears as a scaly, flaky, itchy rash on the face (especially around the nose and eyebrows), chest, or back. It often develops during times of stress, may accompany severe scalp dandruff, and usually requires professional treatment.

Prickly Heat (Miliaria) A burning, itching, stinging rash, prickly heat results from unevaporated perspiration oversaturating the skin, blocking sweat ducts, and forcing trapped germs and perspiration to leak into skin tissues. Other possible instigators include adhesive bandages and airtight baby pants. Wearing a tight, wet swimsuit all day can waterlog the skin to cause a similar rash known as "bikini bottom."

Sometimes called heat rash, the eruptions tend to affect body sites such as armpits, chest, or back, where sweat collects. When Mort H. developed a three-inch band of prickling rash around his waist during his first summer as a parcel-delivery driver, he faced a dilemma because wearing a belt with his uniform was mandatory. Mort resolved the problem by keeping a well-stocked gym bag in his van. Several times each day he stripped to the waist, wiped the irritated area with rubbing alcohol, smoothed on talcum powder, and donned a clean undershirt before replacing his outer shirt.

Folk healers recommend rubbing heat rash with watermelon rind or applying witch hazel or a solution of baking soda and water, then dusting with arrowroot, cornstarch, rice flour, or whey powder. Aloe vera gel is a soothing itch controller. Creams or lotions that could further block pores are not advised. Wearing loose-fitting clothing, taking cool showers, and applying astringents and absorbent powders, usually clears the condition within a day or two.

Diet and Supplements (see note on page xii)

Extremely low-protein or low-fat diets may induce eczematous dermatitis that can be countered by increasing dietary protein and/or adding 1 to 3 tablespoons of vegetable oil daily (or taking supplements of primrose oil or EPA fish oils).[98, 151, 276] Drinking a glass of milk containing 2 teaspoons of blackstrap molasses twice each day for 2 weeks (or 1 teaspoon of apple cider vinegar per cup of water three times daily and sponging the irritated area with a little of the mixture) reportedly has cleared stubborn cases of hand eczema.[42, 262] To help clear chronic dermatitis, nutritionists suggest a glass daily of any combination of these juices: alfalfa sprouts, apple, beet, carrot, celery, cucumber, lettuce, parsley, red grape, spinach. Taking a daily multivitamin-mineral plus separate supplements has cleared longstanding cases of eczema.[301]

Vitamin A In the form of beta carotene, 50,000 to 75,000 IU daily for 1 month, then 25,000 IU as maintenance.

B Complex One high-potency tablet one to three times a day. A deficiency of any of the B vitamins can cause dermatitis. Eating acidophilus yogurt or taking acidophilus capsules contributes to the body's manufacture of the B vitamins. Brewer's yeast, an excellent source of the vitamins, can be stirred into milk or juices, taken in tablet form, or mixed with milk or water and applied topically for itch relief. Additional B_2 and B_6 may be needed to correct cracks at eye or mouth corners, or scaling around the ears, forehead, nose, or mouth. When combined with 500-milligram supplements of vitamin C, 50 milligrams of B_6 plus 100 milligrams of pantothenic acid have an antihistamine effect that may alleviate atopic dermatitis.

Vitamin C 1,000 to 3,500 milligrams in divided daily doses. Studies show that vitamin C improves, sometimes clears, and helps prevent recurrences of either dermatitis or prickly heat.[50, 98]

Vitamin E 100 to 600 IU daily, especially beneficial when combined with a liberal supply of calcium, vitamin D, and magnesium.

Tissue Salts Three tablets *each* 3X Ferr. Phos. and Nat. Phos. three times a day. If pustules contain hard matter, take an equal amount of both Calc. Phos. and Silicea. For eruptions with clear fluid, take Nat. Mur.; for thick white contents, take Kali. Mur.[64, 65]

Zinc 15 to 50 milligrams daily for 3 months, then 15 milligrams daily. Under medical supervision, severe or chronic cases have responded to extremely high doses of zinc plus vitamin C.[228, 317]

Folk Remedies

For localized patches of rash, poultices of grated raw potato, pastes of baking soda and water or cornstarch and vinegar, or cold compresses of any of the following liquids can be applied at frequent intervals: milk, water with 1 teaspoon of baking soda per cup, chaparral tea, oatmeal water (made by simmering ½ cup oatmeal in a quart of water and straining out the solids), or the liquid from a pan of boiled watercress. If the itch is widespread, lukewarm baths with baking soda, cornstarch, or colloidal oatmeal (or regular oatmeal or wheat bran secured in cheesecloth) are soothing. For all rashes except prickly heat, each water treatment should be followed by a lubricating application of a fragrance-free emollient such as petroleum jelly. Turn-of-the-century practitioners advised mixing five drops of carbolic acid with each ounce of petroleum jelly to make the "carbolated vaseline" now sold in drug stores.

Aloe Vera Gel One of the oldest remedies for irritated skin, aloe vera relieves both itching and pain and is believed to speed healing.

Herbs Sip as teas or take in capsules, burdock, chickweed, dandelion, pau d'arco, red clover, sarsaparilla, or yellow dock. Burdock, chickweed, or red clover are considered the most effective herbal treatment for eczema when 2 cups of the teas are taken internally each day and another cup sponged over the eruptions.[150] Herbalists also suggest a poultice of crushed chickweed or plantain leaves; an ointment of powdered turmeric blended with coconut oil; or pastes of dry slippery elm and strained chaparral tea plus a spoonful of olive oil, or of powdered goldenseal mixed with honey and vitamin E oil.

Stress Relief and Mental Imagery

The discomforts of skin eruptions can be intensified by anger, anxiety, or frustration. In one study, 76 percent of the cases of hand eczema were found to be emotionally triggered.[112] Practicing one of the relaxation techniques described in the Introduction may help reduce stress-induced reactions. While in a relaxed state, visualizing the skin as rash-free and imagining the cooling comfort of a midnight swim may allay burning, itching sensations and encourage healing.

Sources (see Bibliography)

2, 6, 16, 17, 29, 42, 47, 50, 64, 65, 66, 75, 87, 98, 109, 112, 116, 135, 137, 144, 148, 150, 151, 176, 177, 186, 201, 218, 228, 254, 255, 256, 262, 276, 281, 283, 293, 294, 300, 301, 311, 312, 313, 317

Diabetes

First described in Egyptian hieroglyphics 3,500 years ago, diabetes is due to a metabolic dysfunction in which genetic predisposition plays a role. Normally, ingested carbohydrates are converted into glucose (sugar) by the body, then the pancreas produces enough of the hormone insulin to allow receptors in the cells to absorb the sugar from the blood for immediate use as energy or for storage. Type I (insulin-dependent or juvenile diabetes), which affects about 10 percent of all diabetics, is considered a hereditary autoimmune disease that first appears during childhood, demolishes insulin-producing cells in the pancreas, and requires treatment with insulin injections. In type II (non-insulin-dependent, adult- or maturity-onset diabetes mellitus), which develops gradually after the age of 40 and usually is due to improper diet, inactivity, and excess weight, insulin is produced but the receptors in the cells fail to remove sugar from the blood.

Tests show that the number of insulin receptors and their sensitivity decreases with obesity and increases as weight is lost.[75] When weight is maintained slightly below the "ideal" on the height-and-weight charts, many diabetics find that their own insulin production is adequate. Oral drugs prescribed for type II diabetics are not insulin replacements; they stimulate pancreatic production of insulin and educe glucose levels.

The goal of a diabetic regimen is to maintain blood sugar and blood fat as close to normal as possible. Blood-sugar swings between high glucose and fat levels (which can lead to complications such as heart disease, kidney failure, and nerve damage) and low blood sugar (temporary hypoglycemia that can cause shakiness, mental confusion, and coma) necessitate both professional and home care. Hypoglycemic episodes usually can be corrected by eating a small piece of candy or by drinking half a glass of orange juice or apple juice, or regular soft drink to temporarily elevate the blood sugar. If the sweet is taken more than an hour before the next meal, a few bites of food containing protein or fat as well as carbohydrates should be

134

eaten to prevent a rebound recurrence of the symptoms. Suggested snacks include crackers or rice cakes and cheese, peanuts, or peanut butter on bread.[94]

Diet

Diabetic diets require customization according to individual caloric and nutritional needs, and dietary alterations should have the approval of the attending physician. Recommendations have undergone many changes. In 1797, a diet of nothing but meat and rancid fat was believed to be the solution; in 1900, an all-oat cure was tried in Germany;[307] but before the isolation of insulin in 1921, all carbohydrates were severely limited and a diagnosis of diabetes meant death within a few months or years.[112] For the 1990s, the American Diabetes Association (ADA) and other authorities advise a diet with 50 to 60 percent of the daily calories from carbohydrates, 15 to 20 percent from protein, and less than 30 percent from fat. Dividing the day's calories among six small meals or three meals and three snacks evenly spaced throughout the day helps stabilize glucose levels, especially when each one contains both carbohydrates and protein.[186] The carbohydrates in all foods are transformed into blood sugar; the speed with which the conversion is accomplished makes a decided difference in the amount of insulin required.

Simple Carbohydrates These include cakes, candy, and pastries. Although rapidly assimilated, simple carbohydrates can be tolerated in modest amounts by most diabetics when consumed along with a regular meal. Although alternative sweeteners like sorbitol or fructose reach the bloodstream more slowly, they can elevate both glucose and triglyceride levels if used to excess by people with low insulin reserves. Noncaloric substitutes (aspartame, saccharin) have been approved for diabetics but should not be used by children or by women who are pregnant or lactating.[293, 300]

Complex Carbohydrates These include the starches in vegetables, dried beans, and whole grains. Complex carbohydrates take longer to digest and, because of their fiber content, help stabilize blood sugar.

Soluble and Insoluble Fibers Found in vegetables, legumes, grains, nuts, and fruits, these fibers slow the digestive process to prevent a rush of sugar into the blood, improve glucose tolerance, and in many cases, can dramatically reduce insulin requirements when 10 to 15 grams are included with each meal.[300] To prevent abdominal distress, increase fiber consumption gradually and drink at least eight glasses of water daily. A tablespoon of psyllium stirred into a glass of water or tomato juice and taken 20 minutes before meals adds soluble fiber and can be especially beneficial in a weight-loss program.[151] Glucomannan or guar gum, taken with a large glass of water and swallowed quickly before it thickens, also provides fiber and acts as a fat mobilizer.[17] Large amounts of caffeine-containing beverages can elevate blood sugar levels. Alcohol is metabolized like fat and if taken on an empty stomach by insulin users can cause a hypoglycemic reaction. Even when imbibed with food by diabetics whose symptoms are under control, no more than two alcoholic drinks per day are advised.[94, 186]

Fat Intake of fat should consist of no more than 10 percent saturated fat from meat and dairy products; as much of the remainder as possible should be monounsaturated from canola or olive oil. Saturated fats may interfere with insulin function; studies show that monounsaturates have the opposite effect—actually lowering blood sugar levels as long as total fats are kept below 30 percent of the daily calories.[254]

Supplements (see note on page xii)

Supplements, which should be taken only with medical approval, allow diabetics to compensate for their increased need of nutrients without violating their special diets.[177]

Vitamin A 10,000 to 25,000 IU daily of preformed vitamin A. Many diabetics are unable to convert the beta carotene from fruits and vegetables into the vitamin A that contributes to healing and eye health.

B Complex One or two comprehensive tablets daily to assist with carbohydrate metabolism. Vitamins B_1, B_2, B_6, B_{12}, and pantothenic acid help stimulate insulin production.[98] Inositol (available as a supplement or from lecithin) protects against diabetic nerve damage. Niacin potentiates the beneficial effects of chromium, but high doses should be taken only under the guidance of a physician.

Vitamin C 1,000 to 4,000 milligrams in divided doses each day. Diabetics lose vitamin C more readily than nondiabetics, and this vitamin is needed to help fight infection, heal wounds, and encourage the production of insulin.

Calcium and Magnesium 800 to 1,500 milligrams of calcium and 500 to 750 milligrams of magnesium in divided daily doses to maintain pancreatic health and help protect against retinal problems.[14, 17] With the physician's approval, increasing the amount of magnesium to 1,600 to 3,500 milligrams daily may be beneficial.

Chromium 200 micrograms daily to improve glucose tolerance and increase the effectiveness of insulin by restoring sensitivity to the insulin receptors in the cells.[151, 201]

L-Carnitine and L-glutamine 500 milligrams of these amino acids; taken twice daily on an empty stomach.[17]

Manganese Up to 50 milligrams daily to collaborate with chromium in improving glucose tolerance.[109]

Tissue Salts Nat. Phos. and Nat. Sulph. are suggested for diabetics. Two to four tablets of each in the 6X potency may be taken twice daily to stimulate pancreatic action.[64]

Zinc 15 to 30 milligrams daily to prolong the effects of insulin and to improve wound healing.[228, 234]

Exercise

Regular exercise is both prevention and treatment—sedentary people are three times more likely to develop type II diabetes than those who are physically active.[204] For diabetics, medically approved exercise can lower blood sugar and improve glucose tolerance. Rhythmic, repetitive muscular movement is the most beneficial—walking for half an hour five to seven times a week is the favored activity. As a general rule, persons who are taking insulin should exercise an hour after eating and keep a snack of raisins or a container of fruit juice available to offset possible hypoglycemic episodes resulting from lowered blood sugar. Type II diabetics who are trying to lose weight may prefer to exercise before meals to reduce appetite.

Folk Remedies

To help regulate blood sugar levels, herbalists suggest teas of blueberry leaf, buchu leaf, dandelion root, goldenseal, juniper berry, uva ursi, or yarrow. Onions (or green onion-garlic oil) have been found useful for lowering blood sugar. Eating fresh garlic or taking deodorized garlic capsules with each meal lowers glucose levels in some cases and helps suppress the yeast infections that often beset diabetics. Taking a capsule of cayenne with each of three daily meals also helps bring down high blood sugar levels.[150, 293]

Nerve Pressure and Massage

To stimulate insulin production and distribution, once a day press or massage any of these points for 30 seconds to 2 minutes.

- ○ The underside of the protuberance at the back of the skull just above the neck.

- ○ The tip of each elbow (with the arms bent); the center of the palm, then the thumb and the two fingers next to it, on each hand.

- ○ Just below the front of each knee, where the separate bones can be felt.

- ○ The pad under the little toe on the right foot, then a strip across the sole of each foot midway between the center of the arch and the pad beneath the big toe.

Sources (see Bibliography)

6, 14, 17, 24, 28, 31, 46, 47, 48, 49, 50, 51, 56, 59, 60, 64, 75, 94, 98, 109, 112, 123, 138, 147, 150, 151, 164, 166, 177, 186, 190, 201, 204, 208, 228, 231, 234, 254, 293, 294, 300, 307, 312

Diaper Rash

The ammonia in urine, especially when combined with feces, irritates skin and promotes diaper rash. In severe cases, especially following antibiotic therapy, the yeast fungus *Candida albicans* multiplies in moist creases of the diaper area to cause thrush, which is characterized by a "baking-bread" odor and flaky white patches in the red rash. Oral thrush (white splotches covering a newborn's tongue and mouth) can be acquired during birth if the mother has a vaginal yeast infection but seldom appears after the first month.[17, 296]

Home treatment usually clears diaper rash within a few days. If it persists or if additional irritation develops, however, a pediatrician should be consulted. Observing the guidelines for preventing diaper rash sometimes serves to correct the problem.

○ Change diapers frequently. Gently cleanse the area and dry thoroughly—a hair dryer set on low is less irritating than a towel when skin is inflamed. Dust with powder or apply a protective coating of lotion or petroleum jelly.

○ Avoid air-excluding disposable diapers or plastic pants. The bacteria responsible for diaper rash are anaerobic—they thrive in an airless atmosphere and are destroyed by exposure to oxygen. Leave the baby diaperless on a sheet-covered waterproof pad whenever possible.

Diet and Supplements (see note on page xii)

Giving older infants ¼ to ⅓ cup of cranberry juice daily reduces irritation by leaving an acid residue in the urine.[293] Limiting the amount of meat in the baby's diet may help curtail the production of ammonia in the urine. A deficiency of vitamins A, B, C, D, E, or K, or of unsaturated fatty acids (UFA) can instigate diaper rash. Nursing mothers can add a tablespoon of vegetable oil to their salads for the UFAs and take a daily multivitamin-mineral. With the pediatrician's approval, the infant can be given a liquid supplement—thrush may be caused by a lack of vitamin A or of the B-complex vitamins.

Topical applications of dietary supplements may reduce pain, speed healing, and prevent recurrence if applied at the first sign of redness. Blending the contents of vitamin A and D capsules with vitamin E oil and smoothing it over the baby's bottom has been effective in many cases and is less likely to provoke an adverse reaction on tender skin than is oral vitamin E squeezed from a capsule. However, applying vitamin E from 400 IU capsules or lecithin from 1,200 milligram capsules after each diaper change has cleared recalcitrant diaper rash in 3 days.[41, 42]

Margot F. had been eating yogurt and taking acidophilus capsules to guard against a recurrence of her vaginal yeast infection. When her baby developed a yeasty-smelling diaper rash on a Friday night, she utilized *Lactobacillus acidophilus* to relieve his discomfort before the doctor's office opened on Monday. Three times a day, she mixed the contents of an acidophilus capsule with the water for her son's bottle and once daily after a bowel movement inserted one of the capsules into his rectum after lubricating it with petroleum jelly.

Folk Remedies

When laundering cloth diapers, adding 2 tablespoons of vinegar to each gallon of water for the final rinse reduces irritation from the ammonia in urine. If thrush is suspected, diapers should be boiled to destroy the yeast spores and avoid reinfection.

"Brown Powder" Plain flour, well browned by stirring in a heavy skillet over medium heat, can be dusted on the affected area with every diaper change and was a pioneer remedy for the irritating rash. Ozark grannies still crush and sieve the little mud houses made by dirt dauber wasps, then use the powder to relieve the pain of diaper rash and cure babies' sore bottoms.

Cornstarch Dusted on with each diaper change, cornstarch helps absorb ammonia and keep the baby dry. Mixing 2 tablespoons of finely powdered camomile, comfrey, or goldenseal with ¼ cup of cornstarch is believed to help control yeast fungus and speed healing. Applying a salve made from cornstarch and petroleum jelly is another option.

Powdered Turmeric   Either applied dry or mixed with coconut oil for an ointment, this remedy is used in tropical countries.

Aloe Vera Gel, Almond Oil, or Herbal Ointments   Made from powdered mullein leaf or slippery elm blended with olive oil or wheat germ oil, these are other time-tested favorites.

Garlic   Not only does garlic guard against bacterial infection, but, researchers report, it is highly successful in killing *Candida albicans*.[318] If garlic does not irritate the baby's skin, garlic water may be used as a wash; garlic oil (diluted if desired) can be applied directly to the sores; or, for thrush, garlic capsules can be inserted in the baby's rectum.[176]

Sources (see Bibliography)

16, 17, 28, 41, 42, 75, 98, 135, 150, 176, 192, 256, 264, 268, 281, 293, 296, 300, 312, 313, 318

Diarrhea

The frequent, watery stools and abdominal cramping of diarrhea can be instigated by anything that interferes with the normal solidification of fecal material. Acute diarrhea that self-corrects after a day or two is usually caused by contaminated food or water or by a virus but may be triggered by food allergy, antacids containing magnesium hydroxide, antibiotics or other medications, overindulgence in alcohol or caffeine-containing beverages, overuse of laxatives, extreme fatigue or stress, or excessive consumption of sorbitol (a sugar substitute that can pull liquid into the intestines from the bloodstream).[29] Since acute diarrhea is part of the body's defense system for getting rid of unwanted substances, most doctors advise allowing the discomfort to run its course for 6 to 12 hours before taking antidiarrheal drugs. Recurrent short-term bouts of diarrhea may be instigated by anxiety or nutritional deficiencies that can be alleviated with relaxation techniques (see Introduction) and improved diet. Medical evaluation should be obtained to rule out a serious disorder if diarrhea continues to recur, if any bout persists for more than 2 or 3 days, if blood or mucus appears in the stools, or if fever is present.

Beverages

First-Aid Tip To prevent dehydration—particularly in infants, the elderly, and the chronically ill—replenishing lost fluids is of vital importance. The U.S. Public Health Service suggests combining 8 ounces of fruit juice with ½ teaspoon natural sweetener and a pinch of salt in one glass; and mixing 8 ounces of carbonated or boiled water with ¼ teaspoon baking soda in another glass, then alternating sips from each glass. Simpler solutions include mixing a teaspoon of sugar and ¼ teaspoon *each* baking soda and salt with a cup of water;[148] or, for infants as well as adults, dissolving 1 teaspoon sugar and a pinch of salt in a quart of water. The rice water diarrhea cure first advised in 3,000-year-old Sanskrit has achieved scientific approval—mothers in third-world countries are being trained to prepare a rehydrating rice-salt solution strained from 2 handfuls of rice and 1 teaspoon of salt boiled with 1 quart of water. Americans have had equal success with the water from cooked barley or oatmeal plus a teaspoon of sugar. Raw honey is not advised for babies because of the danger of botulism, but it and lemon may be added to adult portions of the liquid.[56, 176, 313] Drinking 2 teaspoons of cornmeal or cornstarch stirred in a cup of boiled water is a folk remedy for stopping diarrhea within an hour or two.[150, 312]

Other fluids should include broths and juices as part of the 2 quarts per day recommended for adults. Nutritional consultants suggest lemonade, orangeade, or any combination of apple (for adults only; it sometimes worsens diarrhea in children), carrot, celery, papaya, parsley, fresh pineapple, and spinach juices.[6, 218] Lactose intolerance (an inability to digest milk sugar) is responsible for some cases of chronic diarrhea that clear when milk is avoided or when lactase supplements are taken.[254] For the lactose tolerant, especially children, the anti-infectious agents in milk fat can help conquer chronic diarrhea. Major studies confirm milk fat's ability to destroy bacterial toxins in the intestinal tract and show that adding milk fat "cures" many cases of chronic diarrhea in skim-milk users.[56]

Warm or room temperature liquids are more readily assimilated than are iced drinks, which tend to stimulate intestinal contractions. Herbs believed beneficial for occasional bouts of diarrhea include basil, camomile, cinnamon, ginger, peppermint, red raspberry leaf, sage, slippery elm, thyme, and turmeric. Hourly doses of peppermint tea plus 2 tablespoons of onion juice (from grated onion squeezed through cheesecloth) are a folk cure for diarrhea. Babies can be given ½ teaspoon red raspberry leaf tea every 4 hours; or, after each elimination, 2 tablespoons of a pint of scalded milk blended with 1 tablespoon slippery elm tea; or of a puddinglike mixture of 1 teaspoon slippery elm in molasses and water.[176]

Diet

Rice, bananas, and applesauce (preferably made in a blender from raw apples) make up the diet most often prescribed for controlling acute diarrhea. Folk healers brown the rice in a dry skillet before cooking, and sprinkle it with cinnamon before eating. Some authorities advise avoiding dairy products and eating nothing but clear soups and gelatin desserts until the diarrhea subsides. Others suggest high-protein, low-residue custards, junkets, cheeses, and soft-cooked eggs to "bind" the bowel. An alternative 2-day regimen is to eat only raw or lightly steam-fried vegetables—plus oat bran or rice bran if desired—for their fluid-binding fiber.[17, 305] Eating yogurt or taking acidophilus-pectin capsules helps restore beneficial flora and regulate the digestive tract—⅓ cup of skim-milk yogurt daily has cured diarrhea in infants.[56]

Chronic diarrhea cleared for some children after dietary fats like margarine and peanut butter were increased to 40 percent of total calories.[294] Eliminating milk and wheat products plus apples, corn, peaches, pears, and potatoes for a few days may identify chronic-diarrhea-causing culprits when the foods are individually reintroduced. A diet high in soluble fibers and pectins from fruits, vegetables, and cooked grains such as barley, buckwheat, millet, oats, and rice assists in the formation of bulky stools and provides nutrients not found in the bulking agents sometimes prescribed for chronic diarrhea.[201]

Supplements (see note on page xii)

Diarrhea flushes water-soluble vitamins and minerals out of the body and allows little nutrient assimilation from foods. For adults a daily multivitamin-mineral plus additional supplements may help speed recovery and avoid a "wiped out" aftermath.

B Complex One comprehensive tablet daily, plus 50 milligrams *each* B_1 and B_6, 100 milligrams *each* niacinamide and pantothenic acid, and 400 micrograms of folic acid. This combination has produced rapid improvement in acute attacks and cleared some longstanding cases of chronic diarrhea.[6, 87]

Vitamin C 1,000 to 3,000 milligrams, more if well tolerated, in divided daily doses to help combat allergic reactions and infections.

Calcium and Magnesium 1,500 milligrams of calcium to aid in normal stool formation and 500 to 1,000 milligrams of magnesium for adults (100 milligrams for infants) to assist calcium uptake. A deficiency of either mineral may trigger the onset of diarrhea or cause it to continue.[281]

Potassium 100 to 1,000 milligrams for several days unless potassium-rich bananas are being consumed.

Tissue Salts For frequent, gushing stools, take alternating doses of 6X Calc. Phos., Calc. Sulph., and Ferr. Phos. each hour. Add Mag. Phos. if the diarrhea is accompanied by flatulence and abdominal cramping. For diarrhea caused by emotional upsets, take three tablets of 3X Kali. Phos. each hour. If stools are foul-smelling, add three tablets of Silicea. For stools containing undigested food, take three tablets of 12X Ferr. Phos. each hour.[64, 65]

Folk Remedies

Intended for quick relief, home remedies are often effective.

Carob Clinical studies show that 1 teaspoon to 1 tablespoon of fiber- and pectin-rich carob powder stirred into milk or water and taken at frequent intervals controls 60 percent of infectious diarrhea and 90 percent of noninfectious cases.[71] For infants or toddlers, the carob can be given in a bottle or blended with applesauce or pudding.

Carrots Old-fashioned carrot soup moved out of the folklore realm when hospital tests showed that "baby food" carrots corrected diarrhea in 24 hours or less for adults as well as infants, and that adding a little carob powder increased the benefits.[150, 234]

Charcoal Activated charcoal tablets or capsules effectively mop up diarrhea-causing toxins but are not advised for constant use because they also absorb essential vitamins and minerals.[42, 313]

Garlic Whether eaten raw or swallowed in deodorized capsules three times a day, garlic is a natural antibiotic that can reduce intestinal inflammation and often makes diarrhea disappear in a very short time.[17, 150]

The first four remedies have been scientifically corroborated. Other folk remedy favorites follow.

Alcohol Sipping blackberry brandy or blackberry wine is a time-honored cure credited with halting diarrhea within the hour. Other alcohol-based remedies include brandy or wine in which cinnamon sticks or whole allspice or cloves have been steeped (adults take ¼ to

½ cup; children, 1 tablespoon diluted with water). Or, to be taken by the spoonful by all ages: 1 cup *each* cherry brandy and rum simmered with ¼ pound brown sugar and an ounce of peppermint; or equal amounts of rum, molasses, and olive oil simmered to the consistency of honey.

Apple Cider Vinegar   Add 1 tablespoon vinegar and 1 teaspoon salt to ½ cup warm water, sip slowly, and repeat in 30 minutes if necessary. Or mix 1 tablespoon *each* black pepper and salt, stir in ½ cup *each* vinegar and water, then take by the tablespoonful every half hour.

Bread   Combine 2 tablespoons honey with 1 teaspoon bee pollen granules, spread on whole-grain bread, and eat slowly. Or soak 1 slice dry rye bread in 1 cup boiled water for 15 minutes; strain, then sip the liquid.

Cold or Hot Packs   Some natural healers place an ice pack on the middle and lower back for 10 minutes, remove it for 10 minutes, then replace it for 10 minutes. Others prefer 30-minute hot packs on both the lower back and the abdomen. In the early 1800s, great relief was assured if flannel was moistened with brandy or whiskey, sprinkled with a mixture of all available spices, and placed over the bowels.[69]

Spices   Simmer ¼ teaspoon cinnamon and ⅛ teaspoon cayenne pepper in a pint of water for 20 minutes, then drink ¼ cup of the liquid every 30 minutes. Or mix ¼ teaspoon allspice, cinnamon, and/or nutmeg in a cup of pekoe tea or scalded milk; sweeten with brown sugar and add a tablespoon of brandy or a pinch of cloves, if desired; then sip slowly. Or try Aunt Ruby's peppery remedy. With five children and six grandchildren of her own, she is the health-emergencies expert for the neighborhood. When Tiffany's diarrhea attacked before morning recess, Aunt Ruby brought her home from school, scalded a cup of milk with a teaspoon of butter, sprinkled it liberally with black pepper, and said "Drink this." Tiffany felt like Alice in Wonderland, but the mixture was so effective that the diarrhea was under control by the time her mother picked her up after work.

For Chronic Diarrhea   Squeeze half a lemon or lime into a glass of milk and drink each morning and evening. Or eat a small dish of fresh or frozen blueberries with two or three meals each day. Or incorporate a spoonful of carob powder with each meal. Or take a teaspoon of ground nutmeg four times a day.

Nerve Pressure and Massage

○ Press or massage below the fingernails (on the side nearest the thumb) of the index and middle finger on each hand; then the hollow of each inner elbow, 1 inch to the outside of center.

○ With the thumb or the heel of the hand, deeply massage the navel and a spot 1½ inches directly below it; then massage just below the front of each kneecap to the outside of the shinbone.

○ On both feet, press or massage the web of skin between the big toe and the one next to it; then stimulate a point just in front of the heel on the bottom of each foot.

See also **Traveler's Diarrhea**

Sources (see Bibliography)

6, 10, 17, 20, 29, 42, 49, 51, 56, 57, 64, 65, 69, 71, 75, 76, 87, 92, 98, 101, 109, 135, 148, 150, 164, 168, 172, 176, 186, 201, 202, 218, 234, 254, 255, 256, 262, 281, 283, 284, 293, 294, 300, 302, 305, 312, 313

Diverticulosis and Diverticulitis

Diverticulosis signifies the presence of small pouches or hernias (diverticula) protruding into the abdomen from the colon. Approximately half of the American population past middle age has diverticulosis, but most people are unaware of the condition unless it is detected by an X-ray examination for other problems. Irritable bowel syndrome (see page 271) sometimes coexists with diverticulosis and can cause bloating, pain in the lower abdomen, and alternating episodes of constipation and diarrhea.

Diverticulitis, a complication suffered by 5 to 10 percent of patients with diverticulosis, occurs when waste material or food particles trapped in diverticula become infected.[186] Diverticular disease can result in short, severe attacks or in a long-term but milder malady with periods of pain in the lower left portion of the abdomen and frequent loose stools followed by constipation. In rare cases, infected diverticula rupture, spill their contents into surrounding tissue, and cause peritonitis (infection of the abdominal lining). Medical evaluation is required for diagnosis and should be immediately obtained if symptoms include bloody diarrhea, fever, or nausea and vomiting.

Diverticulosis may be hereditary and appears to be related to aging, as colon walls thicken to increase internal pressure and escalate the incidence of diverticula. Diverticulitis, however, is not an inescapable adjunct of growing older. Dietary adjustments lower the chance of developing diverticulosis and help prevent existing diverticula from becoming infected.[147]

Diet

Fiber is the key to bowel health. Diverticular disease is rare in fiber-eating third-world nations. It became prevalent in the United States only

148

after the advent of processed, low-fiber foods and was worsened by the low-residue diet prescribed prior to 1970. Now the preferred treatment calls for gradually building up daily fiber intake to between 30 and 45 grams. High-fiber foods include barley, brown rice, fruits and vegetables, legumes, and whole-grain cereals and breads. Insoluble fiber from wheat bran or corn bran, and the skins of fruits and root vegetables, is the most effective.

As explained in the *Berkeley Wellness Letter* (April 1992), current dietary guidelines provide approximately 20 grams of fiber. Supplementing them with wheat bran can make an important difference. Studies show that 90 percent of patients hospitalized with diverticular disease experience marked relief of symptoms when 2 or 3 teaspoons of wheat bran are included with each of three fiber-rich meals every day.[147] According to a report in the *Johns Hopkins Medical Letter* (September 1991), ninety out of one-hundred patients in another study remained symptom-free on this regimen for 5 to 7 years after leaving the hospital. Clinical tests also show that members of the cabbage family (broccoli, brussels sprouts, and cauliflower, as well as cabbage and sauerkraut) have colon-healing capabilities,[58] but allergenic sensitivities may preclude their use by everyone. High-fiber popcorn, seeds, nuts, and foods containing them should be thoroughly masticated because fragments might lodge in diverticula and instigate inflammation. Individuals with chronic diverticulitis may need to avoid fatty, sugary, and highly spiced foods as well as seeds and nuts. While recovering from diverticular attacks, eating baby food or transforming roughage into "softage" by pureeing fruits, vegetables, and cooked cereals in an electric blender may relieve discomfort and encourage healing.

Fiber absorbs moisture to produce soft, bulky stools that reduce the work of colonic muscles when eliminating waste; minimizes bowel thickening; and prevents the constipation and straining that forces new hernias to balloon out into the abdomen and fills existing diverticula with fecal material. If constipation does occur, natural remedies (see "Constipation") are preferable to laxatives or enemas, which can further irritate the bowel.[293, 300]

Ample fluid intake (at least eight glasses per day) assists fiber's performance and prevents dehydration of intestinal material and hard-to-pass stools. Nutritionists advise a glass of fresh cabbage or carrot juice daily. Herbalists suggest teas of camomile, red clover, slippery elm, or yarrow. The caffeine in coffee, pekoe tea, chocolate, and some soft drinks tends to irritate the intestines, but one alcoholic drink a day relaxes the colon and may improve diverticular difficulties.[293]

Supplements (see note on page xii)

Taking acidophilus capsules with each meal aids the growth of friendly flora to destroy putrefactive bacteria in the intestines. Three alfalfa tablets a day provide vitamin K for healing; two odorless garlic capsules at mealtime are recommended for their antibiotic effect. Glucomannan supplements, taken before meals, may help prevent accumulations in colonic pouches. Glucomannan is a water-soluble fiber derived from the root of the Japanese Konjac plant. It is available in health food stores. Naturopathic physicians recommend a daily multivitamin-mineral plus optional supplements.

Vitamin A In the form of beta carotene, 25,000 IU daily to protect and heal the lining of the colon.

B Complex One comprehensive tablet daily to reinforce beneficial intestinal bacteria.

Vitamin C with Bioflavonoids 3,000 to 8,000 milligrams in divided daily doses to strengthen the collagen lining of the colon and reduce inflammation.

Vitamin E 100 to 800 IU daily beginning with the lower amount and increasing the dosage 100 IUs per week to protect the membranes lining the colon.

Exercise

Moderate exercise, such as daily walks, aids bowel regularity and is beneficial both for prevention and treatment of diverticular disease. Bent-knee sit-ups and stretching exercises help tone abdominal muscles so there is less strain during bowel movements.

Nerve Pressure and Massage

○ Once each day, press or massage just in front of each ear at the end of the cheekbone.

○ Beginning in the center of the lower third of the palm of each hand, press and massage the area in a clockwise spiral. Use the same movement to massage the soles of both feet from the edge of the heel pad to the ball of the foot.

○ Press or massage each shinbone below the knee, then just below the outside anklebone on each foot.

Sources (see Bibliography)

6, 17, 42, 44, 47, 56, 58, 75, 87, 98, 101, 111, 112, 147, 150, 151, 164, 176, 177, 186, 189, 201, 234, 244, 249, 255, 281, 293, 300, 305

Dizziness and Vertigo

Also described as lightheadedness, faintness, unsteadiness, or loss of balance, dizziness is a common complaint. Healthy people may experience lightheadedness from fatigue; food deprivation; grief; over-the-counter antihistamines, painkillers, or sleeping pills; excessive smoking; or overindulgence in alcohol. Allergy or fluid retention can cause dizziness due to pressure from swollen blood vessels near the ear. Diabetics and hypoglycemics suffer lightheadedness from insulin imbalance. Postural hypotension (momentary dizziness after suddenly getting up from a sitting or lying position) is due to a lapse in the delivery of blood to the brain. Carbon monoxide from traffic fumes can instigate dizzy spells by inhibiting the oxygen-carrying capacity of the blood. Dade P. barely escaped disaster the day he rode his bicycle to work. Pale-faced and disoriented, he staggered into the office after pedaling 5 miles on busy streets. An hour's respite in uncontaminated air restored Dade's equilibrium, and he restricted future biking to little-used country roads. Leah T. had an expensive encounter with carbon monoxide when she waited beside her car while it was being repaired and tested. Attributing her wooziness to weariness, Leah pulled out into the street and demolished her radiator along with a detour sign she was too befuddled to notice.

Vertigo is defined as the illusion of movement, either of self or of the surroundings, when there is no actual motion. The spinning sensation usually results from disturbance of the balance-controlling chambers (labyrinth) in the inner ear. Positional vertigo, generally lasting less than a minute, is one of the most common forms. It can be triggered by tilting the head to look up, or by abruptly turning over in bed. A frequent cause of longer-lasting vertigo is labyrinthitis (the medical term for inflammation of the inner ear), which is instigated by a viral infection like the flu or mumps and normally clears up as the illness subsides. Alcohol or drugs such as antihypertensives, aspirin, opiates, oral contraceptives, and quinine may set off vertigo through a toxic effect on the labyrinth. Chronic or recurrent conditions can result from abnormal glucose metabolism, anemia, hard earwax touching the eardrum, high cholesterol levels, or high or low blood pressure. Vertigo often produces sweating and nausea and may be accompanied by dizziness, faintness, or ringing in the ears (see "Ménière's Disease" and "Tinnitus").

Avoiding abrupt moves may preclude postural dizziness or positional vertigo. Fainting may be forestalled by sitting down and leaning forward with head between the knees to rush a supply of blood to the brain. Severe or recurrent dizziness or vertigo warrants medical evaluation and treatment to determine and correct the underlying cause. Occasional episodes may be combated by staring at a stationary object (like a picture on the wall) to steady a whirling world, or by lying quietly with eyes closed and taking a nonprescription motion sickness tablet.[148]

Diet

Clinical studies show that many cases of dizziness can be corrected with a calorie-reduced diet low in sugar and fat.[147, 186] Low-protein diets are sometimes responsible for dizziness due to abnormal heart rhythm (arrhythmia) that halts blood flow to the brain for a few seconds.[29] Although drinking a glass of orange juice may overcome a brief bout of lightheadedness, snacking on sweets and refined carbohydrates can cause dizziness when blood sugar plunges following the temporary surge of energy.

Supplements (see note on page xii)

A daily multiple, containing minerals as well as vitamins, may be beneficial—shortages, particularly of manganese or potassium, can cause dizziness and vertigo.[28, 256] Attacks of vertigo following antibiotic treatment may be reduced by taking acidophilus capsules with each meal (or eating acidophilus yogurt every day) to help restore the body's manufacture of B vitamins.

B Complex One comprehensive, high-potency tablet daily, plus an optional 50 to 100 milligrams of niacin with each meal. Deficiencies of any B vitamin may instigate dizziness or vertigo; niacin (or niacinamide) has reduced some cases of vertigo without adverse side effects.

Vitamin C   1,500 to 4,500 milligrams in divided daily doses to help improve circulation and for its antioxidant properties.

Calcium and Magnesium   800 to 1,500 milligrams plus 500 to 750 milligrams of magnesium (some researchers recommend 600 to 1,200 milligrams of calcium plus 1,200 to 2,400 milligrams of magnesium) in divided daily doses to improve circulation and help regulate heartbeat.

Vitamin E   400 to 800 IU daily to improve circulation and help neutralize the harmful effects from traffic fumes and other environmental pollutants.

Lecithin   Two capsules with each meal. Lecithin contains the choline and inositol essential for effective nerve function, and for some patients with high blood pressure, it has eliminated chronic dizziness in a few weeks.[86, 87]

Tissue Salts   Two of these 6X-potency tissue salts may be taken every 2 hours during acute episodes, then once daily for a few days after the condition is alleviated. Kali. Phos. for postural hypotension or positional vertigo; Mag. Phos. if dark spots float in front of the eyes; Nat. Phos. for nausea, alternated with Nat. Sulph. if the dizziness or vertigo is accompanied by a bitter taste in the mouth.

Exercise

According to a report in *Longevity* (March 1991), high-impact aerobics can damage the inner ear and lead to dizziness or vertigo. After the worst of an attack is over, however, low-impact aerobics like walking actually hasten the departure of the discomfort.[186] As explained in the June 1991 issue of *Health After 50*, practicing balance-restoring, antidizziness exercises while problem-free may allow the body to develop compensatory measures that will help prevent future attacks.

- ○ Look up and down, then from side to side twenty times each.
- ○ While sitting, turn shoulders to the left and to the right ten times each, then lean forward to touch the floor twenty times.
- ○ While standing, bend forward and backward twenty times with eyes open, then repeat with the eyes closed.

○ Walk across a room five times with eyes open, then repeat with the eyes closed.

Folk Remedies

An old remedy for persistent dizziness was to cook crabapples until mushy, then eat a teaspoonful each hour. A cup daily of ginger tea (1 teaspoon ground ginger in hot water) or strong catnip tea is said to clear chronic dizziness or vertigo. Other suggested herbs are camomile, cayenne, dandelion, ginkgo biloba, peppermint, spearmint and wood betony.

Nerve Pressure and Massage

For Dizziness or Vertigo   Pinch the area between the eyebrows. Or massage both thumbs (or big toes) with a squeezing, rolling motion. Or press and massage the palm of each hand just below the fingers with a back and forth motion. Or press and massage the top of each foot 2 inches toward the arch from the web between the big toe and the second toe.

To Stop a Fainting Spell   Press hard between the nose and the upper lip. Or press and massage the center of the palm of each hand. Or press the fingernails into the pads of both thumbs.

Sources (see Bibliography)

6, 17, 28, 29, 51, 58, 63, 65, 75, 86, 87, 98, 109, 111, 147, 148, 151, 159, 186, 207, 244, 254, 256, 281, 283, 294, 313

Dry Skin

Whether instigated by environmental irritation, an inherited inability to retain moisture in the skin, or the slowing cellular processes due to aging, the basic cause of dry skin is insufficient water, not lack of oil. Moist, dewy-fresh skin is a byproduct of the body's internal cooling system, which sends water up through the lower layers of skin to evaporate from the surface. When the external humidity drops below 30 percent, evaporation exceeds natural replenishment. Room humidifiers and houseplants help offset the harm from dry indoor heating or refrigeration. Applying a sunscreen before winter as well as summer outings slows evaporation and guards against the drying effect of ultraviolet light. Drinking six to eight glasses of water each day prevents physical dehydration, but imbibing excessive amounts cannot correct dry skin.[293] Rehydration is best accomplished by saturating the epidermis with water and sealing its surface to reduce evaporation.

Bathing

Showering or soaking in comfortably warm water for 5 to 15 minutes permits penetration into the deepest layers of the skin. Lengthy immersion, however, increases dehydration by leaching out moisture. Hot water, excessive sweating, and steam baths float away the skin's moisturizing factor. For those with extremely dry skin, experts advise alternate-day bathing, particularly during winter-itch months, when dry, cold air and frigid winds intensify the problem. Mineral oil or vegetable oil may be smoothed over dry areas before showering. Soothing moisturizing agents can be swirled in a tub: bath oil or castor oil (which emulsifies in water), commercial colloidal oatmeal (ground oatmeal, lanolin, mineral oil), 3 cups of whole milk (Cleopatra bathed in camel's milk), 1 cup of apple cider vinegar, or 1 tablespoon of glycerin or honey—with or without 2 tablespoons of bee pollen grains. Dryness-promoting bath salts or bubble baths are not recommended.

Cleansing

Soaps are moisture robbers. They strip off natural oils, contain caustic alkali, and, according to a report in *Longevity* (January 1992), may eventually cause microscopic cracks that allow moisture to escape through the skin's topmost layer. Superfatted soaps are less irritating than pure soap or detergent/deodorant bars. Many dermatologists recommend soap-free cleansing lotions or bars and suggest that parched faces be thoroughly cleansed only at night, then freshened with a cool-water rinse in the morning.

For nondrying makeup removal, wipe with cotton balls or pads dunked in vegetable oil or whole milk plus a few drops of castor oil, or smooth on white vegetable shortening or egg mayonnaise and remove with facial tissue or a damp cloth. Oatmeal (regular, quick-cooking, or colloidal) or rice bran can be tied in a soft cloth and swished in water for a bath scrubber or facial cleaner. "Washing" with heavy cream or plain yogurt is an old-fashioned substitute for soap. More complex washing liquids of ⅓ cup whole milk whirred in a blender with one quarter of a peeled avocado or cucumber can be stored in the refrigerator for several days. Incorporating a teaspoon of bee pollen grains with any cleanser is believed to nourish and moisturize skin cells.[302] All cleansers should be rinsed off with lukewarm water.

Toning

Astringents are never advocated for dry skin; alcohol-free aftershave lotions are available for men. Toners—originally designed to remove any alkalizing soap residue—are optional. For those who enjoy an after cleansing swish of freshener, suggested liquids are rose water plus ½ teaspoon glycerin per cup; witch hazel diluted with an equal amount of distilled water; or the blended and strained mixture of a peeled cucumber, ¼ cup water, and ½ teaspoon olive oil.

Moisturizing

Moisture preserving rather than moisture providing, moisturizers are most effective when smoothed over skin that is still damp from bathing or cleansing. Misting with a half-and-half mixture of aloe vera gel and water (or with plain water) before applying a facial moisturizer boosts hydration. Holding a warm, moist washcloth over the face for 3 minutes after moisturizing increases penetration.

Air-excluding emollients (fat-containing substances) lubricate the skin while sealing in the recently acquired water. Humecants (moistening ingredients such as glycerin) attract water to the skin's surface. Simple, inexpensive emollients are considered as beneficial as their costly cosmetic counterparts. Petroleum jelly is one of the best and most widely used moisturizers.[184] Mildred E., an octogenarian with only enough expression lines to give her face character, has never experimented with exotics. When asked for the secret of her baby-soft skin, Mildred answers, "There isn't any. If I'm wearing makeup, I remove it with petroleum jelly. Then I just wash with soap and water, swipe on a little rose water, and use more petroleum jelly as a moisturizer and night cream."

Mineral oil, olive oil or any vegetable oil, egg-rich mayonnaise, and kitchen-concocted blends are also excellent dry-skin moisturizers. For a super-rich moisturizer, mix 3 tablespoons *each* canola, olive, and safflower oil with 1 tablespoon almond oil and 1 teaspoon glycerin. Louisa L., an efficiency expert who combines dishwashing with an arthritis-easing treatment, has an equally time-saving system for pampering her sensitive skin and defeating the dry flakies. After her nightly bath, she wraps up in a gigantic beach towel to blot excess water; smooths aloe vera gel over her face, arms, legs, feet, and hands; then lightly coats her face and throat with the moisturizer she makes once a month: 3 tablespoons *each* honey and wheat germ oil blended with 2 tablespoons *each* glycerin and witch hazel, and 1 tablespoon rose water.

Moisturizing Masks

To deep-moisturize desert-dry skin after cleansing, pat any of these masks over the throat and face (except for the eye area) and wait 10 or 15 minutes before rinsing off.

○ Ripe avocado, mashed and applied as is or mixed with an egg yolk, or with equal amounts of ripe banana or sour cream.

○ Egg yolk, plain, or whisked with 1 tablespoon honey and 1 teaspoon vegetable oil or with 1 teaspoon *each* glycerin and bee pollen grains.

○ Heavy cream, or 1 tablespoon *each* light cream and honey, or a half-and-half blend of honey and mashed banana, or ½ cup cocoa powder mixed with 1 tablespoon olive oil and enough heavy cream to make a soft paste.

Diet and Supplements (see note on page xii)

A nutritious diet emphasizing fruits, vegetables, and whole grains is important for healthy, moist skin. Severely restricted low-salt or low-fat diets sometimes cause dry skin. Using kelp as a salt substitute compensates for the iodine lost by avoiding iodized salt; taking a primrose oil capsule with meals provides essential fatty acids. Many skin-care experts suggest a daily multivitamin-mineral plus optional individual supplements.

Vitamin A In the form of beta carotene, 25,000 IU daily to increase cell renewal rate.

B Complex One comprehensive tablet daily. Deficiencies of B_1, B_2, biotin, or pantothenic acid can instigate dry, flaky skin and scaliness around the nose and mouth.[98, 151]

Vitamin C 500 to 5,000 milligrams in divided daily doses. Essential for production of the skin's natural oil coating, the body's supply of vitamin C is depleted by factors such as oral contraceptives, smoking, and stress.[276]

Zinc 15 to 50 milligrams daily—a deficiency can cause rough, dry, scaly skin.[40]

Sources (see Bibliography)

16, 17, 29, 40, 46, 47, 49, 50, 53, 74, 98, 99, 108, 109, 111, 112, 150, 151, 177, 184, 276, 293, 300, 302, 312, 313

Earache (Otitis Media)

Although a painful ear may be caused by impacted earwax or water in the ear (see "Ear Problems"), otitis media (inflammation of the middle ear) usually results from fluid buildup or obstruction of the Eustachian tube connecting the middle ear with the back of the nose and throat. Allergies may be responsible for abnormal production of fluid, or germ-laden mucus may enter the Eustachian tube during upper-respiratory disorders and be forced into the middle ear by sneezing or vigorous nose blowing. Children are especially susceptible to earache—approximately half of them develop otitis media before the age of 5.[244] Supine bottle feeding may clog an infant's Eustachian tube, or pressure from enlarged adenoids may prevent normal drainage. Children or adults with recurrent ear infections may benefit from moisturizing dry indoor air with a humidifier and taking an over-the-counter nasal decongestant before bed each night to dry up excess ear fluid. When an earache strikes, applying heat, keeping the head upright, chewing gum, or sipping liquids helps clear the Eustachian tube and relieve pain. Medical help should be obtained if the earache persists or is accompanied by a reddish discharge or a temperature over 102 degrees.

Diet and Supplements (see note on page xii)

Food allergies often instigate children's ear infections by promoting mucus production and swelling in the Eustachian tubes. A study of over 100 youngsters with chronic otitis media revealed that 78 percent were sensitive to foods such as corn, milk, peanuts, and wheat. By eliminating the allergens from their diets, 86 percent of those who were allergic were cleared of ear problems (*Pediatric News* 25, no. 2, 1991). If antibiotics are prescribed for an infected ear, eating acidophilus yogurt daily (or taking acidophilus capsules with each meal) during the treatment may forestall a recurrence by replenishing the body's beneficial bacteria.

During an ear infection, nutritionists suggest the following supplements to help speed healing. Dosages should be reduced for children and given only with a physician's approval.

Vitamin A   In the form of beta carotene, 50,000 IU daily.

B Complex   One comprehensive 50-milligram tablet three times a day.

Vitamin C   1,500 to 5,000 milligrams daily in divided doses.

Vitamin E   400 to 600 IU daily.

Zinc   One 10-milligram lozenge three times a day for 5 days.

Tissue Salts   Three 12X-potency tablets can be taken each hour for several hours: Ferr. Phos. for throbbing pain after exposure to cold or wet; to relieve a congested Eustachian tube, alternate with Kali. Mur. Take Nat. Mur. if the ache is accompanied by a roaring sound in the ear; substitute Nat. Sulph. if there is ringing in the ear; use Kali. Phos. for an elderly person if there is dullness of hearing with a humming sound in the ear.

Folk Remedies

For pain relief, herbalists suggest sipping meadowsweet or willow bark tea, combined if desired. Both teas contain aspirinlike compounds so should not be given to children because of the risk of Reye's syndrome, a neurological disease. For a nasal spray believed to relieve earache, mix 1 teaspoon *each* glycerin and salt in a pint of warm water. Several times a day, spray each nostril until the liquid begins to drip into the back of the throat, then spray the throat.

Drops   (Fluids should not be dropped in the ear if there is a possibility that the eardrum is ruptured.) A few drops of warm castor oil, garlic oil, or olive oil can be placed in the ear. The contents of a garlic oil capsule, garlic powder, or garlic or onion juice may be added to the olive oil (combining olive oil with the contents of a vitamin E capsule and a garlic perle is said to have an antibiotic effect);[150] or the juice from freshly grated ginger can be mixed half-and-half with sesame oil. To increase effectiveness, a drop of lobelia tincture can be added after any of the oils. Liquid squeezed from roasted cabbage stalks, a few drops of warm honey blended with bee pollen granules, or warmed vodka, are other options.

Cotton Dip a small cotton ball in a half-and-half mixture of glycerin and witch hazel, insert it in the ear and plug with a fluff of cotton.

Heat A hair dryer set on warm and held 18 inches away from the ear is a healthful replacement for the old remedy of blowing mouthfuls of tobacco smoke into an aching ear. A heating pad or a foam cup containing a paper towel soaked in hot water, then squeezed out and held over the ear are other modern methods of providing warmth. Earlier ear warmers include table salt heated in a skillet, wrapped in cloth, and placed between the ear and a pillow; poultices of hot camomile or slippery elm tea held over the ear with dry cloth; or, for severe pain, a paste of dry mustard, flour, and water or egg white spread on gauze and placed behind the ear—soaking the feet at the same time in a pan of hot water with a tablespoon of dry mustard is said to increase the benefit. Hot, roasted onion is another old favorite for "drawing out" pain. Tie onion slices over the ear or make an onion earmuff by cutting a large onion in half, scooping out the center, and heating the shell in the oven.

Nerve Pressure and Massage

◯ Pull at the earlobe for 10 seconds, then gently massage around the outside of the ear, including hinge of the jawbone in front and the mastoid bone behind the ear.

◯ Roll a narrow strip of gauze into a tight cylinder, place it in back of the last tooth on the side of the aching ear, and bite down on it for 5 minutes. Repeat every 2 hours until the pain is relieved.

◯ On the same side as the aching ear, exert firm pressure on the tip of the fourth finger for 5 minutes. Or massage the little toe, the one next to it, and the sole of the foot directly beneath them.

Sources (see Bibliography)

2, 6, 17, 26, 41, 57, 59, 60, 64, 65, 75, 85, 92, 98, 112, 135, 148, 150, 164, 168, 186, 195, 203, 213, 244, 264, 281, 284, 293, 302, 312, 313, 317

Ear Problems

Whether the problem arises from excess earwax, a visiting insect, pressure from altitude alterations, or discomfort from trapped moisture, the old rule regarding treatment still applies: Nothing smaller than an elbow should be pushed past the entrance to the ear canal. Even a cotton-tipped swab can harm delicate tissues or force hardened earwax against the fragile eardrum.

Earwax

Medically termed cerumen, earwax is secreted by glands in the outer ear to cleanse and moisturize the lining of the external canal and to protect the inner ear by serving as a barrier against germs, moisture, dust, and other debris. If there is a deficiency of the wax (indicated by dryness and itching), a cottonball dipped in almond oil can be inserted in the outer ear canal. Itchy ears may be relieved by inserting a few drops of apple cider vinegar and waiting 30 seconds before tilting the head to let the liquid drip out.

Normal secretion of cerumen is encouraged by jaw movement during eating, talking, and yawning. These same motions usually cause wax to work itself out of the ear after it becomes laden with impurities. Then the waxy flakes either fall out during sleep or may be wiped out of the outer ear with a washcloth. If surplus cerumen accumulates, it can harden into plugs near the eardrum to cause a feeling of fullness or ringing in the ears (see "Tinnitus") as well as muted hearing. If allowed to remain, pollutants can build up in the wax and increase susceptibility to bacterial or fungal infection. People who do not have a perforated eardrum may be able to remove excess earwax with this two-step remedy: (1) For soft earwax, twice daily for 2 or 3 days put a few drops of hydrogen peroxide in the affected ear. To soften hardened earwax: substitute drops of almond oil, olive oil, or sesame oil, and plug the ear with cotton. (2) To flush wax out of the ear, gently squirt warm water (folk healers recommend using a weak saltwater solution) into the ear with an ear syringe. Tilt the ear down to allow liquid and wax to drain out, then insert a few drops of rubbing alcohol to absorb any remaining water and sterilize the ear canal. For tightly packed wax plugs, the procedure may need to be repeated several times, or professional treatment may be required.

Insects

First-Aid Tip An intruding insect may be enticed into exiting by tilting the ear toward the sun or toward a flashlight in a dark room. A ripe apple or peach held close to the ear may appeal to a bug that is not attracted by light. If the intruder is leery of leaving or is entrapped in earwax, a teaspoon of warm vegetable oil poured into the occupied ear and held there for a few moments may immobilize and/or free the unwanted visitor so that it flows out with the oil when the ear is tilted downward—pulling the ear backward and upward straightens the canal to ease the passage. If the bug refuses to budge, pouring warm water into the ear (with the ear tilted up) may float it out. If not, medical assistance should be obtained to perform the eviction.

Pressure Problems

Normally, the Eustachian tubes connecting the back of the throat to the middle ear equalize pressure between the ear and the external environment. Not designed for the rapid changes encountered during air travel, high-altitude motoring, or scuba diving, these passageways can experience a vacuum effect that produces echolike hearing and an uncomfortable feeling of fullness in the ears. Chewing gum, moving the jaw from side to side, sipping liquids, staying awake and sitting upright during descent, sucking on mints, or yawning assists the muscles controlling the Eustachian tubes. Allergies, colds, or upper-respiratory ailments can impede Eustachian tube function by swelling the mucous membranes. Individuals suffering from any of those disorders may benefit by taking a time-release decongestant prior to anticipated altitude changes or by using a nasal decongestant spray when the cabin pressure increases during airplane descent.

"Popping" the ears relieves pressure distress by opening the Eustachian tubes. The ear-popping Valsalva maneuver calls for pinching the nostrils shut, taking a mouthful of air, closing the mouth, and either puffing out the cheeks or using cheek and throat muscles to force air up into the back of the nose. Small children may be able to help themselves by blowing up a balloon or two; babies can be given a bottle of formula or water to encourage frequent swallowing to help keep the pressure-equalizing passages open.

Swimmer's Ear

A bacterial or fungal infection of the outer ear canal, swimmer's ear (otitis externa) can result from watery contacts other than swimming. Shampooing, showering, or profuse sweating can leave water in the ear canal to become a breeding medium for microorganisms. According to a report in the October 1991 issue of *Prevention,* water can also make earwax swell and plug the ears. People who wear hearing aids are advised to remove them occasionally to permit the evaporation of accumulated moisture.

Wet ears can be dried with the corner of a towel or with a hair dryer set on low and held 18 inches away from the ear. If water enters the ear canal, inserting a few drops of rubbing alcohol or a half-and-half mixture of alcohol and white vinegar will make the water evaporate and, at the same time, destroy infectious agents and restore the acid balance of the skin to prevent itchy ears.

When the discomfort of swimmer's ear develops, experts estimate that 80 percent of the cases can be cured by using the alcohol-vinegar drops three times a day.[300] Medical help should be sought if the drops instigate burning or sharp pain, if symptoms persist for more than a few days, if the disorder is accompanied by fever, or if there is discharge from the ear. People prone to ear infections may need to insert a few drops of jojoba oil or mineral oil, or wear earplugs (or cottonballs coated with petroleum jelly and gently tucked into the outer ears) while showering, shampooing, or swimming.

Sources (see Bibliography)

17, 29, 49, 75, 92, 98, 108, 111, 112, 135, 148, 150, 186, 202, 244, 255, 264, 281, 293, 294, 300, 312, 313

Fatigue

The daily weariness affecting millions of Americans is usually due to everyday energy sappers—lack of exercise, lack of rest, poor nutrition, stress—and can be alleviated with home remedies. Constant fatigue that persists for months (especially if accompanied by enlarged lymph glands, fever, joint pain, sore throat, or unusual thirst) warrants medical evaluation. It could signify an undetected illness such as anemia, chronic fatigue syndrome (CFS—once derided as psychosomatic "yuppie flu," now considered a bona fide disorder), diabetes, Epstein-Barr virus, hypoglycemia, hypothyroidism, mononucleosis, or systemic yeast infection (candidiasis).

Adequate sleep (6 to 8 hours is average) is essential, but sleeping too much can cause mental and physical lethargy. Alcohol is an energy depressant unless limited to one or two drinks imbibed with food.[177, 293] Although nicotine is a mild stimulant, smoking is an energy robber because it limits the amount of oxygen the blood can process. Shallow breathing, which utilizes only the upper portion of the lungs, is another potential cause of chronic fatigue. Taking a few deep breaths each hour promotes oxygenation of the blood and has a revitalizing effect.[321] Losing excess weight at the rate of no more than 2 pounds per week may reverse an energy drain for obese people. Getting out into daylight and opening the drapes while indoors helps prevent SAD (seasonal affective disorder), which, as explained in the January 1992 *Berkeley Wellness Letter,* can be responsible for lethargy and depression from lack of winter sunshine.

Diet

Complex carbohydrates from fruits, vegetables, and whole grains are the most efficient energy producers. Grapes, garlic, and onions were ancient remedies for tiredness. Low-fat protein foods stimulate the production of mentally energizing chemicals. Simple carbohydrates from sweets and white- flour products provide a brief spurt of energy then trigger weariness from lowered blood sugar levels and release of serotonin, a soothing chemical. Fats or excessively large meals can create lethargy by slowing digestion. Many people find that reserving refined carbohydrates and desserts for the last meal in the evening and eating six high-protein, complex-carbohydrate snack-meals throughout the day keeps energy levels at their peak. Skipping breakfast or other meals can lead to chronic fatigue. So can crash diets, which not only force the body to burn its reserves but also slow the metabolic rate and cause the body to function poorly.[51, 186]

Iron deficiency, even without anemia, is a common cause of chronic fatigue. Iron is most easily absorbed from meats, and as reported in *Harvard Health Letter* (March 1991), adding small amounts of meat to an otherwise meatless meal nearly doubles the absorption of iron from other sources such as corn, dark leafy greens, dried fruits, egg yolks, legumes, and whole wheat. Cooking in cast-iron pans and consuming vitamin C-rich foods also increases iron assimilation. Iron or potassium supplementation, other than that provided by a daily multiple, is advised only under medical supervision. Potassium-rich foods include apricots, bananas, dried fruits, and fresh vegetables.

Beverages offer energy-boosting options. A cup of coffee may dispel morning doldrums, but no more than two caffeine-containing drinks per day are recommended. Fresh fruit and vegetable juices are natural energizers that can be "fortified" into energy elixirs. Suggested combinations include a glass of orange or grapefruit juice whirred with 1 teaspoon brewer's yeast and ½ teaspoon *each* wheat germ and bran (incorporating 2 tablespoons of instant nonfat dry milk adds protein plus calcium); tomato juice stirred with 1 or 2 tablespoons of brewer's yeast; ½ cup each grape juice and orange juice (or a half-and-half mixture of carrot and pineapple juice) blended with a teaspoon of bee pollen or 1 teaspoon *each* brewer's yeast and lecithin granules; or ⅓ cup *each* cabbage, carrot, and celery juice blended with 2 tablespoons of wheat germ.

Nora J. had been enjoying the energy lift she got from the brewer's yeast and milk she drank for breakfast to control the osteoarthritis in her fingers. When the demands of her new job left her tired by midmorning, Nora resolved her energy crisis by transforming her usual mixture into an all-day energizer. Each morning, she blended 2 cups of skim milk, ⅓ cup instant nonfat dry milk, ¼ cup *each* brewer's yeast and protein powder, 1 tablespoon lecithin granules, and a piece of fruit or a few tablespoons of orange juice concentrate. She drank half a cup with her breakfast and poured the remainder into a thermos to sip every hour or so at work to augment the energy boost provided by breakfast and her lunchtime salad.

Supplements (see note on page xii)

A daily multivitamin-mineral is often advised because mild deficiencies of almost any vitamin or mineral can instigate chronic fatigue. Severe cases may benefit from additional daily supplements.

Vitamin A   In the form of beta carotene, 25,000 IU.

B Complex   One or two comprehensive tablets plus sublingual B12.

Vitamin C with Bioflavonoids   3,000 to 8,000 milligrams in divided doses.

Minerals   Essential for the production of energy, up to 1,500 milligrams of calcium and 750 milligrams of magnesium per day are recommended by some nutritionists.[17] Some experts recommend reversing the proportions of calcium and magnesium. A sluggish thyroid may be stimulated by the iodine in a glass weekly of tomato-celery juice containing ¼ teaspoon of kelp granules.[305] The lethargy produced by a mild zinc shortage may be corrected by taking up to 50 milligrams daily.[256]

Exercise

Although overexercising or working out strenuously every day can create chronic fatigue, sedentary lifestyles and prolonged physical inactivity are more common causes of weariness. Aerobic fitness regimens call for 30-minute walks or workouts three times a week. As explained in *Men's Health* (December 1991), however, energy levels rise with an increase of ordinary muscle movements—parking a block away from the store, standing up and moving around while talking on the telephone or watching the news on television, and taking brief "exercise breaks" several times a day. According to a report in the January 1992 *Annals of Internal Medicine,* a brisk 10-minute walk not only boosts energy more effectively than eating a candy bar, but the benefits last an hour longer. Vigorous exercise such as performing 25 jumping jacks, running-in-place for 2 minutes, or trotting up and down a flight or two of stairs provides a quick pick-me-up by nearly doubling the body's intake of oxygen and speeding it through the veins and by converting blood fats into blood sugar for energy.[177]

Folk Remedies

"Tired blood" is not a modern misfortune—it was described by Egyptian physicians in 1500 B.C.—and some ancient remedies for fatigue are being vindicated by scientific studies. Brazil nuts, chia seeds (eaten by Native Americans for round-the-clock stamina), soybeans, sunflower seeds, and tomato seeds have been found to contain similar amino acids and energy-producing proteins.[151, 313] *Longevity* (January 1991) reports that tests with over 3,000 patients indicate that energy is increased by sleeping with a magnet (four times stronger than those used to hold memos on the refrigerator) attached to the head, then being exposed to bright light for half an hour after awakening.

Bee Pollen Taking up to 2 teaspoons of bee pollen granules (or 750 milligrams in tablets) in divided doses daily is believed to increase physical and mental energy.[150]

Herbs Taken in capsules or sipped as teas, effective herbs include alfalfa, bayberry, black cohosh (the principal component of Lydia Pinkham's famous compound), blessed thistle, cayenne, dandelion, fennel, ginger, ginkgo biloba, ginseng, gotu kola, guarana, licorice root, red clover, and yellow dock.

Showers and Baths Cascading from a shower, water emits energizing negative ions. Alternating 2 minutes of hot with 30 seconds of cold is effective for some people. Others prefer a cool shower or tepid tub soak. Herbalists suggest looping a cheesecloth-encased bag of herbs over the shower spray or steeping ½ cup of herbs for 20 minutes and pouring the strained liquid into the bath water to increase the benefits. If desired, the solids can be tied in cheesecloth to use as a bath scrubber. Suggested mixtures include equal parts of alfalfa, comfrey, orange peel, and parsley; or of basil, bay leaves, and fennel; or of juniper, rose geranium, and rosemary.

Nerve Pressure and Massage

One ancient theory holds that tiredness "collects" on the inside of the elbows and the back of the knees and that slapping these areas will reenergize the body. Acupressurists and reflexologists offer other options.

○ Stand up straight and rock from toes to heels a dozen times, inhaling and lifting the arms straight up while rising on the balls of the feet, exhaling and extending the arms straight down while rocking back on the heels.

○ Rub and squeeze the earlobes and the ridges of the ears.

○ For 15 seconds each, press or massage the following points: the center top of the head, the pit of the stomach, and 1½ inches toward the elbow from the wrist on the inside of each forearm.

○ Press and massage completely around the tip of each thumb and the inside of the hands across the fleshy mounds at the base of the last three fingers, the palm of the right hand below the last two fingers, and the palms of both hands at the top of the thumb pad below the index finger. For added benefit, the corresponding areas on the feet may be pressed and massaged in a similar manner.

Stress Management

Studies have found that people who are anxious or depressed are seven times more likely to suffer from chronic fatigue than those without these emotional problems and that an accumulation of unrelieved minor stresses can be as debilitating as a major upheaval.[105, 293] New interests and challenges can unleash energy; deep breathing and physical exercise both relax tension and revitalize. Practicing relaxation techniques (see Introduction) combined with positive mental visualization of increased vitality often combats the fatiguing buildup of daily stresses.

Sources (see Bibliography)

17, 19, 26, 46, 48, 49, 51, 53, 75, 86, 98, 105, 108, 109, 150, 151, 164, 176, 177, 186, 201, 204, 205, 244, 255, 256, 265, 281, 293, 294, 295, 304, 305, 312, 313, 319, 321

Fingernail Problems

Fingernail changes or abnormalities are often the result of nutritional deficiencies but can be caused by injuries, illness, or external mistreatment. Composed almost entirely of hardened protein (keratin) and sulfur, nails derive optimum nourishment from a balanced diet with adequate protein, vitamins, and minerals. Insufficient iron may be responsible for lengthwise ridging; weak, pale, thin, flat, or spoon-shaped nails; or nails that break, chip, crack, or peel easily. Dietary iron is better assimilated from meat, poultry, fish, and eggs (which are also complete proteins and rich in sulfur) than from plant sources such as dried fruits, leafy greens, legumes, and nuts, which, along with gelatin, are incomplete proteins. Brussels sprouts, cabbage, dried beans, garlic, and onions supply dietary sulfur. Medical approval is advised before taking iron supplements other than the amount provided by a daily multimineral (see note on page xii).

To strengthen nails, herbalists suggest drinking a cup or two of horsetail or oat straw tea each day and soaking the fingertips in a bit of the brew for 10 minutes. Nightly nail soaks in any warm vegetable oil or nut oil help restore flexibility to brittle nails and help correct problems with soft or splitting nails. Excess oil should be wiped off with a tissue, and the hands should not be washed until the following morning.

Avoiding lengthy immersion in water, and wearing protective gloves when using detergents or household cleansers help prevent the fragility, peeling, splitting, or loosening that can occur as nails dry and shrink after softening and swelling from absorbed liquid. Rubbing petroleum jelly or other moisturizers into the nails and cuticles before and after bathing or swimming helps offset potential harm. Adding a few drops of castor oil to a bottle of nail polish remover and washing with soap and water immediately after using it helps counteract the drying effect on nails and cuticles.

Cuticles protect the nail base from harmful bacteria or fungi. Pushing them back each time hand lotion is applied prevents drying and cracking

171

without the hazards of cutting them or using cuticle removers. Rubbing fresh lemon juice on the cuticles is said to strengthen them. If a hangnail develops, it should be softened with water or lotion before being snipped off with manicure scissors. Coating the area with vitamin E from a pierced capsule speeds healing. Frequent hangnails may indicate that protein, vitamin C, and folic acid are undersupplied. Overexposure to water or paper (which absorbs oil from the skin) are other possible instigators. Faye R. had her first encounter with hangnails when she agreed to proofread and index a friend's manuscript. After 2 days of full-time paper handling, her hands were painfully dry and splits had formed in the cuticles of several nails. Determined to complete the project, Faye took remedial measures. With promptings from a kitchen timer, she washed her hands every hour and alternated applications of aloe vera gel and a vitamin-enriched hand cream. Relief was almost immediate, and by the time the assignment was finished, Faye's cuticles were smooth and pliable.

Brittle, Weak Nails These may be corrected with additional dietary protein and iron, a daily multivitamin-mineral, 25,000 IU of beta carotene, a B-complex tablet, and 800 milligrams of calcium plus 500 milligrams of magnesium (with medical approval, up to 1,600 milligrams of magnesium). Studies show that daily supplementation with 2.5 milligrams of the B vitamin biotin increases nail thickness by at least 25 percent.[49] Taking 1 tablespoon desiccated liver powder or 2 tablespoons of brewer's yeast stirred into tomato juice once a day has restored nail health for some individuals; others have benefited from two capsules daily of evening primrose oil.

Brittle nails that separate in layers may indicate a deficiency of either iron or B vitamins and may benefit from the tissue salt Silicea. Eating sunflower seeds and taking 15 to 50 milligrams of zinc each day has stopped nails from peeling and made them more flexible within 2 or 3 months.[2]

Splitting nails due to a lack of stomach acid may improve when betaine hydrochloride tablets are taken with each meal.[17] Folk healers suggest soaking the nails in diluted apple cider vinegar, eating half a dozen raw almonds every day, and consuming generous amounts of garlic and raw cucumber or cucumber juice. Beauty experts advise filing dry nails from the outside toward the center and beveling the tips to discourage splitting.

Constantly breaking nails that do not improve with home remedies may be an indication of poor circulation or thyroid gland dysfunction requiring medical attention.[300]

Soft, Weak Nails Excessive contact with water or the chemicals in nail cosmetics, or an inadequate diet may be responsible for this problem. Taking 1,000 milligrams of dolomite daily for a month has strengthened frail nails for people with calcium and magnesium deficiencies.[301] Folk remedies include nibbling sunflower seeds, eating an extra carrot every day, and swallowing a teaspoon of apple cider vinegar with each meal. Coating polish-free nails with fresh lemon juice, vinegar, or white iodine are other options. Occasionally, soft nails are a sign of a thyroid disorder.

Horizontal Ridges and Furrows Called Beau's lines, these move upward and grow out with the nail in five or six months. They usually result from an episode of severe illness or stress but may be caused by a chronic B-vitamin deficiency, or by an injury or the pressure of manicure tools at the base of the nail. Recurrent ridging during menstrual cycles may be prevented by consuming adequate protein, vitamin A, and brewer's yeast.

Longitudinal Ridges and Furrows These can be an indication of iron-deficiency anemia, or of insufficient vitamin A, B vitamins, and calcium. In many cases, however, the lengthwise lines are either hereditary or gradually develop after the age of 40 because of slowing cell reproduction.

Pitted Nails Those resulting from deficiencies of protein, calcium, or sulfur can be corrected by upgrading the diet. Pitting may occur in conjunction with psoriasis or alopecia areata (patchy hair loss); or, according to a report in *Modern Medicine* (57, 5:57), pitting or beading may indicate the presence of muscular inflammations or rheumatoid arthritis.

Spoon Nails Nails that are depressed in the center and raised at the edges may be caused by injury to the nail, but these and pale nails most often occur in older children and in middle-aged women because of iron deficiency or anemia. The nails usually return to normalcy when the diet is adequate or the anemia is treated.[75, 300]

White Spots Common in children and teenagers, white spots in fingernails are attributed to everything from telling fibs or acquiring a new sweetheart to minor injuries, pockets of air, and mineral deficiencies. Dr. Carl Pfeiffer[228] and other holistic practitioners recommend daily supplements of calcium (800 milligrams), magnesium (500 milligrams—with medical approval, up to 1,600 milligrams), and zinc (15 to 50 milligrams). A Vermont folk remedy calls for stirring 1 teaspoon *each* apple cider vinegar and honey in a glass of water to accompany each meal.[172]

Fungus Found under and around the fingernails, fungus may be instigated by artificial nails (which can trap moisture, bacteria, and fungi under the nail) or by antibiotic treatment that leads to insufficient "friendly" bacteria in the body.[17, 111] Taking a B-complex tablet plus 15 milligrams of zinc every day and acidophilus capsules with each meal may rectify the problem. Soaking the nails in a strong solution of vitamin C crystals and water twice a day and squeezing vitamin E oil under the nails has hastened improvement in some cases.

Sources (see Bibliography)

2, 13, 17, 42, 45, 49, 50, 53, 64, 65, 75, 82, 86, 87, 98, 111, 162, 172, 186, 226, 228, 254, 255, 256, 262, 276, 281, 293, 300, 301, 304, 312, 313, 317

Flatulence

An average adult generates 2 gallons of flatus (intestinal gas) daily and expels 2 cups of it rectally; the remainder is reabsorbed into the body.[112] Some of this flatus is swallowed air that is not belched up and wends its way to the intestines, but most gas is a byproduct created by colonic bacteria as they ferment foods that have not been digested and absorbed higher up in the digestive tract. Flatulence (abnormal gassiness), sometimes accompanied by abdominal bloating and pain from bubbles of gas trapped in a fold of the colon, is due to excessive amounts of swallowed air or to a larger-than-normal quantity of flatus being produced in the bowel.

One common cause is lactose intolerance (the inability to digest the natural sugar in milk), which can be overcome by taking supplements of the missing enzyme, lactase. Certain foods are known for their gas-engendering tendencies, but individual reactions differ and much depends on the efficiency of the digestive system. Constipation can step up fermentation by slowing the passage of food through the gastrointestinal tract. Overeating can overwhelm digestive enzymes, leaving partially digested food to be turned into gas. Inadequate mastication sends hard-to-digest chunks on to the intestines for fermentation. Chewing with the mouth open draws in extra air, as does gum chewing, smoking, and gulping carbonated beverages. Taking baking soda for indigestion can produce an abnormally high flatus content in the intestines. Anxiety and stress increase air swallowing and slow digestion, allowing more time for flatus production. Allergies, inadequate nutrients, or medications such as bulk-forming laxatives, cholesterol-lowering drugs, and tranquilizers can instigate or increase flatulence.

Excessive gas is more likely to be a social embarrassment than a symptom of serious illness. Making dietary adjustments, dining in a relaxed atmosphere, and practicing deliberate relaxation (see Introduction)

175

during periods of stress often remedy flatulence, but medical advice should be obtained if the condition is chronic or is accompanied by severe pain.

Diet and Supplements (see note on page xii)

Freedom from flatulence depends on proper digestion and absorption of foods by enzymes and digestive acids, beneficial intestinal flora, and the contractions (motility) of the stomach and intestines. Beginning meals with a salad and ending them with fresh fruit is believed to aid digestion. Both fresh papaya and pineapple contain enzymes that contribute to complete digestion and the avoidance of gas. When fresh papaya is not available, papaya tablets or digestive-enzyme supplements may prove helpful. The lactic-acid organisms from acidophilus milk, yogurt, or capsules reinforce the beneficial intestinal bacteria to inhibit gas production.

Eating high-fiber foods is essential for health and the avoidance of constipation, but their addition should be accomplished gradually and be accompanied by adequate fluids to prevent excess gas production from their insoluble fibers. No one food generates gas for all people at all times, but beans foster flatus for almost everybody. Studies show, however, that 90 percent of the offending compounds can be removed by soaking the legumes in tap water for 12 hours, then draining, rinsing, and cooking the beans with fresh water.[293] Also known for engendering gas are brussels sprouts, cabbage, carrots, celery, eggplant, onions, and some fruits (apples, apricots, bananas, citrus fruits, prunes, raisins). Other flatulence-causing culprits include dairy products, breads, fatty foods, pastries, potatoes, and wheat germ. Refined carbohydrates such as white flour and sugar (or the sugar substitute sorbitol), especially when combined with proteins, can contribute to gassiness.

B-Complex Vitamins These are necessary for adequate production of stomach acid; for carbohydrate, fat, and protein metabolism; and for the maintenance of motility in the gastrointestinal tract. In addition to taking a B complex tablet daily, supplements of 50 milligrams of B_1, B_6, and niacinamide, plus 200 micrograms of folic acid, may be helpful. Pantothenic acid is the most vital B vitamin for control of flatulence. Besides assisting in digestion, it improves intestinal peristalsis. Taking 50 to 100 milligrams of pantothenic acid after each meal has relieved flatus and distension for which there was no physical cause, and hospital studies show that 250 milligrams of pantothenic acid daily either prevent or relieve postoperative gas pains.[98]

Tissue Salts For flatulence with cramps, take three 6X tablets Mag. Phos. dissolved in a little hot water. If the condition continues, take three tablets of 6X Calc. Phos. Repeat both at frequent intervals until relieved. For flatulence with a sour taste in the mouth, take three tablets of 6X Nat. Phos. For flatulence with discomfort in the chest, take 3X Calc. Fluor. and Kali. Phos. alternately, at frequent intervals, while the condition lasts.[64, 65]

Exercise

Walking or other aerobic activity stimulates intestinal motility and helps break down large gas bubbles. If distension is a frequent problem, exercises such as bent-knee sit-ups help improve abdominal muscle tone. To relieve pain and ease out flatus trapped in the colon, sit on the floor with knees drawn up and rock back and forth. Or lie flat and slowly bring knees up to the chest and back down, massage the abdomen with a circular motion, then bring the knees up and down again. Or lie on the painful side, draw up the opposite knee, and roll from side to side.

Folk Remedies

Referred to as carminatives, cures for "escaping wind" have been searched for since the days of Hippocrates. Charcoal is a centuries-old remedy that has been rediscovered. Taking two activated charcoal tablets or capsules before and immediately after eating flatulence-causing foods may prevent gas by binding to the offending substance or by absorbing the flatus when it is formed.[186] Charcoal also reduces existing bloating and cramps by soaking up excess gas and transporting it out of the system. However, charcoal should not be used daily or be taken within an hour of dietary supplements or medications because it can bind with and inactivate needed nutrients or therapeutic drugs.[151] Lucille M. was troubled with odoriferous intestinal gas that caused cramping. She tried to avoid flatulence-causing foods but still had to munch charcoal tablets to relieve painful episodes. Lucille's little daughter was so accustomed to seeing her mother doubled over with flatulence that when she saw a stooped-over ancient on the street, her comment was, "Poor man, gas." Lucille has conquered her problem by combining an assortment of remedies. Taking acidophilus capsules with each meal plus some bee pollen every day inhibits the odor production. Vitamin C supplements create an acid environment antagonistic to gas-fomenting microbes, and with a daily B-complex tablet plus a charcoal capsule before a suspect meal, she can even indulge in an occasional bowl of chili by degassing the beans according to an old folk formula: Add 1 teaspoon of powdered ginger to the cold water covering dried legumes, bring to a full boil, let stand for an hour, drain and rinse, then cook in fresh water.

Digestive Aids Sipping diluted lemon juice or a mixture of 2 teaspoons *each* apple cider vinegar and honey in a glass of water with each meal are used to improve digestion and reduce the formation of flatus. After consuming gas-producing foods, eating watermelon or sipping a cup of hot water in which 2 tablespoons of grated fresh citrus peel has steeped for half an hour is said to overcome flatulence problems. Taking two mustard seeds with a glass of water before breakfast, then gradually building up to twelve seeds a day is an old remedy for chronic flatulence. Once the gassiness is under control, the number of seeds can be gradually reduced to one or two daily.

Heat Old-fashioned remedies included covering the abdomen with a towel wrung out of a mixture of hot water and brandy with a pinch of salt, or with a poultice of oats simmered in vinegar. A heating pad or hot-water bottle may be equally effective for allaying a bout of gas pain.

Herbal Teas Either singly or in combination, these carminative teas are used to stimulate digestion, decrease putrefactive bacteria, and improve intestinal motility: allspice, anise, cardamom, camomile, caraway, catnip, cinnamon, cloves, coriander, dill, fennel, ginger, nutmeg, parsley, peppermint, sage, savory, slippery elm, and yarrow.

Spice Compounds To be taken by the spoonful, these compounds include ¼ teaspoon *each* catnip, cinnamon, fennel, and sage steeped in ½ cup boiling water for 10 minutes; or ¼ teaspoon *each* ground cardamom, cinnamon, cloves, and nutmeg simmered in 2 cups wine, strained, and mixed with 1 cup brown sugar. Either compound may be diluted with warm water, if desired.

Nerve Pressure and Massage

○ Press and massage the center of the top of the head, then press upward on the center of the skull at the back of the neck.

○ Press or massage 1 inch to the left of the center of the chest.

○ While lying down, use a fist to press in front of the right hip bone, then up to the rib cage, across, and down to left side of the stomach.

Sources (see Bibliography)

6, 10, 17, 28, 29, 47, 51, 57, 60, 64, 65, 75, 87, 89, 92, 98, 101, 108, 109, 111, 112, 116, 135, 144, 147, 148, 150, 151, 164, 172, 186, 187, 202, 230, 252, 254, 255, 283, 284, 285, 293, 294, 300, 302, 312, 313

Fluid Retention (Edema)

Water, which is constantly being exchanged between blood and tissues, accounts for approximately three-fifths of body weight. Formerly called dropsy when it affected the entire body, edema refers to abnormal fluid retention in the tissues. A disturbance in fluid balance may be evidenced only as weight gain until the excess fluid in the body becomes apparent as swelling and puffiness. Obesity, pregnancy, or an occupation requiring standing for long periods may cause swollen legs and feet. Waterlogged tissues often afflict women during their menstrual cycles because of fluctuating hormone levels. Allergies or certain medications may be responsible for fluid retention. Persistent or chronic episodes of edema could be indications of heart, kidney, bladder, or liver disorders and should be investigated by a physician.

Regular aerobic exercise—cycling, swimming, walking—helps maintain fluid balance by improving vascular tone. Wearing support hose and elevating the feet several times a day may benefit people troubled with puffy ankles. Although prescription diuretics may be required in some cases, remedying the cause and relieving edema by natural methods whenever possible avoids the unpleasant side effects that can accompany continued use of diuretics.

Diet

Medical nutritionists have found that fluid retention unrelated to serious physical conditions usually can be rectified by dietary measures. The regulatory mechanisms controlling water balance within the body can be disturbed by a lack of protein, an overabundance of sugar and refined carbohydrates, or too much sodium (which allows fluid to penetrate cells, causing some of them to burst and create edema) in relation to potassium (which prevents sodium from entering the cells).[14] Since sodium deficiency

180

can be dangerous, many physicians advise increasing dietary potassium with fruits and vegetables (especially apricots, bananas, and dried legumes) and limiting rather than eliminating salt.

Foods with diuretic properties include apples, asparagus, beets, carrots, celery, cucumbers, grapes, green beans, horseradish, lettuce and other leafy greens, melons, onions, parsnips, pineapple, and pumpkin. Raw beet juice (made from the leaves as well as the beets) or pear juice is also believed helpful, as is the juice of one lemon in a cup of hot water. If desired, the water in which asparagus, celery, or turnips are cooked may be combined with the juices. Regular coffee and tea are mild diuretics, but indulging in more than 6 or 7 cups a day can be responsible for a form of edema that disappears when decaffeinated products are substituted.[4, 201]

Supplements (see note on page xii)

Insufficient calcium, vitamin D, or B vitamins can lead to fluid retention. In addition to a daily B-complex tablet, individual supplements are often beneficial. Prolonged deficiencies of B_1 can cause edema in the legs and feet.[109] Heightened estrogen levels occurring during the menstrual cycle, when pregnant, or when taking oral contraceptives increases the need for B_6. The dosage required to relieve edema varies from 25 milligrams to 200 milligrams in divided daily doses, with the mega amounts administered under medical supervision. Vitamin C (500 to 5,000 milligrams in divided daily doses) and 100 to 400 IU of vitamin E are beneficial for maintaining fluid balance by promoting the kidney's excretion of excess water and sodium.

> **Minerals** One multimineral tablet daily. Extra supplements of potassium are advised only with a physician's approval and should not be taken with potassium-conserving diuretics. Research studies show that increased dietary potassium plus supplementation with 800 milligrams of calcium and 500 milligrams of magnesium (which encourages cell retention of potassium) relieves fluid retention;[13] other researchers advise increasing the proportion of magnesium to 1,600 milligrams for this purpose.
>
> **Tissue Salts** Four 6X tablets of Nat. Sulph. every 4 hours until relieved. Taking two or three tablets of 6X Silicea each day has been helpful in some cases; Nat. Mur. has been of benefit for others.

Folk Remedies

Corncob Tea Simmer two or three fresh corncobs (from which the corn has been removed) in a quart of water for an hour. Drink two or three cups of the strained liquid during the day.

Garlic Take four garlic capsules daily to stimulate fluid elimination.

Gin Fill a jar with crushed, fresh spearmint leaves, cover with gin, and let stand for a day. Or combine ¼ cup bruised juniper berries with ¼ cup *each* crushed caraway and fennel seeds, add 2 cups gin and ½ cup water, and cover and steep for several days. Either of the mixtures should be strained and taken by the tablespoon three or four times a day. Or take 3 tablespoons gin (mixed with orange juice, if desired) and repeat the dosage in an hour or so. If the condition is not remedied, this treatment should be discontinued. (Note: These gin remedies are not recommended for recovering alcoholics, or for persons with blood sugar problems or liver disorders.)

Herbs Drink 1 or 2 cups daily of alfalfa, burdock, camomile, cornsilk, dandelion, fennel, horsetail, marshmallow, skullcap, or uva ursi. For a potassium-rich diuretic said to relieve edema within an hour, add 1 cup chopped fresh parsley to 1 quart boiling water, cover, and steep 40 minutes. Strain and drink a cup with each meal. Parsley seed or parsley root tea is believed equally effective.[150, 176]

Honey and bee pollen granules Mix half-and-half and take by the tablespoonful or stir into fruit juice.

Pumpkin, squash, or cantaloupe seeds For a native American remedy for edema, simmer a handful of the crushed seeds in a quart of water for half an hour, then drink several cups of the strained liquid each day.

Nerve Pressure and Massage

❍ Press or massage the center of the breastbone, then hook the middle fingers under the bottom of the ribs on both sides and press the slight notch approximately one-third of the distance up toward the lowest end of the breastbone.

❍ Press and massage a point 4 inches up from the anklebone on the inside of each leg.

Sources (see Bibliography)

4, 6, 13, 14, 15, 17, 56, 64, 65, 66, 75, 86, 87, 92, 98, 109, 135, 143, 144, 147, 148, 150, 151, 164, 173, 176, 201, 202, 203, 205, 218, 225, 229, 254, 256, 264, 265, 281, 294, 302, 304, 313, 316, 317, 320

Food Poisoning

"Ptomaine poisoning" is an obsolete term encompassing food poisoning caused by any of more than twenty kinds of foodborne bacteria or the toxins they generate. Salmonellosis, the most common form, increased from 740,000 reported cases in 1970 to an estimated 4 million in 1991.[300] This rise is attributed to the feeding of antibiotics to food animals (which speeds their growth but promotes the development of antibiotic-resistant bacteria from the strains present in the intestinal tracts of all animals—eggs and unpasteurized milk also harbor the bacteria) and to mechanical methods of evisceration, especially of poultry, that introduce the salmonella into the meat.

Other causative organisms include Campylobacter (in fish, fowl, meat, and raw milk), Ciguatera (in large reef fish), Vibrio (in shellfish), Trichinella (in pork), Clostridium botulinum (from improperly canned foods or oxygen-deprived foods like foil-wrapped baked potatoes left out overnight), and the "cafeteria germ" (Clostridium perfringens), which grows rapidly in large portions of food or in meat or poultry dishes allowed to cool slowly. Staphylococcus is carried on human skin and in airborne droplets from coughs or sneezes; Shigella also is passed on by food handlers with poor personal hygiene. When cream-filled pastries, potato salad, or cooked high-protein foods are contaminated through unsanitary handling, the bacteria multiply at room temperature and produce poisonous toxins.

Bacterial contaminants are odorless, tasteless, and invisible; large colonies may develop without obvious food spoilage. Visible molds that grow on foodstuffs, even when refrigerated, can produce mycotoxins or poisons. According to the U.S. Department of Agriculture, small spots of mold can be safely removed from jams and jellies, hard cheeses, hard salami, smoked turkey, and the surface of firm vegetables. Other moldy foods—including dairy products, bacon, canned ham, sliced lunch meat, grains, nuts, dried legumes, and soft vegetables—should be discarded. So should potatoes that have begun to sprout. The green shoots have high concentrations of solanine, which infiltrates the potato, is not destroyed by cooking, and can cause hallucinations for days after recovery from the food poisoning.[29]

Prevention

Despite the presence of potentially harmful organisms, most food poisoning is preventable through personal control. Eating yogurt or drinking acidophilus milk every few days bolsters the beneficial bacteria in the intestinal tract and encourages an ample internal supply of B vitamins to protect against foodborne contaminants. In addition, yogurt bacteria spin off substances that help squelch intruders such as salmonella and staphylococcus.[56] Dwight O. credits acidophilus combined with a folk remedy for saving him from frequent bouts of food poisoning. With an overly sensitive digestive system, Dwight often got sick after group dinners that left other participants symptom-free. On the advice of a friend, he began eating yogurt once a week. Then, before consuming any of the fare at the next picnic, he took two acidophilus capsules plus an old-fashioned preventive, 2 teaspoons of apple cider vinegar in a glass of water. It worked. Now Dwight plays it safe by taking the combo before indulging in any questionable food.

Sanitation Proper food handling reduces the potential for foodborne illness. Besides washing the hands before touching food, hands, cutting boards, and utensils used in preparing raw fish, meat, or poultry should be cleaned with hot water and soap before contact with other foods.

Temperature control Most bacteria hibernate at temperatures below 40 degrees Fahrenheit, revive and multiply in temperatures between 45 and 150 degrees, and perish at temperatures above 165 degrees. Exceptions are the botulism-causing toxins in home-canned foods, which take 20 minutes of boiling to kill, and staphylococcus bacteria, which are not destroyed by cooking. Frozen meats should be defrosted slowly in the refrigerator, quickly in a microwave oven, or, securely wrapped, in hot water in the sink. Turkey should be stuffed just before cooking. If returned to the refrigerator, the warm stuffing can activate bacteria in the surrounding meat before cold penetrates to the center of the bird. Foods being marinated should be kept in the refrigerator, and as explained in *American Health* (June 1992), even tasting raw or undercooked poultry, meat, seafood, or eggs is risky. Leftovers should be promptly refrigerated, then reheated to 165 degrees before serving, because cooked foods can be recontaminated by flies or unsanitary utensils.

Treatment

The cramps, diarrhea, nausea, and vomiting associated with food poisoning develop in half an hour to a week after the contaminated food is eaten and disappear within a few hours or days. The timing, severity, and duration depend on the kind and amount of contamination and on the strength of the individual's immune system. The very young, the very old, and people with chronic illnesses are at highest risk. Medical assistance should be obtained if severe vomiting and diarrhea suddenly appear or if symptoms linger longer than 48 hours. The local health department should be contacted if the source of the distress is a restaurant or commercially canned food.

Unless under doctor's orders to the contrary, the body should be allowed to purge itself of the poison without interference from antidiarrheal medications. Antacids, or the home remedy of baking soda and water, should be avoided during a bout of food poisoning—either can weaken internal defenses by reducing the acids in the stomach that are antagonistic to bacteria.[293] However, taking 6 activated charcoal tablets at the onset of symptoms, and again in 6 hours, assists the body by absorbing toxins and escorting them out of the system,[17] and garlic is a natural antibiotic and detoxifier—two deodorized garlic capsules can be taken three times a day.

Sipping ginger tea, ginger ale, colas, or other soft drinks reduces nausea and helps prevent dehydration by replacing lost fluids. Defizzing carbonated beverages by pouring them back and forth between two glasses avoids the possibility of further aggravating an upset stomach. Clear broth, or fruit juice with a spoonful of honey and a pinch of salt, helps replenish flushed-out minerals as well as liquid. Folk healers suggest burdock root tea, currants or currant juice for food poisoning from meats, and, to alleviate the symptoms from spoiled seafood, a tea made by steeping a chopped ripe persimmon and 1 tablespoon dried horehound herb in a pint of water for half an hour.

Sources (see Bibliography)

17, 29, 41, 44, 56, 75, 98, 108, 111, 112, 148, 149, 150, 171, 172, 176, 204, 207, 231, 234, 255, 256, 264, 277, 281, 283, 293, 294, 300

Foot Odor

Perspiration alone is not responsible for smelly feet. Eccrine sweat glands secrete an odorless, watery fluid on the soles of the feet as part of the body's temperature-regulating system. The amount of perspiration secreted depends not only on external heat but also on internal metabolism and emotions. Excitement, fear, anger, anxiety—all can trigger a wet response. When this liquid is prevented from performing its duty of cooling by evaporating from the skin, bacteria naturally present on skin surfaces take advantage of the moist warmth. The airless atmosphere inside closed shoes provides such an ideal environment for them that bacterial multiplication and decomposition can make feet malodorous after only a few hours.

Daily washing is necessary to remove accumulated secretions and bacteria. Using an antibacterial soap helps guard against future odor. Wearing shoes of breathable materials (leather, canvas, ventilated synthetics), rotating footwear to allow at least a day for drying out, and frequently washing washable athletic shoes help prevent foot odor. Selecting sandals, pumps, or moccasins, and unobtrusively slipping off the slip-ons whenever appropriate give feet a bacteria-discouraging "breather."

The material between foot and shoe plays an important role in odor control. Research reported in the June 1991 issue of *Prevention* reveals that socks fabricated from new synthetic materials (Coolmax, orlon, polypropylene) wick perspiration away from feet instead of merely absorbing the moisture as do previously preferred cotton or wool. People beset by excessive perspiration and foot odor may ameliorate the problem by changing shoes and hose in the middle of the day, by wearing two pairs of socks so the air spaces between layers of fabric will enhance cooling, and by utilizing some of the natural foot odor foilers that follow.

Diet and Supplements (see note on page xii)

Strange as it seems, eating pungent foods like garlic or onions, or spices such as cumin and curry, can cause smelly feet when their odor is exuded through sweat glands in the soles. Eliminating possible offenders one at a time on an experimental basis may prevent unnecessary dietary deprivation. Other tips for controlling external odor from the inside include taking two chlorophyll tablets with each meal and/or supplementing the diet with 500 to 750 milligrams of magnesium and 30 to 50 milligrams of zinc every day.

Homeopathic doctors recommend taking three 6X tablets of the tissue salt Silicea twice daily. B vitamins are another option. As tennis instructor at a health resort, Luke N. was able to keep his foot odor problem under control with soap and water, but it was a bother. He bought socks and athletic shoes by the dozen, showered and changed at least twice a day, and washed the smelly shoes and socks every night. He decided to experiment with supplements after the resident nutritionist mentioned that some individuals require dietary supplements, especially B vitamins, to avoid having unpleasant body or foot odor. Luke began taking a one-a-day multiple and a B-complex tablet each morning plus another B-complex tablet with dinner and was happily surprised by the results. He still showers and changes after a strenuous morning on the courts, but the offensive odor is gone. Luke's shoes can air-dry between wearings, his socks can cohabitate with other garments in the hamper, and a weekly washday suffices.

Folk Remedies

Boric Acid   An ingredient of modern foot odor products, boric acid was dusted inside shoes and stockings during the 1800s, and freshly laundered socks were dipped in a boric-acid solution before being hung to dry.

Rubbing Alcohol   Sponged over clean, dry feet to diminish both perspiration and odor, this is another folk remedy that has been vindicated by recent studies. *The Edell Health Letter* (July 1991) reports that alcohol kills foot bacteria as effectively as prescription-only antibacterial ointments.

Deodorant Washes Witch hazel, diluted vinegar, or white willow bark tea mixed with borax help quell foot odor.

Dry Miller's Bran, Dry Oatmeal, or **Crushed Dried Sage Leaves** These can be sprinkled in shoes as deodorizers.

Zinc Oxide Even more effective than the preceding as a shoe sprinkle, 2 tablespoons of zinc oxide can be blended with ¼ cup *each* cornstarch and fuller's earth; or ¼ cup zinc oxide can be mixed with 1 tablespoon powdered orris root and ½ cup of either cornstarch or talcum powder.

Baking Soda By itself or combined half-and-half with cornstarch or talc, this can be used as a foot powder to deodorize and absorb moisture.

Foot Baths A solution for truly malodorous feet. Soaking time (15 to 30 minutes) and frequency (twice a day to twice a week) depends on the seriousness of the problem.

○ To 2 quarts of water, add 1 tablespoon ammonia; or 2 tablespoons baking soda, or 1 cup of coarse (kosher) salt or tomato juice or vinegar.

○ Steep double-strength horsetail tea or regular pekoe tea; add cold water for a comfortably warm foot bath.

○ For those who are neither diabetic nor suffering from impaired circulation, alternating hot and cold plain-water foot baths for a few minutes each, adding ice cubes and lemon juice to the final cold soak, then concluding with an alcohol rub constricts circulation and reduces both perspiration and odor.

Sources (see Bibliography)

3, 36, 42, 52, 53, 65, 75, 109, 150, 165, 186, 202, 216, 245, 252, 256, 258, 281, 283, 284, 293, 294, 300, 312, 313

Frostbite, Chilblains, and Hypothermia

When exposed to severe cold for long periods, the body hoards heat to keep the vital organs functioning by reducing blood circulation to the extremities—which leaves the nose, cheeks, ears, fingers, and toes vulnerable to frostbite. Affected areas at first redden, tingle or ache, and feel cold. Then, as the skin, blood, and underlying tissues freeze, the area becomes hard, numb, and grayish white. Chilblains (pernio) are swollen, inflamed areas of skin that itch or burn as an aftermath of being frostbitten or as a result of frequent exposure to cold that may not have been severe enough to cause frostbite.

Hypothermia (a condition in which body temperature falls below 95 degrees Fahrenheit) most often occurs in elderly people living in poorly heated homes but can be caused by falling into icy water or wearing damp clothing in a cold environment and may accompany frostbite. Symptoms of hypothermia include drowsiness, failing vision, staggering, mental confusion, and, eventually, unconsciousness.

Prevention

Several studies show that taking massive amounts of vitamin C with bioflavonoids (at least 1,500 milligrams for each 65 pounds of body weight) in divided daily doses helps the body maintain its normal temperature to prevent hypothermia and frostbite.[98, 233]

Dressing defensively precludes most problems caused by environmental cold. Old-fashioned nightcaps and daytime head coverings that protect ears and the back of the neck are recommended—at least one-third of heat lost from the body is from the head.[254] Face masks and goggles protect skiers (the corneas of the eyes are subject to frostbite), an extra pair of shorts may forestall the penile frostbite experienced by cyclists and runners.[111, 300] Moisture-absorbing socks and undergarments covered by a waterproof outer layer reduce the danger of heat loss from damp clothing and windchill. Mittens keep hands warmer than gloves; either offer protection from contact with frozen metal, which can immediately form ice crystals and destroy cell tissue. Smoking during exposure is not recommended because tobacco decreases circulation by constricting blood vessels. If it is not possible to escape from the cold at the first warning of chilliness, covering the face or ears with gloved hands, wiggling the fingers or tucking them under the armpits, or jumping up and down may help restore circulation.

First-Aid Tips Frostbite and/or Hypothermia should have prompt medical attention. No friction should be applied to frostbitten areas—particularly not the archaic remedy of rubbing with snow—and frostbitten parts should not be exposed to an open fire or a radiant heater. The victim should be wrapped with blankets or coats, given warm, non-alcoholic beverages or soup to sip (alcohol provides an artificial feeling of warmth but restricts blood flow), and taken to the nearest medical facility.

Folk Remedies

After professional treatment, home remedies may hasten recovery and relieve the discomfort of frostbite or chilblains.

Aloe Vera Gel This ancient remedy for burns has been shown to reduce frostbite damage.[49, 111]

Alum At bedtime, dissolve 1 tablespoon alum in a basin of hot water. Apply towels wrung out of the mixture to chilblains or frostbitten areas; or soak hands or feet for 20 minutes, then cover with gloves or socks for the rest of the night.

Liquid Applications Sponge the afflicted areas with diluted boric acid, slippery elm tea, witch hazel, or warm vinegar mixed with salt. Wheat germ oil can be painted on with a soft brush to relieve pain and speed the healing of blisters. A before-bed treatment for chilblains is to apply alternate hot and cold compresses for 20 minutes and keep warm overnight. To relieve stinging pain, medical anthropologist John Heinerman[150] suggests this prepare-ahead, paint-on liquid used in the frigid regions of Inner Mongolia: Steep 2 tablespoons whole black pepper and 1 tablespoon *each* grated horseradish and ginger root in

1¼ cups of white wine for a week, then strain and store in a tightly covered jar.

Vegetables For either frostbite or chilblains, apply the inner sides of cucumber peelings, securing them overnight for chilblains, or use the water in which potatoes have been boiled to sponge the areas or provide a hand or foot bath. Gently rubbing frostbitten skin with raw onion or potato slices, or with liquefied raw radishes; or covering the area with room-temperature, cooked, mashed potatoes or turnips is said to relieve pain.

Nerve Pressure and Massage (do not use on a frostbitten area)

○ To help restore inner warmth, rub the area over the kidneys (from the top of the pelvis to the center of the back) for a minute or two.

○ Extend the right arm and use the left hand to massage the triangular hollow between the collarbone and shoulder of the extended arm for 30 seconds; repeat with the other arm. Then press and massage the hollow behind and slightly below each anklebone.

Tissue Salts for Chilblains

To ameliorate discomfort, dissolve three 6X tablets under the tongue each hour or so: Calc. Fluor. if there are cracks in the skin; Kali. Sulph. for broken chilblains leaking fluid; Kali. Mur. for swelling, alternating with Ferr. Phos. for pain and inflammation.

Sources (see Bibliography)

21, 29, 42, 49, 57, 65, 75, 86, 92, 98, 108, 109, 111, 133, 135, 148, 149, 150, 159, 168, 186, 202, 233, 254, 281, 283, 285, 293, 294, 300, 322

Gallbladder Disorders

Inflammation of the gallbladder (cholecystitis) may be provoked by irritation from digestive enzymes, drugs, or infection but most often is caused by gallstones blocking one of the bile ducts connecting the gallbladder to the liver and the small intestine.[281] Bile (composed primarily of cholesterol, lecithin, and mineral bile salts) is constantly produced by the liver to assist digestion, especially of fats, in the upper segment of the small intestine. When no food is present, surplus bile is stored and concentrated in the gallbladder, then squeezed into the intestine as required.

A chemical imbalance in the bile—usually an overload of cholesterol—can precipitate tiny crystals around which solids accumulate into gallstones ranging from the size of a pinhead to an inch in diameter. Predisposing factors include heredity, diabetes, high levels of blood cholesterol—and middle age. Women who have had many children or who are taking oral contraceptives or supplementary estrogen are at highest risk.[177, 254] Studies show that obesity (more than 30 percent over ideal weight) increases the risk of gallstones by 600 percent.[28, 186] However, weight should be lost gradually; fasting or drastic dieting can cause bile to stagnate and create additional stones.

Gallstones may remain symptomless or may merely induce nausea and abdominal discomfort after a large meal. An acute attack, possibly accompanied by vomiting, can be triggered by a stone becoming lodged in a bile duct and causing waves of intense pain to radiate from the upper right side of the abdomen to below the right shoulder blade as the gallbladder contracts in an attempt to expel the stone. If the stone drops back into the gallbladder or is ejected into the intestine and eliminated, the pain subsides. If the blockage continues and/or causes fever or jaundice, medical help should be obtained.

Of the 25 million Americans with gallstones, only about 20 percent experience more than one attack or symptoms severe enough to warrant surgical removal of the gallbladder.[75, 112] The liver can supply bile directly to the intestine after the gallbladder has been removed, but prevention and control of gallbladder disorders through home remedies may be preferable options if approved by a physician.

Diet

While no specific diet is perfect for every patient—some gallbladders react adversely to spicy foods or gassy vegetables like brussels sprouts and cabbage—the basic strategy calls for limiting fats to less than 25 percent of total calories and emphasizing high-fiber fruits, vegetables, and whole grains. Fiber helps avoid gallstone formation by stimulating bile flow from the liver and preventing its resorption. In one study, generous amounts of unprocessed bran not only significantly lowered the cholesterol saturation of bile but also reduced the size of existing stones.[205, 300] Apples, pears, beet greens, and soybeans are considered particularly beneficial. A daily glass of equal amounts of beet juice and lettuce juice (or diluted lemon juice) is said to reduce the size of larger stones.[306] All fresh fruit and vegetable juices are thought to guard against stone formation by liquefying the tiny crystals before they can snowball into gallstones.[150, 305]

Although one alcoholic drink per day has protective value,[75, 109] excess amounts of alcohol, sweets, or white-flour products are metabolized as fats and increase the risk of gallbladder disorders. Cholesterol-containing animal fats are especially suspect. Studies involving over 700 women revealed that vegetarians are only half as likely to experience gallbladder disturbances as are meat eaters.[201, 294] Dietitians suggest using low-fat dairy products, limiting eggs to three a week, having only 3-ounce servings of lean meat or poultry, and tossing salads with lemon juice and canola or olive oil.[147] Patrick N., who had adhered to his diet and had no flareups following his gallbladder attack, discovered that the daily allotment of fats should be distributed among several small meals during the day. When he was declared one of the winners in the sales department's annual steak-or-beans banquet, Patrick skipped breakfast, ate an apple for lunch, then devoured his huge steak and sour-cream-topped baked potato with a clear conscience. The pleasure, however, was short lived. The nausea, pain, and vomiting from midnight on convinced Patrick that skipping and splurging were not worth the discomfort.

Supplements (see note on page xii)

Inadequate bile production or gallbladder malfunction reduces the absorption of fat-soluble vitamins A, D, E, and K and inhibits the conversion of beta carotene (from fruits, vegetables, or supplements) to vitamin A. In addition to 5,000 to 25,000 IU of emulsified vitamin A and 400 IU *each* of vitamins D and E, the following supplements may be beneficial in the treatment of gallbladder disorders.[17, 98]

B Complex   One comprehensive tablet daily, plus 500 milligrams *each* choline and inositol to improve digestion and gallbladder function.

Vitamin C   1,000 to 3,000 milligrams in divided daily doses to hasten the conversion of cholesterol into bile acids and prevent gallstone formation.

Lecithin   One teaspoon to 1 tablespoon of granules or liquid (or the equivalent in capsules) with each meal. Lecithin emulsifies fat, is essential for the maintenance of soluble bile to prohibit gallstones, and may help dissolve existing stones.[2, 151]

Tissue Salts   Dissolve four tablets of 6X Calc. Fluor. under the tongue every 2 hours during an attack.[55]

Folk Remedies

Folk healers report wondrous results with natural remedies, but none of them should be attempted without a physician's diagnosis and approval.

Herbs   Angelica (dong quai), barberry, camomile, catnip, dandelion, fennel, ginger, horsetail, parsley, and peppermint are recommended. Drinking a cup of peppermint tea 1 hour after each of the two largest meals of the day is thought to stimulate bile production following gallbladder surgery.

Lemon Juice   A gallbladder cleanser and stimulant, lemon juice can be diluted with water (3 tablespoons lemon juice to ½ cup water) and taken before breakfast for a week; or the juice of half a lemon may be added to each cup of camomile tea, and 7 cups of the mixture sipped daily for 7 days.

Pain-Relieving Poultices   Mashed watermelon rind; or cloths squeezed out of castor oil, milk, or hot water (with or without the addition of a teaspoon of dry mustard) may be placed over the painful portion of the abdomen and covered to keep warm.

Treatments   Both of these classic remedies utilize olive oil to stimulate bile flow and relieve pain by acting as a lubricant to ease the elimination of gallstones. Incorporating other liquids helps break up or partially dissolve the stones (sleeping on the right side is believed to expedite their exodus) and less than a month of either regimen is reported to remove gallstones that were apparent in X-rays.[42, 150, 312] (1) Begin with 1 teaspoon olive oil in ½ cup grapefruit juice before breakfast each morning and gradually increase the amounts to ¼ cup oil in 1 cup of juice. (Diluted lemon juice or 1 teaspoon apple cider vinegar in ½ cup water may be substituted for the grapefruit juice.) (2) Add 2 tablespoons dried catnip to 3 cups of freshly made burdock tea and steep for 1½ hours before straining. Twice during the day, and just before bed, stir 1 teaspoon *each* lemon juice and maple syrup into a cup of the tea and drink slowly. Then, 10 minutes later, take 1 teaspoon olive oil.

Vegetables   To benefit the gallbladder and help dissolve gallstones; Add ⅓ cup finely chopped raw endive to 3 cups of hot chicory root tea, steep 45 minutes, strain, then drink a cup between meals and 2 hours before bed. Or consume two red radishes a day, either minced with olive oil and lemon juice or whirred in a blender with ½ cup red wine. A Cajun remedy said to expel gallstones in 1 week is to drink 4 or 5 cups of broth made from well-scrubbed potato peelings daily.

Nerve Pressure and Massage

○ Press inward and upward under each cheekbone, 1½ inches out from the earlobe toward the nose.

○ Press downward on the middle of the upper edge of the collarbones.

○ Press and massage 2 inches to the right of the navel, midway between it and the lower ribs.

○ Massage the edge of the right hand just below the little finger, then the outer edge of each foot and the pad under the little toe.

Sources (see Bibliography)

2, 6, 10, 17, 26, 28, 42, 44, 55, 56, 59, 60, 75, 77, 98, 103, 109, 112, 135, 147, 148, 150, 151, 164, 171, 173, 176, 177, 179, 186, 193, 201, 203, 205, 207, 254, 255, 256, 264, 280, 281, 294, 300, 305, 306, 312, 313

Gout

Sometimes termed gouty arthritis, gout is a metabolic disease that usually attacks a big toe but can appear in an ear, heel of the hand, or in any joint, with inflammation, swelling, and excruciating pain from the buildup of needlelike uric-acid crystals. Once regarded as a tribulation of titled noblemen who gorged on rich foods, gout is actually discriminatory only in that over 90 percent of its victims are middle-aged males.[312] Medical diagnosis is important to rule out the possibility of pseudogout, a different disorder that often requires professional aspiration of fluid before treatment.

Heredity plays a role in the selection of gout victims—25 percent of its sufferers have a family history of the disease—but no single cause has been established. Apparently unrelated factors such as emotional stress, diuretics or other prescribed drugs, injuries, and obesity (half of all gout patients are overweight[49]) may provoke an attack or a recurrence of gout. Obese gout sufferers may be able to correct the problem through weight loss, but it must be accomplished gradually—fasts or extreme caloric deprivation can trigger acute gouty attacks.

For temporary pain relief, a cloth-covered ice pack may be applied for 10 minutes at a time and alternated with moist hot-towel compresses, if desired. When a painkilling pill is necessary, one containing inflammation-reducing ibuprofen is advised. Acetaminophen lacks sufficient inflammation-fighting capability, and aspirin inhibits excretion of uric acid.[186]

Diet

Some doctors believe gout results from low blood sugar or inefficient breakdown of proteins and that since at least 50 percent of the uric acid from which the crystals are formed is synthesized by the body instead of being

197

derived from purine-containing foods, dietary restrictions are unimportant.[147] However, meals rich in purines, fats, or concentrated sweets may instigate gout or its recurrence, so most medical authorities advise avoiding the prime purine contributors (organ meats, anchovies, herring, sardines) during an attack. Beer, wine, and other spirited beverages should be imbibed with discretion—they not only increase the production of uric acid, they impair the body's ability to excrete it.[49] If no diet has been prescribed, the general rule is to have no more than three to five servings weekly of these foods with moderate purine content: dried legumes, meats and meat broths or gravies, poultry, seafood, oatmeal, whole grains, asparagus, cauliflower, mushrooms, and spinach. Using generous quantities of other vegetables, fruits, and their juices helps keep uric-acid crystals in solution and facilitates their excretion.

Eating a ripe pear before each meal is an old French remedy; strawberries and cherries (fresh, frozen, canned, or juiced) contain an enzyme that neutralizes uric acid.[17] Willard G. prefers cherries. Despite adhering to a low-purine diet and taking his prescribed medications, Willard's gout flared up so frequently he was forced to move his accounting office into his living room, where he could work with the throbbing toe propped on a pillow. Willard's wife knew he didn't believe in experimenting with home remedies, so when she read that eating a cup of cherries a day had cleared gout symptoms for many people, she didn't mention it. She merely placed a bowl of fresh cherries on his worktable every day with the comment that she had bought several pounds at a bargain price. After a week of "cherry therapy," Willard was able to return to his regular office and agreed to continue eating a few cherries every day—just in case they were contributing to his recovery.

An ample intake of fluids helps flush excess uric acid out of the system. Drinking a total of 3 quarts of liquid a day at the first twinge of discomfort has forestalled some gout attacks. At least one-third of that amount should be water, the remainder made up of fruit or vegetable juices (diluted celery juice or combinations of potato juice with celery, carrot, or beet juice are thought to be especially beneficial), low-fat milk, and herb teas brewed from alfalfa, birch, buckthorn, burdock, celery seed, chervil, comfrey (which folk healers advise using for a foot bath as well as a beverage), corncob (made by simmering fresh cobs for half an hour), elder flower, ginger, hyssop, juniper, parsley, peppermint, plantain, rose hip, rosemary, sarsaparilla, or yarrow.

Supplements (see note on page xii)

Low-purine diets are low in vitamins B, E, and other antioxidants (see Introduction). The following supplements may help prevent the damage from free radicals that can intensify gouty problems.[224]

B Complex One to three high-potency tablets daily, plus 500 milligrams of pantothenic acid in divided doses to assist the body's conversion of uric acid into harmless compounds.[98]

Vitamin C 1,000 milligrams per hour at the onset of a gout attack, then a gradual tapering off to a maintenance dosage of 500 to 3,000 milligrams a day to lower serum uric acid.

Vitamin E 100 IU, slowly increased to 600 or 800 IU daily—a deficiency of this vitamin can contribute to the formation of excessive amounts of uric acid.

Tissue Salts To prevent the formation of uric-acid crystals, take two tablets of 6X Silicea three times each day. During an attack of gout, increase the dosage to three tablets and add an equal amount of Nat. Phos. and Nat. Sulph.

Folk Remedies

Apple Cider Vinegar Two teaspoons *each* vinegar and raw honey stirred in a glass of water and sipped at mealtime is believed to prevent and relieve gout. Liniments prepared by simmering 1 tablespoon cayenne pepper in 2 cups vinegar or by heating the vinegar and stirring in all the salt that will dissolve can be rubbed on afflicted joints. Soaking the painful area in a solution of ½ cup vinegar and 3 cups hot water is also thought to alleviate gouty pain.

Apples Europeans make a tea from dried apple peels and sweeten it with honey. Vermont folk medicine recommends stirring 2 teaspoons honey into a glass of apple juice at each meal. Other folk practitioners promote apple cider as the ideal beverage for those with a "gouty constitution."

Butter and Wine Heat unsalted butter to boiling, add an equal amount of wine, cook until the consistency of an ointment, then rub on the affected area to soothe and heal.

Charcoal Take ½ to 1 teaspoon of activated charcoal powder four times a day, or apply a poultice of warm water mixed with half a cup of the charcoal powder and 3 tablespoons of ground flaxseed to draw out the toxins.

Garlic Eating several cloves of raw garlic each day has been a gout-preventive since the Greco-Roman era (swallowing minced garlic with cherry juice may increase the benefits), and a poultice of cooked garlic may be used to relieve the pain.

Nerve Pressure and Massage

○ Press inward and upward on the underside of the protuberance at the base of the skull.

○ Press just below the center of the nose toward the upper lip.

○ On both hands, press and massage a point on the inside of the pad at the base of the thumb directly beneath the index finger; then on the left palm only, stimulate a point halfway between the base of the little finger and the wrist.

○ Press and massage between the ball of the foot and the bottom of the big toe on the sole of each foot; then on the left foot only, stimulate a point halfway between the base of the little toe and the heel pad.

Sources (see Bibliography)

2, 4, 14, 17, 39, 49, 57, 64, 66, 75, 86, 98, 135, 143, 144, 147, 148, 150, 156, 159, 164, 171, 173, 186, 200, 203, 207, 218, 224, 225, 234, 244, 246, 272, 275, 281, 283, 293, 294, 301, 306, 312, 313, 320

Hair Loss (Alopecia)

Each hair grows from a root encased in a follicle that is nourished by blood vessels. A youthful scalp contains 100,000 to 200,000 hairs—the exact number depending on the number of hair follicles, which is established before birth. Hair grows about half an inch a month for 2 to 6 years, rests (the telogen phase) for approximately 3 months, then falls out and is replaced by a new hair in 3 to 5 months. Normally, 85 percent of the follicles are in the growing phase and 50 to 100 resting hairs are shed daily.

Generalized Alopecia Hair loss that usually reverses when the cause is corrected results when an abnormal number of hairs simultaneously enter the resting phase and all fall out in 3 or 4 months. Causes include anemia, high fever, malnutrition, certain medications, stress, and thyroid disorders. The hormonal changes of pregnancy may extend the growing cycle then cause dramatic hair loss if those hairs go into the telogen phase immediately after the baby is born. Alopecia areata (loss of hair in patches) sometimes corrects itself but may be a symptom of an underlying disease and warrants consultation with a physician.

Localized Hair Loss Traction alopecia can occur when the hair is pulled too tight in braids or ponytails or is frequently set with tight rollers. Friction alopecia can be caused by wearing tight hats or wigs. Barton N. developed a bald strip across the top of his head from the pressure of a heavy earphone radio he wore while jogging and working in the garden.

Androgenic Alopecia This type of hair loss is determined by hormones and genetic inheritance. The most common form is male-pattern baldness—hair loss at temples and crown gradually creating a bald pate with hair only on the sides and back. According to the

Berkeley Wellness Letter (June 1992), this type of hair loss can begin as early as age 20 and affects half of all American men of European origin by the time they reach the age of 50. African Americans, Asians, and Native Americans seldom suffer from androgenic alopecia. Female-pattern baldness—usually evidenced by a widening part line or over-all thinning—affect 20 to 30 percent of women in their 40s and becomes more pronounced after menopause.

Diet and Supplements (see note on page xii)

Hair is composed of protein and minerals and requires a balanced diet with adequate calories for proper nourishment. Foods believed to encourage hair growth include alfalfa sprouts, barley and oats, beans, fish, fresh fruit or vegetable juices, green vegetables (especially sulfur-containing brussels sprouts, cabbage, kale, and watercress), onions, prunes, raspberries, strawberries, and wheat germ. Combining even small amounts of meat with vegetable and grain dishes and cooking acidic foods in cast-iron pots increase the assimilation of iron to help prevent hair fallout. To help compensate for the slowing metabolic processes that make sparse hair a common facet of aging, nutritionists suggest a breakfast "hair tonic": Blend a cup of plain yogurt with half a banana, ½ cup strawberries, 2 tablespoons brewer's yeast (for protein plus B vitamins), and 1 tablespoon unflavored gelatin. If desired, include 2 tablespoons wheat germ, 1 tablespoon lecithin granules (lecithin contains the hair-growth stimulators biotin, choline, and inositol), one egg yolk, and/or a tablespoon of honey.

When Connie V. noticed that her hairline was receding, she knew the probable cause—she had been hiding her baby-fine hair under a snug-fit-ting wig so she could present a stylish appearance at work. As an experi-ment, she started taking a high-potency multivitamin-mineral and, by beginning with 1 teaspoon a day, gradually built up to 2 tablespoons of brewer's yeast in her breakfast juice plus 2 tablespoons in a before-bed glass of milk. Within a month, there was noticeable improvement. Connie no longer wears a wig, and her associates insist that her short-and-bouncy hairstyle is far more flattering, and fashionable, than her previous coiffure.

Vitamin A In the form of beta carotene, 10,000 to 30,000 IU daily to preclude falling hair due to vitamin A deficiency. Taking excessive amounts of preformed vitamin A over extended periods can trigger a type of hair loss that reverses when the supplementation stops.

B Complex   All the B vitamins are important for hair growth. In addition to one or two B-complex tablets daily, individual supplements are sometimes helpful: 1 milligram folic acid; 50 milligrams *each* B_6, niacin, and pantothenic acid; 50 to 200 milligrams biotin; 500 milligrams *each* choline and inositol. Vegetarians may need to take supplemental B_{12}.

Vitamin C with Bioflavonoids   500 to 5,000 milligrams in divided doses, to strengthen capillaries and to assist vitamin E (100 IU gradually increased up to 800 IU daily) in promoting hair growth by improving circulation to the scalp.

L-cysteine and L-methionine   500 milligrams of each of these amino acids taken twice daily with B_6 and at least 1,500 milligrams of vitamin C, may improve hair growth and help strengthen the follicles to prevent premature fallout.

Minerals   One multi mineral tablet daily. Taking an additional 15 to 50 milligrams of zinc is credited with halting hair loss and stimulating new growth in some cases.[40]

Tissue Salts—Taking Calc. Phos., Kali. Sulph., Nat. Mur., and/or Silicea may correct hair-loss problems. The suggested dosage is three 6X tablets dissolved under the tongue twice daily.

External Care

Frequent shampooing keeps the scalp clear of any buildup that might impede the emergence of new hairs and is particularly important for those with androgenic alopecia because scalp sebum contains hormones that may penetrate the skin to accelerate hair loss. Thinning hair requires gentle handling. Towel blotting and air drying are recommended. Vigorous toweling can prematurely dislodge rooting hairs, heat from blow dryers and curling irons can damage the roots as well as the shaft. Brushing (which should be limited to a few gentle strokes on dry hair—not the 100 strokes a day once recommended) and teasing can pull hairs out or break them off in the follicle to inhibit regrowth. Ten minutes of fingertip massage daily, while sitting with the head bent toward the knees or while reclining on a slantboard, brings nourishing blood to the scalp. Rubbing a turkish towel on bald areas until the skin is pink, or using an electric vibrator on bare spots twice each day, has promoted regrowth within 3 months for some individuals.[198]

Folk Remedies

According to a papyrus dated 1550 B.C., Egyptian physicians "cured" baldness by anointing hairless heads with a mixture of crocodile, elephant, lion, and hippopotamus fat. Oriental remedies include spreading grated fresh ginger on bald spots half an hour before shampooing, then washing the hair with water in which snails have been boiled. Folk medicine offers less exotic, and less expensive options.

Apple Cider Vinegar Three times a day, drink a glass of water containing 1 teaspoon of vinegar, and eat a teaspoon of horseradish with each of two daily meals. Twice a day, brush bare spots with a soft toothbrush dipped in vinegar and add a tablespoon of vinegar to a quart of water for the final rinse after each shampoo.

Herbs Once or twice a day, sip a cup of alfalfa, camomile, cayenne, fenugreek, nettle, parsley, rosemary, or sage tea. For a hair rinse, use double-strength burdock, camomile, chaparral, horsetail, nettle, rosemary, or sage tea.

Overnight Treatments A weekly program for hair restoration in a few months calls for massaging castor oil into the scalp the first 2 nights, wheat germ oil for 2 nights, olive oil the next 2. Cover with a plastic bag or sleep cap and shampoo out each morning. After skipping one day, the sequence should be resumed. Substitutes for those oils are aloe vera gel, garlic oil squeezed from capsules, jojoba or sesame oil, lard (plain or mixed half and half with castor oil), equal parts of olive oil and oil of rosemary, onion juice or sliced raw onion rubbed over the scalp, or 2 tablespoons vodka blended with 1 tablespoon honey (onion juice may be added, if desired).

Rub-in Remedies Twice daily, massage the scalp with a tonic prepared by steeping ¼ cup cayenne pepper with 1 ¼ cups vodka for 2 weeks (shaking the bottle every day), then straining through a cheesecloth-lined sieve. For alternatives to rub in once a day, steep onion slices in a cup of brandy for 2 weeks, strain, then add a cup of water. Or steep 1 tablespoon dried nettle with 2 teaspoons *each* camomile, rosemary, and sage in a cup of gin for 2 weeks, strain, then add ½ cup cooled nettle tea. Another daily option is to rub the scalp with equal parts of castor oil and white iodine, then sit in the sun for 15 minutes before washing it off.

Nerve Pressure and Massage

To stop falling hair and stimulate new growth, rub the fingernails of one hand directly across the nails of the opposite hand for 5 minutes. Repeat three times a day.[59]

Relaxation and Mental Imagery

Stress and tension constrict blood vessels in the scalp to impair the delivery of nourishment to hair roots. Severe or prolonged stress may release enough adrenaline to force an abnormal number of hairs into the telogen phase and cause temporary hair loss or may trigger an overproduction of androgen on the scalp and instigate or accelerate male- or female-pattern baldness. Relaxing for a few minutes each day with the techniques described in the Introduction helps relieve stress before hair is harmed. Incorporating a visualization of new hairs growing up from the follicles may speed regrowth.

Sources (see Bibliography)

2, 6, 7, 16, 17, 29, 40, 42, 44, 49, 53, 59, 64, 65, 75, 87, 92, 98, 108, 112, 142, 144, 146, 150, 151, 165, 173, 186, 190, 193, 195, 198, 203, 215, 220, 224, 258, 262, 284, 294, 300, 304, 305, 312, 313

Hay Fever and Sinus Problems

"Allergic rhinitis" is the medical term for the seasonal indisposition known as "catarrhal affection" until given the name "hay fever" during the British haying season of 1820. Perennial allergic rhinitis refers to the year-round variation. Irritated, swollen sinus membranes and postnasal drip often accompany hay fever's itchy eyes, sneezing, and drippy or stuffy nose. Sinus pain persisting longer than 3 or 4 days could be an indication of sinusitis, a bacterial infection requiring medical evaluation. Severe cases of hay fever may also warrant professional treatment—desensitizing shots (allergen immunotherapy) are about 85 percent successful against allergies to dust, grass, ragweed, and trees.[45]

Researchers believe that individuals who develop hay fever have a genetic tendency to produce greater than normal amounts of an antibody that stimulates reactions to substances having no effect on most people. The allergic response causes histamine to be released by the antibodies produced to protect the mucous membranes of the eyes and air passages and makes the capillaries more permeable to the fluid accumulation that accentuates swelling and irritation. Although emotional stress has been known to trigger hay fever attacks, they are nearly always due to airborne allergens.

Air conditioning helps keep pollens out of the house; room air purifiers help remove indoor irritants such as tobacco smoke. Household molds can be partially controlled by cleaning humidifiers at regular intervals and by keeping houseplants mold-free by frequent repotting and the removal of dead leaves. The inhalation of steam from a vaporizer or from a pot of boiling potatoes helps thin mucus so it can be expelled from clogged sinuses. If nasal passages are too dry, saline nose drops may relieve the discomfort. For a homemade saline solution, dissolve ¼ teaspoon salt in ½ cup warm water. Using commercial nasal drops or sprays for longer than a week is not recommended—when discontinued, they may cause a rebound effect of increased congestion that can lead to blocked sinuses and infection.[76, 186]

Diet

Doctors have found that dormant food allergies can be aroused as a result of the stress that hay fever puts on the body's immune system. Chocolate or coffee can intensify the effects of other mild allergies to instigate or aggravate hay fever for some people, but an old English remedy calls for drinking 3 or 4 cups of a mixture of coffee and hot chocolate each day. Persons who are allergic to ragweed may experience similar reactions after eating cantaloupe, cucumber, watermelon, or zucchini. Alcohol, fried foods, salt, sugar, and tobacco are also suspected of contributing to allergic conditions. Eating a small garlic clove (or taking two garlic perles) every 6 hours has been known to relieve congestion caused by hay fever. Some authorities believe that hay fever is due to an excess of fats and concentrated carbohydrates and can be remedied by adhering to a low-fat, sugar-free diet.

To compensate for the body fluids lost through sneezing and nasal discharge, liquid intake should be at least 2 quarts per day. The enzymes in 1 or 2 glasses daily of raw juices in any combination of beet, cabbage, carrot, celery, cucumber, parsley, spinach, and tomato may help neutralize the histamines. Drinking one or two cups of fenugreek, or red clover tea (or taking two capsules of freeze-dried nettle) each day during hay fever season has alleviated symptoms for many people. Alternating 1 day of regular meals with 1 day of nothing but fresh fruits and vegetables and their juices has brought relief for some seasonal hay fever sufferers.[305] Eating yogurt every day (or taking acidophilus capsules with meals) has proven beneficial for others.[17] Deficiencies of protein or of almost any nutrient can increase cell permeability and hay fever sensitivity.

Supplements (see note on page xii)

Individual reactions are so varied that no single supplement can be a universal panacea. For Gayle D. and her friends, a vitamin combination is more satisfactory than commercial antihistamines, with their side effects. Gayle's prescribed medications made her either too drowsy or too tense to cope with her second-grade class. She couldn't hibernate for 3 weeks every spring, so she took antihistamines only at night and endured the days in bleary-eyed, sniffling misery. Then a friend suggested she try taking 500 milligrams of vitamin C with bioflavonoids, 100 milligrams of pantothenic acid, and 50 milligrams of vitamin B$_6$ every few hours. The combination worked so well that she offered to share the magic formula and was a bit abashed to discover that her fellow teachers had already evolved their own variations and that the art teacher doubled Gayle's dosage twice a day when she had hay fever problems.

Because the body's immune system can be weakened by allergic reactions, many doctors and nutritional consultants advise giving it a boost with a daily multivitamin-mineral tablet in addition to any optional supplements.

Vitamin A In the form of beta carotene, 25,000 to 75,000 IU daily for 1 month, then 10,000 to 25,000 IU per day. Vitamin A decreases cell permeability, protects the mucous membranes, and reduces susceptibility to infection.

B Complex One comprehensive tablet daily to compensate for the stress of allergic reactions and to avoid creating deficiencies of other Bs when megadoses of pantothenic acid and B$_6$ are used. Taking brewer's yeast tablets for 2 months in advance of the hay fever season minimizes the problem for some individuals.[312]

Vitamin C and Bioflavonoids 1,000 to 5,000 milligrams of vitamin C, plus at least 100 milligrams of bioflavonoids for each 1,000 milligrams of vitamin C, in divided daily doses, to decrease cell permeability and help detoxify foreign substances entering the body.

Vitamin E 100 to 600 IU daily. Most effective when taken before symptoms begin, vitamin E is believed to repress the release of histamine and reduce the discomforts of hay fever.[98]

Tissue Salts For acute hay fever, alternate doses of 3X Ferr. Phos. and Nat. Mur. each half hour until relieved. For chronic hay fever, take alternating doses of 12X Kali. Phos, Nat. Mur. and Silicea every 2 hours for 2 days, then twice daily. For sneezing, try Linda. C.'s solution. Although she had never had allergy problems, pregnancy produced paroxysms of sneezing at the slightest touch of cool air—especially when she opened the refrigerator door. As uncomfortable as the sneezing bouts were, they were also comical. A friend, unable to resist laughing as Linda attempted to cover her nose while supporting her abdomen with both hands, gave her three tiny pellets to place under her tongue. The sneezes ceased before the friend could explain that the pills were Silicea, a tissue salt, and from then on Linda kept a container of 6X Silicea within easy reach.

Folk Remedies

Eighteenth-century treatments included a diet of foxes' lungs, the application of leeches to draw out evil humors, and smoking mullein leaves in a corncob pipe. Less exotic remedies, like applying a warm washcloth over eyes and cheekbones to alleviate sinus pain or exercising vigorously for 5 minutes to constrict small blood vessels and curtail hay fever symptoms are still being used with success.

Apple Cider Vinegar For nasal drip, three times a day for 4 days drink a glass of water containing 5 tablespoons of apple cider vinegar. Gradually reduce the amounts as the condition clears.

Citrus Peel Each morning and evening take 1 teaspoon grated lemon or orange peel, plain or sweetened with honey. Or soak small strips of orange peel in apple cider vinegar, drain and cook with honey, then eat at bedtime to prevent clogged nasal passages.

Cod Liver Oil or Castor Oil To relieve nasal congestion, each morning take 1 tablespoon of cod liver oil, or stir 5 drops of castor oil into a glass of juice and drink before breakfast.

Horseradish or Onion To help clear sinus passages, each morning and evening take ½ teaspoon prepared horseradish mixed with a few drops of lemon juice. Or cover a sliced, raw onion with 1 cup of water, let stand for 1 minute, remove the onion and sip the water. Or drink a cup of scalded milk containing a tablespoon of grated onion.

Nerve Pressure and Massage

For Sneezing Press directly above the center of the upper lip.

For Hay Fever Symptoms

❍ Use the index fingers to press in an upward direction on both sides of the nostrils.

❍ Press and massage the center of the chest, then a point 1½ inches directly below the navel.

○ Massage the thumbs, index and middle fingers, and the webs between them on both hands. Or rub the tip of each toe, just below the toenail, and massage the bottom of each foot 1 inch from the heel pad toward the toes on the outer edge of the foot.

See also **Allergy**

Sources (see Bibliography)

2, 4, 6, 17, 29, 42, 45, 56, 57, 59, 60, 61, 63, 64, 72, 76, 83, 84, 87, 91, 92, 98, 110, 135, 144, 150, 151, 164, 171, 186, 202, 207, 218, 262, 284, 293, 300, 301, 302, 305, 306, 312, 313, 316

Headaches

Pain in the head usually is caused by contraction of the neck, forehead, or scalp muscles (tension headache), or by constriction or dilation of blood vessels in the brain (vascular headache—see also "Migraine and Cluster Headaches"). Organic headaches may be induced by eyestrain, injury, or an underlying physical disorder. Medical advice should be sought for any headache accompanied by blurred vision, dizziness, or numbness, and for persistent headaches.

The localized misery of a sinus headache may result from an allergic reaction or the stuffiness accompanying a head cold. To relieve the congestion, eat chicken soup (scientifically shown to increase mucus movement).[45] Or sip hot anise, fenugreek, or horehound tea. Or strain and drink the liquid from 1 ½ tablespoons minced chives and ½ teaspoon shredded ginger root steeped for 30 minutes in a cup of boiling water. To help open sinus passages and relieve pain, cover the area with a warm compress. Or massage the bony ridges surrounding the eyes. Or press 1 inch out from each nostril and between the eyebrows, or push up against the roof of the mouth with a thumb. Rarely occurring headaches from infected sinuses require professional treatment.

Tension Headaches Associated with mental or physical stress, tension headaches produce either steady or shooting pain with a feeling of tightness. Warm compresses or a warm bath or shower help relax contracted muscles. Squeezing and massaging taut neck and shoulder muscles is often helpful; pressing the high point of each eyebrow may help relieve pain.

Vascular Headaches These include those from hunger or hangover are evidenced by throbbing pain often in only one area of the head. Constricting the distended blood vessels with cold compresses or ice packs may bring relief; simultaneously immersing hands or feet in hot water may assist by drawing excess blood to the extremities.

Headache provokers range from anxiety, constipation, fluorescent lighting, and lack of sleep or oversleeping to low blood sugar, reactions to foods or medications, stuffy or smoke-filled rooms, sun exposure, or changes in the weather. Anything that affects hormonal balance—anger, extreme exertion, even sexual orgasm—may trigger a headache. Menstrual cycles, oral contraceptives, and estrogen supplements make women especially susceptible to headaches.

Over-the-counter painkillers are considered safe for occasional relief, but prolonged use of aspirin can irritate the stomach, acetaminophen and ibuprofen can adversely affect the liver and kidneys.[76, 300] Since headaches can be caused by an accumulation of factors, self-help remedies may need to be experimented with in combination to be effective.

Diet

Eating at regular intervals and having a bedtime snack help prevent the hunger headaches that can occur when blood sugar levels drop too low. Sweets and refined carbohydrates elevate blood sugar only briefly, so the complex carbohydrates of fruits, vegetables, and whole grains should be stressed. For many people, headaches are triggered by the amino acid tyramine, which is found in aged cheeses, chocolate, fermented foods, freshly baked yeast products, and organ meats.[112] Other often-cited offenders are citrus fruits, eggs, milk, wheat, and food additives such as monosodium glutamate (MSG), the nitrites used to preserve meat, sugar substitutes, and the sulfites used on restaurant salads. Drinking a glass of fresh cabbage, celery, lettuce, or other green-vegetable juice may help neutralize reactions from other foodstuffs. Taking activated charcoal tablets an hour before, and immediately after, consuming suspected headache triggers often brings rapid relief by eliminating the toxic substance.[17]

Ample fluid intake, especially during exercise or heat exposure, helps avoid the dehydration and mineral loss from perspiration that can bring on a headache. Too much caffeine constricts blood vessels, can instigate a headache, and should be abjured during tension headaches. However, persons unaccustomed to caffeine may be able to abort a vascular headache by drinking a cup of black coffee, and those who normally have several colas or cups of tea or coffee every day may develop a headache when caffeine deprivation dilates the blood vessels.

Imbibing one alcoholic beverage may relieve a tension headache by dilating constricted blood vessels, but alcohol should be shunned while a throbbing vascular headache is in progress, and too much is always counterproductive. Hangover headaches may be prevented by eating foods containing protein and unsaturated fats prior to and during indulgence—according to *Clinical Research* (April 1992), saturated fats can extend the duration of alcohol's unpleasant effects—and by drinking only light-colored alcohol. As explained in *Men's Health* (December 1991), substances called congeners in red wine and dark liquors can cause hangovers without any alcohol. Drinking a glass of noncarbonated liquid with each ounce of alcohol and having a snack plus a B-complex tablet with a glass of water before retiring compensates for alcohol's diuretic effect and its destruction of B vitamins. If a morning-after headache does appear, coffee and foods high in fructose (honey or fruit or tomato juice) help dissipate the misery.[112]

Supplements (see note on page xii)

Vitamin A In the form of beta carotene, 25,000 IU daily may correct recurring tension headaches due to overuse of the eyes.

B Complex One comprehensive tablet daily to help maintain normal blood vessel dilation. Taking 50 milligrams of niacin at the onset of a tension headache may produce a prickly flush but may relieve the congestion by dilating the capillaries and blood vessels. If fluid retention is responsible for a headache, taking 50 milligrams of B6 often helps remove excess water.[98]

Vitamin C with Bioflavonoids 1,000 to 5,000 milligrams in divided daily doses. Stressful conditions, toxic substances, or painkillers reduce the absorption of vitamin C yet rapidly use up large amounts of it. In some cases, taking 500 milligrams of C every hour has relieved headaches.[98, 313]

Calcium and Magnesium 1,500 milligrams of calcium plus 1,000 milligrams of magnesium (some researchers suggest 1,500 milligrams of magnesium and 750 milligrams of calcium) in divided daily doses to aid muscle relaxation and act as tranquilizers.

Tissue Salts Three 6X tablets dissolved under the tongue each half hour until the condition is relieved: Ferr. Phos. for a throbbing headache; Kali. Sulph. for a generalized tension headache; Mag. Phos. for sharp, shooting pain; Mag. Phos. and Kali. Phos. for a frontal headache.

Exercise and Posture

A program of regular exercise plus a habit of sitting and standing tall with shoulders relaxed help prevent headaches. Mild exercise at the first warning sign of a tension headache may forestall its development. Hunching over a desk or sitting in an awkward position for prolonged periods can contract neck muscles and lead to a headache. Marlys L. "cured" the headaches she experienced every day at the office by training herself to nestle the phone on alternate shoulders and by making a few simple moves. At least once an hour, she sat up straight and slowly turned her head all the way to each side, lowered chin to chest, then tilted her head back as far as it would go. In privacy during her breaks, Marlys placed her palms against her chest, stuck her elbows out and circled them forward and backward three times to stretch and relax the tense muscles.

Folk Remedies

Burying haircut clippings under a rock may not prevent headaches, but some of the folk healers' prescriptions have been scientifically vindicated. The herb feverfew has been found effective for vascular headaches. Eating raw almonds or unsweetened strawberries, or drinking meadowsweet or white willow bark tea may relieve headache pain because they all contain salicylates (the painkilling compound in aspirin).[16, 313]

Apple Cider Vinegar Taking 3 tablespoons of apple cider vinegar with 1 tablespoon of honey, or drinking a glass of water mixed with 1 tablespoon *each* vinegar and honey, at the onset of a headache has achieved anecdotal success.[172] Saturating a bandanna with vinegar and rolling it into a cylinder to tie around the head above the eyebrows is said to reduce the painful pressure.

Herbs Tucking rolled-up marjoram or mint leaves in the nostrils was a sixteenth-century headache nostrum. Drinking a cup of tea (or taking herb capsules) and resting in bed for an hour has more aesthetic appeal. For general relief: angelica (dong quai), basil, camomile, catnip, fenugreek, marshmallow, passion flower, peppermint, sage, rosemary, or thyme. A combination of fenugreek and thyme is recommended for sinus and vascular headaches. Black cohosh is suggested for women with pain in the back of the head.

Lemon Stir a tablespoon of lemon juice into a cup of hot pekoe tea, or add the juice of one lemon to a glass of warm water and stir in a teaspoon of baking soda, then sip slowly while rubbing the white portion of fresh lemon rind over the forehead and temples.

Poultices and Compresses Bind slices of raw apple or potato, a paste of powdered ginger and water, or wilted beet or mint leaves on the forehead. Or place moistened baking soda, crushed garlic, or shredded horseradish or onion between pieces of gauze and apply to the back of the neck and the bend of the elbows for half an hour. Or cover the forehead with a cloth squeezed out of hot thyme tea or a cup of cool basil tea to which 2 tablespoons of witch hazel have been added.

Nerve Pressure and Massage

To abort a fledgling headache or hasten the departure of a full-grown one, press or massage any or all of the following points.

- ○ The center of the top of the head; the depressions in front of the upper part of the ears; and the hollows at the back of the head on each side of the spine.
- ○ The middle of both shoulders, about 1 inch toward the back.
- ○ The back of each hand where the bones of the thumb and index finger meet; then the crease on the inner wrists, in line with the little fingers.
- ○ Two inches down from the outside of each kneecap, and the depression behind the anklebone on each leg.
- ○ The top of both feet an inch above the web between the first and second toes, and the bottom of each foot between the base of the third toe and the ball of the foot.

Relaxation

Regular use of any relaxation technique (see Introduction) helps avoid the stress buildup that can trigger headaches. When a headache does occur, it may be possible to "wish" it away, or at least lessen its severity, by taking a few deep breaths, relaxing tense muscles, visualizing a peaceful scene, and concluding with the affirmation that the entire body will feel refreshed and pain-free following the period of relaxation.

Sources (see Bibliography)

16, 17, 26, 29, 45, 46, 47, 56, 58, 59, 60, 64, 65, 69, 75, 76, 98, 102, 108, 111, 112, 144, 147, 150, 151, 164, 172, 176, 177, 179, 186, 201, 202, 212, 218, 235, 236, 238, 244, 255, 256, 260, 265, 281, 293, 294, 297, 300, 305, 312, 313

Hearing Loss

Conductive hearing loss, due to interference with the transmission of sound waves to the inner ear, is usually correctable. The cause may be anything from a benign cyst, eardrum damage from an injury or the pressure of a deep-water dive, earwax or fluid in the ear (see "Ear Problems"), to otitis media (a middle-ear infection) or otosclerosis (a disorder of the tiny bones in the middle ear). In perceptive (sensorineural) hearing loss or nerve deafness, sounds that reach the inner ear are not transmitted to the brain. Formerly regarded as a degenerative problem that develops with age, most perceptive hearing loss is now considered to be noise induced—and it is rapidly increasing among people of all ages. A study reported in *American Health* (February 1992) found that 13 percent of high school seniors and 7 percent of the second graders tested had noise-induced hearing loss—whereas, 10 years earlier, only 3 percent of the students in grades 2 through 12 had impaired hearing.

Loud noise damages delicate inner-ear hair cells that translate sounds into nerve impulses; repeated exposure results in hearing loss.[98] Even an accumulation of low-level sounds from air conditioners, appliances, background music, and outside traffic can be hazardous to hearing. The potential harm from noise depends on duration as well as on intensity, which is measured in decibels (dB). The risk from exposure is magnified by alcohol, which impedes the protective contraction of inner-ear muscles, and by smoking, which reduces the amount of oxygen reaching the ear's blood vessels. Normal conversation registers 50 dB; a vacuum cleaner or washing machine, 75; a food blender, blow dryer, electric razor, or city traffic, 85; power lawn mowers or symphony orchestras, 90 to 105; amplified rock concerts, car stereos or headsets, power boats, stadium sporting events, or rifle shots, 110 to 140 dB.

The Occupational Safety and Health Administration (OSHA) permits workplace exposure to 90 dB of noise for 8 hours a day, 100 dB for 2 hours, or

115 dB for 15 minutes. Audiologists believe 75 dB to be the "safe" limit for extended periods and advise the use of ear protectors whenever the sound level exceeds 90 dB—the point at which it is necessary to raise the voice to carry on a conversation. Protective earplugs or earmuffs can provide up to 35 decibels of noise reduction without blocking desirable exterior sounds.

Medical evaluation is warranted whenever hearing loss becomes noticeable because conditions or medications unrelated to the hearing process may be responsible. High cholesterol, diabetes or hypoglycemia, infections, kidney trouble, low thyroid function, and rheumatoid arthritis have been linked to hearing impairment, as have antibiotic treatment, large doses of aspirin, and heart or blood pressure medicines.[75, 255]

Diet and Supplements (see note on page xii)

Diet as well as quiet can affect hearing health. Drinking two glasses daily of a mixture of fresh carrot and citrus or pineapple juice is believed to provide enzymes that energize sensory receptor cells to help restore hearing.[305] Excess dietary fat or cholesterol can adversely affect hearing by impeding blood flow to the inner ear. Clinical studies show that hearing acuity improves by as much as 30 decibels with a high-fiber, low-fat diet and worsens when fatty foods are added.[147, 312] Arnie E. knew he had a high-frequency hearing loss—he couldn't hear the warbling ring of the alarm clock—but did not arrange for a hearing test until the lower tones on the television began to fade away. His appointment was postponed because of a severe stomach upset that turned out to be a gallbladder attack. By sticking to a low-fat diet and taking three 1,200-milligram lecithin capsules with each meal, Arnie not only avoided gallbladder surgery but regained his ability to hear low tones.

Vitamin A   In the form of beta carotene, 25,000 IU daily. Otosclerosis, which is sometimes treated with injections of vitamin A, may be slowed or improved with oral supplements.

B Complex   One comprehensive tablet daily. Taking an additional 100 milligrams of niacinamide with each meal and incorporating 1 to 3 tablespoons of brewer's yeast with foods or beverages has improved hearing for some patients.[98]

Vitamin C   1,000 to 5,000 milligrams in divided daily doses, plus 400 IU of vitamin E a day is believed to improve hearing by increasing the amount of blood and oxygen reaching the ears.

Minerals   One daily multimineral that includes glutamic acid and 750 milligrams of magnesium. Researchers have found that loud noise lowers the amount of magnesium in the ears and that lack of this mineral constricts blood vessels and increases hearing impairment.[108] Deficiencies of other minerals—especially manganese, potassium, and zinc—are also associated with hearing loss.

Tissue Salts   For chronic impairment not caused by bone damage, take two three-tablet daily doses, alternately, of Kali. Mur., Kali. Phos., Kali. Sulph., and Silicea. If the Eustachian tubes are swollen, substitute Nat. Mur. for the Kali. Phos.

Exercise

Regular exercise such as walking or swimming may reduce hearing loss by improving blood circulation to the ears, but according to a report in the *New England Journal of Medicine* (February 1991), the jarring force of high-impact aerobics may increase the impairment by disrupting transmission of information from the ears to the brain.

Folk Remedies and Tips

Mixing 2 teaspoons *each* apple cider vinegar and raw honey in a glass of water to sip with each meal is a folk medicine prescription for preserving good hearing and reversing many types of hearing loss. The nightly insertion of a cotton ball saturated with of almond oil is thought to correct hearing loss caused by abnormally dry ear passages. Ear drops reported to restore hearing include castor oil, onion juice, or half-and-half blends of almond oil (or olive oil) and garlic oil or of wine and fresh cabbage juice. Recent studies show that twice-daily doses of 80 milligrams of ginkgo biloba (an herb used medicinally in China for 5,000 years) improves age-related deafness more effectively than standard medical therapy.[51]

When attending concerts or sporting events, experts advise escaping from the noisy environment for 5 minutes each hour to allow the ears to recuperate. If turning down the background noise of radios, televisions, or busy restaurants is not feasible, selecting a location near sound-absorbent surfaces such as drapes and upholstered furniture diminishes the decibels. For high-frequency hearing loss, adjusting the bass and treble tones of the radio or television may be more effective than turning up the volume.[99]

Nerve Pressure and Massage

○ For several minutes several times a day, bite down on a wad of cotton or a pencil eraser placed behind the last tooth on each side of the jaw. Follow with finger pressure against the floor of the mouth for an equal period, then with brief pressure against the roof of the mouth and the back of the tongue.

○ Once a day, use the fingernail of the left middle finger to lift the nails on the third and fourth fingers of the right hand for 1 minute each.

○ Two or three times a day, massage the tips of both ring fingers and their knuckles; then gently press the tips of all the fingers with the teeth of a comb.

○ Once each day, massage the soles of the feet just beneath the third, fourth, and little toes.

Sources (see Bibliography)

2, 26, 29, 49, 51, 58, 59, 64, 65, 75, 87, 98, 99, 108, 111, 112, 147, 164, 171, 177, 186, 202, 203, 213, 220, 244, 255, 281, 293, 294, 300, 305, 312, 313

Heartburn and Hiatal Hernia

Heartburn, the burning sensation that begins in the lower chest and may extend to the throat, occurs when gastric acids backflow through the sphincter (ring of muscle) separating the stomach from the esophagus. During the digestive process, this lower esophageal sphincter normally opens to permit food to enter the stomach, then quickly pinches itself shut. The malfunction that allows gastroesophageal reflux (heartburn) occurs when this sphincter is inappropriately relaxed or is weakened by age so that it cannot close completely, or when pressure is exerted by constrictive clothing, an overly full stomach, pregnancy, or obesity. Occasionally, a hiatal hernia, a portion of the stomach bulging upward through the diaphragm (the sheet of muscle dividing chest and abdomen), is responsible for heartburn. Research shows that at least half the population has this structural abnormality, yet few suffer from heartburn, and many people with heartburn do not have hiatal hernias.[10, 177]

Antihistamines, oral contraceptives, tranquilizers, and other drugs promote heartburn for some people. Drinking alcohol or smoking relaxes the esophageal sphincter and can contribute to heartburn. Vigorous aerobic exercise can cause gastric acids to spill over into the esophagus. Bending over or lying down after a meal encourages gastric reflux. If it is necessary to recline, lying on the left side is recommended. A study reported in the March 1992 issue of *American Health* showed that left-siders experienced only half as much reflux as right-siders. Taking a sedative to sleep through the pain is not recommended because acids allowed to remain in the esophagus can lead to precancerous erosion of its lining. The reflux fluid should be neutralized as quickly as possible. Swallowing saliva (which can be increased at least eight times by chewing gum)[313] or sipping plain water may wash away the displaced gastric juices. Drinking a little milk or papaya juice, or chewing a calcium carbonate or papaya tablet usually douses the fire in a burning esophagus.

Occasional occurrences of heartburn are not considered dangerous unless the discomfort is accompanied by nausea, pallor, shortness of breath, or sweating, in which case immediate medical attention is required to preclude the possibility of a heart condition. Persistent or chronic heartburn that does not respond to home remedies also warrants a medical examination. Prolonged use of antacids can cause bowel irregularities, allow fluid retention, interfere with the body's absorption of nutrients and medications, mask potentially serious illness, and result in disorders of the bones or kidneys.[76, 177, 186]

Grace E. began having heartburn when she plunged into painting after the death of her husband. With a picture always in progress and no necessity for preparing regular meals, she didn't bother about eating until the light faded in the evening, then ate heartily. A visit to the doctor produced a diagnosis of hiatal hernia and a pamphlet of suggestions for minimizing heartburn occurrences. Daytime problems disappeared when she ate several snack-meals, but she still experienced some nighttime distress. Rather than hire someone to put 6-inch blocks under her bed so gravity could help keep the acid where it belonged, Grace stuffed old telephone books and pillows under the head-end of the mattress. Success! No more being awakened by burning sensations in her chest.

Diet and Supplements

Slowly eating small, frequent meals in a relaxed atmosphere helps assure the efficiency of the lower esophageal sphincter. Hurried eating encourages air swallowing, which can result in heartburn. As the swallowed air warms to body temperature it expands, rises to the top of the stomach, and can take acids along with it if belched into the esophagus. For this reason, burp inducers like baking soda or peppermint tea are not recommended for heartburn sufferers.[98, 112]

Not drinking any liquids 30 minutes before, during, or after meals may allow the digestive enzymes to perform at full strength and prevent heartburn. Sugar may be a source of irritation, particularly when taken on an empty stomach in the form of candy or soft drinks. Certain foods—most commonly citrus juices, cabbage, onions, and tomato products—ignite heartburn for some individuals; the culprits usually can be identified through experimentation and then avoided.

A fiber-rich diet prevents constipation and the straining for evacuation that can push the stomach upward, aggravate a hiatal hernia, and contribute to heartburn. Low-fat, high-protein foods such as dried beans, fish, skinless chicken or turkey breast, and skim milk improve the muscle tone of the sphincter.[186] Fatty foods increase acid production, delay digestion, and prompt the release of hormones that open the esophageal valve.[47, 111] After-dinner liqueurs, chocolate candies or mints, and caffeine-containing beverages can further relax a loose lower sphincter to light heartburn's fire.

For all heartburn, but especially when the pain goes through to the back, take frequent doses of three tablets *each* Ferr. Phos. and Nat. Mur. in the 6X potency.

Folk Remedies

Mealtime preventives for the heartburn-prone include eating a daily serving of green peas, or a bowl of cooked buckwheat groats or oatmeal each morning; or sipping a glass of water containing 2 teaspoons of apple cider vinegar with each meal (an equal amount of honey may be stirred in, if desired); or drinking a glass of milk before or after eating.

To relieve the distress of heartburn, folk healers suggest thoroughly chewing and swallowing a teaspoon of dried, grated citrus peel; a stick of raw carrot or celery, or a kiwi fruit; a spoonful of uncooked oat flakes; or hot, buttered raisin toast sprinkled with cardamom and cinnamon. Other options include drinking "lettuce water" prepared by blending two iceberg lettuce leaves with ¾ cup of water; taking two capsules of powdered ginger; eating a teaspoon of brown or white sugar or a piece of horehound candy; or sipping anise, caraway, peppermint or slippery elm tea. Slowly drinking ½ cup water with a teaspoon of lemon juice or swallowing a tablespoon of lemon juice or apple cider vinegar is said to stop heartburn for people whose stomachs do not produce enough acid—taking betaine hydrochloride tablets after meals is sometimes advised to compensate for the lack of stomach acid.[17]

Nerve Pressure and Massage

Press or massage a point 1 inch to the left of the center of the chest for 10 seconds, release for 10 seconds, and repeat three times.

Sources (see Bibliography)

10, 17, 28, 29, 42, 47, 49, 64, 75, 76, 87, 98, 109, 111, 112, 135, 148, 150, 152, 164, 171, 177, 186, 201, 202, 203, 214, 240, 254, 255, 262, 287, 294, 300, 304, 305, 306, 312, 313

Heat Disorders

Under normal conditions, the cooling effect of perspiration evaporating from the skin dissipates excess body heat. Overexposure to external heat, especially if compounded by the internal heat generated during physical activity, can cause dehydration and mineral depletion from excessive sweating and can result in heat cramps or heat exhaustion. If the body's heat-regulating system fails, a life-threatening heatstroke can occur.

Preventive Guidelines

○ If moving to or visiting a hotter climate, allow time for the body to adjust. It takes 1 to 3 weeks of gradually increasing exposure for full acclimation.[75]

○ Avoid exertion during the hottest part of the day, especially if the air is humid. Diabetics, the elderly, and people who are obese or are taking beta blockers, diuretics, or tranquilizers are at risk for heat-related problems,[186, 254] and they are advised to alternate 30-minute cooling-off periods with equal amounts of heat exposure.

○ Wear lightweight, loose-fitting clothing to allow air circulation; a broad-brimmed hat and heat-reflecting light colors if in the sun. As suggested in *American Health* (February 1992), placing a wet handkerchief under a ventilated hat will air-condition the head on hot, dry days.

○ Drink extra fluids. Increase salt consumption unless prone to high blood pressure. Under average circumstances, the body loses and needs to replace 2 to 3 quarts of water daily—more than a quart can be lost in perspiration during an hour's activity in a hot environment.[291]

Diet and Supplements (see note on page xii)

Perspiration carries away electrolytes (dissolved minerals such as calcium, magnesium, potassium, and sodium). A balanced diet accentuating fresh fruits and vegetables and supplemented with a daily multi-vitamin-mineral helps supply replacements. Salty foods provide sodium. Salt tablets are not recommended; they hold fluid in the stomach instead of releasing it for perspiration production.[293]

The fiery foods favored by natives of torrid regions have been found to improve heat tolerance. Cayenne and other hot peppers first stimulate, then desensitize internal heat detectors so that body temperature drops. Chewing honeycomb, or occasionally biting a chunk of gauze-wrapped granulated honey tucked next to the cheek like chewing tobacco, is another body-cooling remedy verified by scientific studies.[150]

To help prevent heat disorders during physical activity on a hot day, drink one or two glasses of water or nonalcoholic, caffeine-free liquid before exposure; several additional ounces each 20 minutes while in the heat; and another glass while cooling down. The rapid metabolization of alcohol raises body temperature, and, like caffeine, alcohol is a mild diuretic that speeds dehydration.[47] Fruit juice or tomato juice helps replenish lost electrolytes, as does the addition of ¼ teaspoon of salt to each glass of water during prolonged heat exposure.

Heat Cramps

Due to excessive fluid loss through perspiration, heat cramps usually attack legs, arms, or the abdomen during or shortly after strenuous exercise in a heated environment. The painful paroxysms occur in firemen and skiers wearing insulated garments, as well as in outdoor laborers and leisure-time players. To relieve the spasms, relax in a cool spot while sipping ½ cup of cool liquid every 15 minutes for an hour. Adding ¼ teaspoon salt to 8 ounces of fruit juice or tomato juice speeds recuperation. Gently massaging and stretching the cramped muscles may bring immediate relief.

Heat Exhaustion

Formerly called heat prostration, heat exhaustion results from body fluid depletion. It may signal its approach with queasiness, fatigue, or faintness, or may strike in full force up to half an hour after exposure.

Characteristic symptoms are clammy skin with profuse sweating, dizziness, blurred vision, shallow breathing, nausea, and headache. If promptly treated, heat exhaustion is usually transient, but if symptoms worsen or last longer than an hour medical help should be obtained.

First-Aid Tips Recline in a cool place with the feet elevated. Cool the body by applying cold, wet cloths or taking a cool bath. Alcohol- or caffeine-containing beverages are not advised, but ½ cup of cold (not iced) liquid should be sipped every 15 minutes for an hour—ginseng root, licorice root, or peppermint tea is recommended by herbalists. To replenish electrolytes as well as fluid, stir ¼ to 1 teaspoon salt in 8 ounces of water; or ¼ teaspoon baking soda and ⅛ teaspoon salt in a glass of lemonade; or drink fruit juice or tomato juice. Homeopathic practitioners advise taking three 12X tablets of the tissue salt Nat. Mur. with each of the half-cups of liquid. To improve respiration, alternating doses of the same potency of Ferr. Phos. is suggested.

Heatstroke (Sunstroke)

Whether preceded by heat exhaustion symptoms or appearing abruptly, a life-threatening heatstroke can occur when the body's internal cooling mechanism malfunctions. Perspiration ceases, internal temperature rises, and the skin becomes hot and dry. (Sweating may continue, however, in the exertional heatstroke sometimes suffered by athletes.) Pulse and respiration speed up. There may be nausea and vomiting, mental confusion, and if not treated, possible brain damage.

Medical assistance should be obtained as quickly as possible. In the interim, the head should be kept elevated; body temperature should be lowered by removing outer clothing and placing ice packs at the neck, armpits, and groin; and the skin cooled with alcohol rubs or cold, wet cloths. If rectal temperature is above 106 degrees Fahrenheit, total immersion in cold water and continuous massage is recommended to help get cooler blood to the brain. Cold applications should be stopped when the temperature drops to 101 degrees, and repeated if the temperature rises again.[148] If the victim is conscious, cool liquids should be sipped as for heat exhaustion.

Sources (see Bibliography)

42, 47, 53, 63, 64, 65, 75, 108, 111, 148, 149, 150, 159, 184, 186, 254, 255, 281, 291, 293, 294, 322

Hemorrhoids (Piles)

Dilated rectal veins are an age-old complaint. It is said that the Philistines were plagued with piles after capturing the Ark of the Covenant and that Napoleon might have won the Battle of Waterloo had his hemorrhoids allowed him to mount his horse on the day he planned to begin the battle. Many of the estimated 80 percent of Americans with hemorrhoids become aware of the problem only when the bulging veins protrude from the anal opening, rupture to cause bleeding, or occur as painful external varicosities. As explained by Sidney E. Wanderman, M.D., in the book *Hemorrhoids* (Consumer Reports Books, 1991), internal membranes lack pain-sensitive nerve fibers; external varicosities are dense with pain nerves. Although rarely a precancerous condition, professional diagnosis and treatment is warranted when there is severe pain or frequent bleeding.

Genetic inheritance and increasing age are predisposing factors, but most hemorrhoids result from undue pressure on the anal veins from sitting or standing for long periods, frequent lifting of heavy objects, pregnancy, or obesity. The primary cause, however, is constipation. Straining to pass a bowel movement or sitting on a toilet for more than 5 minutes at a time forces tissue near the anus to become engorged with blood. Overuse of enemas or laxatives can destroy the body's normal ability to eliminate waste and can instigate or worsen hemorrhoid problems. To gently cleanse the anal area after each bowel movement, premoistened baby wipes, facial tissues impregnated with moisturizing cream, or toilet tissue dampened under the faucet is recommended.

Baths

A daily warm-water bath helps shrink swollen veins, control inflammation, and reduce the itching of hemorrhoids. For a sitz bath treatment in a tub, sit with knees raised—or feet elevated on the sides of the bathtub—in

6 inches of water for 10 to 45 minutes two to four times a day. Sitz baths may be more beneficial when ¼ cup epsom salts or witch hazel is added, or when a cup of cornstarch or several cups of strong camomile or white oak bark tea are swished in the warm water. If a bath is impractical, a towel squeezed out of any of the solutions and applied for 20 minutes may bring relief.

Diet

A high-fiber diet with lots of liquids may prevent hemorrhoids from developing and will soothe the symptoms of existing ones by forming soft, bulky stools that pass without aggravating tender tissues. In addition to drinking six to eight glasses of water daily and increasing the proportion of fruits, vegetables, and whole-grain products, it may be beneficial to augment each meal with 2 or 3 teaspoons of wheat bran, corn bran, or rice bran, or with a psyllium supplement.

Foods reputedly helpful for hemorrhoids include apples, all members of the cabbage family, carrots, lima beans, papayas, parsnips, plums, prunes, pumpkin, sweet potatoes, and winter squash. Eating a boiled leek or a serving of fried onions or onion soup every day is an 1870's remedy for persistent hemorrhoidal bleeding. Carrot juice and okra juice are believed to promote healing. Any combination of juices from apples, beets, celery, citrus fruit, cucumbers, pineapple, and spinach is also considered beneficial.

Supplements (see note on page xii)

Ointments containing vitamins A and D or E may be helpful for lubrication and relief of pain. Oral supplements have been found to benefit many hemorrhoid sufferers.

Vitamin A In the form of beta carotene, 25,000 IU daily to promote healing.

B Complex One comprehensive tablet daily, plus 10 to 50 milligrams of B6 with each meal to improve digestion and reduce stress on the rectum.

Vitamin C with Bioflavonoids 1,000 to 5,000 milligrams in divided daily doses to strengthen capillaries in the veins near the anus and to aid healing.

Calcium and Magnesium 800 to 1,500 milligrams of calcium plus 500 to 750 milligrams of magnesium to assist normal blood clotting. With medical approval, altering the amounts of these minerals to 600 to 800 milligrams of calcium plus 1,200 to 1,600 milligrams of magnesium may be beneficial.

Vitamin E 400 to 800 IU daily. Vitamin E is believed to improve circulation, promote normal blood clotting and healing, and help prevent or dissolve blood clots in hemorrhoidal varicosities. To augment oral supplements, vitamin E oil or wheat germ oil (which contains vitamin E), or liquid lecithin can be applied to external hemorrhoids. For painful internal hemorrhoids, pierced capsules may be used as suppositories, or an ounce of vitamin E oil or wheat germ oil can be injected into the rectum with a baby syringe.

Tissue Salts Unless otherwise indicated, take hourly doses for an acute condition, three or four daily doses for chronic hemorrhoids.

- For painful or bleeding hemorrhoids, take two tablets of 6X Ferr. Phos. every 10 minutes until the condition improves, then every hour or so, and apply an external compress of three tablets dissolved in hot water.
- If accompanied by low back pain, take 12X Calc. Fluor. internally and dissolve three tablets in ½ cup warm water to use as an external lotion. If the pain is sharp, take 6X Mag. Phos.

Exercise

Moderate exercise, such as walking, improves circulation and helps keep anal blood vessels from overinflating. Passive exercise—reclining on the left side for 20 minutes at least twice a day—decreases the pressure that pregnancy or obesity puts on rectal veins. The knee-chest position (achieved by kneeling with shoulders on the floor and elevating the buttocks) relieves gravitational pull on hemorrhoidal muscles.

Folk Remedies

Folk healers advise applying petroleum jelly ½ inch inside the rectum before each bowel movement and, at bedtime, applying a coating of petroleum jelly blended with witch hazel. As reported in the January 1991 issue of *Health After 50*, many experts believe petroleum jelly or plain zinc oxide is as effective as products formulated specifically for hemorrhoid relief and is free of their side effects—preparations containing local anesthetics or vasoconstrictors may oversensitize the affected area if used on a regular basis. Folk medicine offers many other options.

Aloe Vera Gel Apply the gel to external hemorrhoids, or to relieve bleeding, insert a suppository cut from a peeled aloe leaf.

Apple Cider Vinegar To stop anal itching and "cure" chronic hemorrhoids, stir a teaspoon of vinegar in a glass of water to sip with each meal, then use another glass of the same mixture for external applications throughout the day.

Fruit To reduce irritation and help stop bleeding, wrap a tablespoon of finely chopped raw cranberries in cheesecloth (or drench a cotton ball with papaya juice), insert in the painful area, and replenish after an hour.

Herbs Cayenne tea is thought to relieve hemorrhoids by stimulating circulation. Stoneroot is believed to strengthen hemorrhoidal veins when two capsules are taken between meals twice daily during acute attacks, once a day for maintenance. Flax seed, rose hips, slippery elm, or white oak bark teas can be sipped every 4 hours, applied externally, or injected into the rectum 2 tablespoons at a time with a baby syringe. Teas of goldenseal, gotu kola, or yarrow can be used as external poultices to reduce swelling and alleviate pain.

Ointments and Poultices An ice pack or cold-water compress may ease discomfort. Castor oil, cocoa butter, or cod liver oil can be used to coat inflamed tissue. Some folk practitioners suggest simmering strained white oak bark tea until thick, then combining it with an equal amount of white vegetable shortening. A poultice of chopped green onions cooked in white vegetable shortening can be applied at bedtime. Another option is simmering 2 tablespoons of smoking tobacco with ¼ cup butter and applying the strained liquid three times a day.

Potato or Cucumber To reduce pain and swelling, make a suppository from a raw potato (coat it with vitamin E oil, if desired) and insert it overnight. An unpeeled cucumber slice may be used in the same manner 3 times a week.

Witch Hazel One of the ingredients approved for hemorrhoid preparations by the Federal Drug Administration, witch hazel shrinks external hemorrhoids and has been utilized for hundreds of years to alleviate itching, bleeding, and pain. As a soothing substitute for toilet paper, small squares of soft cloth can be moistened with a mixture of witch hazel and glycerin. Joel F. uses witch hazel ice to keep his hemorrhoidal flareups under control at work. Commercial products and a "doughnut" cushion failed to relieve his misery, so Joel freezes witch hazel in little medicine cups, wraps each one in a square of soft cloth, and stores them in a container in the lunchroom freezer-refrigerator. Every hour or so during the day, he presses the cloth-covered ice against his throbbing posterior to shrink and numb the swollen veins.

Nerve Pressure and Massage

○ Use the handle of a tablespoon to press down on the center of the tongue as far back as possible without gagging; maintain pressure for 2 minutes. Then push down on the depression at the hollow of the throat at the center of the collarbones and, at the same time, push up on the tip of the coccyx (tailbone). Maintain pressure for 10 seconds, release for 10 seconds, and repeat three times.

○ Massage the outer edges of the inside of both hands with a press-and-roll motion. Then use the thumbs to massage the center of the inside of the arms about one-third of the way between the wrist and the elbow.

○ Massage all around the heels on both feet, pressing in toward the bone and down toward the heel pad. Then massage the cord on the back of each leg from just above the heel to the calf.

Sources (see Bibliography)

2, 10, 17, 26, 42, 44, 47, 51, 57, 58, 59, 60, 64, 65, 72, 75, 98, 101, 109, 111, 135, 144, 147, 150, 151, 168, 171, 176, 186, 201, 202, 225, 240, 244, 254, 256, 262, 268, 278, 280, 284, 293, 294, 300, 304, 306, 312, 313

Hepatitis

Acute viral hepatitis has three principal types. Type A (infectious hepatitis) is liver inflammation caused by a virus in fecal matter that can be transmitted by direct person-to-person contact, by infected food handlers, or through water polluted with human sewage. The hepatitis B virus lives in blood and other body fluids. Formerly called serum hepatitis because of its transmission through blood transfusions before development of tests for the virus, it is now mainly spread by sexual contact (especially among homosexuals), intravenous needle or razor sharing, or contaminated ear-piercing or tattoo equipment. Type C is a blood-borne virus that can be transmitted by transfusions as well as by the same means as type B, except for doubt regarding its spread through sexual contact. Either the B or C virus can be transmitted from an infected mother to her baby during birth.

Characteristic symptoms of hepatitis are a flulike illness, tenderness in the right upper part of the abdomen, and jaundice (yellowing of the skin and the whites of the eyes). Type A is highly contagious during the 2-to-6-week period before symptoms develop, and for 8 days after the onset of jaundice.[75] Gamma globulin (infection-resisting substances extracted from human blood) injections, which enhance immunity for about a month, are advised before traveling to areas where hygiene is poor and immediately after any known exposure. Hepatitis B and C, potentially more serious than type A, have an incubation period of a few weeks to a few months. Immunization with hepatitis B vaccine is recommended for health care personnel and others at high risk. For those who have not been vaccinated, a shot of hyperimmune globulin provides protection if taken within a week after known exposure.

Chronic or toxic hepatitis may be due to incomplete recovery from viral hepatitis or may be caused by liver damage from alcohol abuse, chemicals like those used in dry cleaning, reaction to medications, or by an autoimmune disorder. Although the liver is capable of healing and regenerating itself, all types of hepatitis warrant medical monitoring to prevent spread of the infection or the development of cirrhosis. Drug therapy is available for cases that do not improve with rest, wholesome diet, and avoidance of alcohol, tobacco, and other toxic substances.

Diet

One of the liver's functions is to remove useless or toxic chemicals ingested with food, as well as those inhaled or absorbed through the skin. Minimizing its chores by avoiding processed foods containing chemical additives, and building up its detoxifying capacity with a nutritious diet, can hasten recovery. Eating small, frequent meals lightens the liver's load. Apples, carrots, citrus fruits, collard and turnip greens, parsley and fresh leafy greens, red beets and their tops, strawberries, summer squash, and tomatoes are considered especially beneficial. Meats and dairy products put added strain on the liver, not only because it must produce bile to assist digestion of their fats but because animal fat contains concentrated pollutants.[201] Cold-pressed vegetable oils are advised for dressing salads and cooking.

Alcohol has a toxic effect on the liver. Recovery from liver damage requires total abstention until liver function tests are completely normal.[254] Distilled water, herbal teas, skim milk, and natural juices should be substituted for coffee, pekoe tea, and soft drinks. If jaundice is present, drinking a glass of carrot juice plus 8 ounces of any combination of apple, beet, celery, citrus, cucumber, or grape juice daily is suggested.[218, 305]

Supplements (see note on page xii)

Nutritionists and holistic practitioners recommend a daily multi-vitamin-mineral that includes 15 milligrams of zinc, plus therapeutic amounts of individual supplements to provide nutrients essential for the metabolic work of the liver.[17, 98, 201]

Vitamin A Preferably in emulsion form, 10,000 to 25,000 IU. Persons with liver problems have difficulty converting the beta carotene from foods or supplements into vitamin A.

B Complex One or two comprehensive tablets to assist liver function. Additional supplements of B6 and folic acid may be helpful. Clinical studies show that taking 1 to 3 grams of choline speeds recovery from all types of hepatitis—apparently by repairing the membranes of liver cells.[151] Lecithin, which contains choline, helps improve liver function. The suggested dosage is 1 or 2 tablespoons of granules or the equivalent in capsules. As Janice K. discovered, brewer's yeast is another source of liver-helping B vitamins. After a week of uncomfortable isolation due to infectious hepatitis, she concocted an updated version of the "fortified milk" advised by Adelle Davis in *Let's Get Well.*[87] Every morning she blended ¼ cup *each* brewer's yeast and sugar-free protein powder with a quart of skim milk, then accompanied each of three daily glasses of the mixture with 100 milligrams of pantothenic acid and 1,000 milligrams of vitamin C. With the final glass at bedtime she took a B-complex tablet and another thousand milligrams of vitamin C. Within a few days, Janice noticed improvement, and she astounded her physician by being totally "clear" in 3 weeks instead of the 5 or 6 estimated at the time of the diagnosis.

Vitamin C with Bioflavonoids   3,000 to 5,000 milligrams in divided doses to assist the liver's detoxification efforts and act as an antiviral agent.

L-cysteine and **L-methionine**   500 milligrams twice daily. These sulfur-containing amino acids help detoxify the hepatotoxins.[17]

Tissue Salts   Three 6X tablets of Nat. Sulph. dissolved under the tongue twice a day to aid liver function and the disposal of toxins.

Unsaturated Fatty Acids   Primrose oil, as directed on the label, to combat liver inflammation.

Folk Remedies

Old-fashioned cures for liver ailments and jaundice include drinking three glasses daily of water mixed with 2 teaspoons *each* apple cider vinegar and raw honey, or one glass a day of fresh beet or carrot juice.

Castor Oil Packs   Placed over the liver area and kept warm, these may relieve discomfort.

Herbs   Recent research has verified the value of several herbs: licorice root for chronic viral hepatitis; milk thistle or wormwood (two capsules of either, twice a day) for a detoxifying, liver-protective effect; St. John's wort for antiviral activity against hepatitis B.[150, 151] Other herbal specifics for liver problems are barberry, black radish, dandelion, goldenseal, red clover, and yellow dock.

Lemon There is anecdotal evidence that drinking the juice of half a lemon in a cup of hot water each morning and evening improves liver function.[173]

Nerve Pressure and Massage

❍ Press inward and upward on the notch in the bone under the center of each eyebrow.

❍ Press or massage 1 inch below and to the right of the center of the chest; then, in line with the center of the chest, press against the rib directly under the right armpit.

❍ Once each day use a firm, rolling motion to massage the outer edge of both hands near the base of the little fingers. On the right side only, massage the fleshy pads of the thumb and the big toe, the middle of the palm directly below the fourth finger, and the sole of the foot 2 inches from the base of the fourth toe.

Sources (see Bibliography)

6, 10, 17, 21, 37, 58, 59, 65, 75, 87, 98, 112, 135, 144, 148, 150, 151, 164, 168, 172, 173, 176, 195, 201, 202, 203, 205, 218, 226, 244, 254, 255, 256, 262, 284, 305, 306

Hiccups

The telltale "hic" results from sudden closure of the throat following a spasmodic contraction of the diaphragm due to irritation of the phrenic or vagus nerves. Hiccups (singultus) can occur for no apparent reason or may be triggered by eating or drinking too rapidly or too much, by a fit of laughter, or by nervous tension. Hiccuping that persists longer than 24 hours may indicate underlying disorders requiring medical attention. Most episodes, however, are short-lived annoyances—and hiccup-annihilating methods abound.

Counterirritation

Shout or sing as loudly as possible.

Place an ice pack over the stomach, or hold ice cubes under the Adam's apple or on the back of the neck, or swallow tiny bits of crushed ice.

Cover the diaphragm with a towel wrung out of hot water or with a poultice of ½ cup vinegar and ½ teaspoon cayenne pepper thickened with wheat flour.

Use a cotton-tipped swab to tickle the soft section in the back of the roof of the mouth. Or take a whiff of smelling salts.

Drowning

Gargle for 1 minute with hot or cold water.

Drink a glass of water while clenching a pencil with the back teeth, or place a piece of silverware in the glass and hold the metal handle against the temple while drinking.

Light a wooden match, blow it out, drop it in half a glass of water, then swallow the water—but not the match. Or dissolve three 6X tablets of the tissue salt Mag. Phos. in a tablespoon of hot water (or under the tongue); for persistent hiccups after hasty eating, alternate with doses of Nat. Mur.

Without stopping, drink a glass of cold beer, pineapple juice, or water containing a teaspoon of apple cider vinegar.

Sip a small glass of orange juice, sugar water, or vermouth; or a cup of hot apple juice, or caraway or dill tea. For babies, dissolve ½ teaspoon sugar in ½ cup water, or mix ½ teaspoon honey with a diluted mixture of catnip and fennel or peppermint tea.

Swallow a teaspoon of honey, onion juice, or vinegar.

Force Feeding

Eat a teaspoon of dry white sugar or a spoonful of brown sugar moistened with vinegar. Or eat a teaspoon of peanut butter, a slice of orange, or a pickled pepper.

Chew activated charcoal tablets, dill seeds, or fresh mint leaves.

Eat small pieces of soda cracker or stale bread, chewing each bite ten times, or eat a half cup of dry bread crumbs.

Suck a lemon wedge coated with salt or sprinkled with angostura bitters, vinegar, or Worcestershire sauce.

Nerve Pressure and Massage

Compress the chest by leaning forward or by pulling up the knees. Or interlock the fingers at the back of the neck and, with the head tipped back, push in with the thumbs under the edge of the jawbone. Or while leaning backward with the head hanging down from a bed or sofa, clasp the hands behind the neck. Or pull out on the tongue by holding it with a strip of gauze.

For 30 seconds, massage the hollow at the back of the neck with the fingers, then rub the diaphragm with the palm of the hand. Or use the heel of the hand to massage upward from the navel to the base of the breastbone with slow, circular movements.

Exert 30 seconds of pressure or massage on any of the following areas: the center of the upper lip, the middle of the tongue, the small depression in the breastbone 2 inches below the hollow of the throat, the soft pad at the base of each thumb, the thumbs and the next two fingers on both hands—including the webs of skin between them—the center bottom of each foot between the ball of the foot and the arch.

Suffocation

Hold the breath as long as possible, swallowing whenever a hiccup approaches. Or blow and rebreathe ten times with a paper (not plastic) bag held over the nose and mouth.

Regurgitation

If all else fails, induce vomiting by holding a finger down the throat.

Sources (see Bibliography)

2, 26, 29, 57, 59, 63, 64, 65, 75, 109, 111, 112, 135, 148, 153, 159, 164, 176, 186, 202, 247, 254, 255, 262, 284, 293, 306, 311, 312, 313

High Blood Pressure (Hypertension)

Called the silent disease because it seldom evinces early symptoms, hypertension plagues an estimated 60 million Americans. Blood pressure readings with a sphygmomanometer (a cuff connected to a pressure-measuring device and placed around the upper arm) determine the degree of hypertension. The higher figure (systolic pressure) is the force of blood against artery walls when the heart beats. The diastolic (lower number) refers to the pressure exerted while the heart relaxes between beats. Between 110/70 to 140/90 is considered normal. Systolic pressure between 140 and 159, with the diastolic registering 90 to 105, is mild hypertension. The severity of high blood pressure is graded according to the diastolic reading with 105 to 120 considered moderately severe, and a consistent reading of greater than 120, severe hypertension.[78] Since blood pressure fluctuates with the time of day as well as with physical or emotional stress, diagnosis should not be made from a single reading. In addition to periodic professional screenings, self-testing with an electronic blood pressure monitor may be wise—especially for "white coat hypertensives" who experience dramatic elevations in blood pressure when in the presence of medical personnel.

High-risk factors for the onset of the disease are heredity (a family history of high blood pressure doubles the chances of developing it),[300] race (black Americans are one-third more likely to develop hypertension than are white Americans), and age and sex (high blood pressure usually first occurs in men under the age of 55; in women over the age of 55). In the United States, two-thirds of the people between 65 and 74 are hypertensive; in many other countries, blood pressure does not increase with age. Factors influencing or aggravating blood pressure include too high a consumption of salt, fat, stimulants, or alcohol; smoking; stress; and too little exercise.

Chemicals in oral contraceptives, artificial sweeteners, and diet pills elevate blood pressure for some individuals. Excess body weight is a factor in 60 percent of all cases of hypertension. A study reported in the *Journal of the American Medical Association* (September 1990) showed that hypertensives weigh an average of 29 pounds more than people with normal blood pressure. For many of the overweight, each 2 pounds of weight loss results in a one-point drop in both systolic and diastolic readings.[111]

Diet

Excess sodium causes fluid retention, which exerts pressure on blood vessel walls and contributes to hypertension; potassium helps the body excrete the surplus. Both nutrients are present in natural foods and a two-to-one or three-to-one ratio of potassium to sodium can be maintained by consuming several servings of potassium-rich edibles daily—supplementary potassium should be taken only when medically advised.

Potassium-Sodium Comparison Chart*		
	Potassium	Sodium
1 medium baked potato with skin	844	16
1 cup fresh orange juice	496	2
1 medium banana	451	1
1 cup skim milk	406	126
3 fresh apricots	314	1
3 ounces broiled sirloin steak	306	53
3 ounces sole, baked with lemon juice	286	101
1 raw salad tomato	255	10
3 ounces roast chicken breast	220	64
½ cup frozen, chopped broccoli	167	22
1 cup regular or quick oatmeal	131	2
*Expressed in milligrams; from *USDA Nutritive Value of Foods*.[130]		

Salt, at 2,123 milligrams of sodium per teaspoon, is the ingredient that upsets nature's balance. The typical American diet contains 19,000 milligrams of sodium per day—at least twice as much as is considered acceptably healthful and far more than the 1,000 milligrams per 1,000 calories (up to 3,000 milligrams of sodium) advised by some authorities.[294] Much of this sodium comes from hidden sources—75 percent of it, according to the March 1993 *Berkeley Wellness Letter.* A raw apple, for instance, has 159 milligrams of potassium with no sodium; a slice of apple pie contains 476 milligrams of sodium and 126 milligrams of potassium. One-half cup of instant pudding has 440 milligrams of sodium and 176 milligrams of potassium.

For the approximately 50 percent of hypertensives who are salt sensitive, sodium should be limited to less than 500 milligrams per day. To accomplish this without deprivation, utilize low-sodium products; bake, broil, microwave, or steam unsalted natural foods (a potato loses 50 percent of its potassium when it's boiled); and table-season with herbs, granulated kelp, or a half-and-half mixture of salt and a potassium-containing salt substitute.

Also pertinent to blood pressure control is the nutritional guideline for fat consumption (30 percent of daily calories, at least one-third from monounsaturated canola, olive, or peanut oils). In some studies, a low-fat diet proved more effective than salt reduction for lowering blood pressure.[177] Unsaturated fatty acids (UFA) from two or three weekly servings of saltwater fish, or capsules of primrose oil or EPA may lower blood pressure by dilating blood vessel walls.[17, 150] Increasing dietary fiber also helps keep blood pressure down by controlling insulin levels; minimal amounts of concentrated sweets are recommended because blood sugar imbalances are closely associated with hypertension—adding sugar to a high-salt diet increases blood pressure much more rapidly than the high-salt diet alone.[248]

Since the two to four points of elevation from a cup of coffee disappear after 3 hours, caffeine is no longer forbidden for most mild to moderate hypertensives,[186] but stimulating beverages should be limited to two cups of coffee or four cups of tea or caffeine-containing soft drinks per day. Although small amounts of alcohol are permissible, imbibing more than two drinks daily is so detrimental that overindulgence is regarded as one of the most common instigators of hypertension.

Supplements (see note on page xii)

When taken in addition to a daily multivitamin-mineral, the following supplements have shown excellent results in reducing high blood pressure for many individuals.

B Complex One comprehensive tablet twice daily to improve circulatory function and act as a natural tranquilizer. Lecithin contains the B vitamins choline and inositol, which are believed to help decrease blood pressure by preventing fatty deposits in the arteries and by dilating blood vessels. Suggested dosages vary from three 1,200 milligram capsules to 3 tablespoons of lecithin granules daily.

Vitamin C with Bioflavonoids 1,000 to 5,000 milligrams to maintain the health of blood vessels and improve the potassium ratio by assisting in sodium excretion.

Vitamin E 100 IU daily, increased by 100 IU each month to a total of 400 IU daily for decreasing the need for oxygen and thus improving heart function.[17]

Calcium and Magnesium 1,000 to 2,000 milligrams of calcium plus 500 to 750 milligrams of magnesium in divided daily doses to calm nerves, help regulate heart contractions, and encourage sodium excretion. Studies indicate that calcium lowers blood pressure only for people who are salt sensitive.[231] With medical approval, some hypertensives may benefit from 1,000 to 2,000 milligrams of magnesium plus 500 to 1,000 milligrams of calcium. In some cases, positive results have been obtained in less than a month when a tablespoon of powdered whey (available in health food stores) was taken in ½ glass of water three times a day.[72]

Zinc 10 to 50 milligrams daily to increase blood circulation and help compensate for stress.

Tissue Salts Two or three 3X-potency tablets, two or three times daily, of Ferr. Phos. (to increase the amount of oxygen reaching the cells) and Silicea (to improve circulation).

Exercise

Studies show that people who maintain their physical fitness are 34 percent less likely to develop hypertension than are the sedentary.[105] For those who already have the disease, there is encouraging evidence that regular aerobic exercise, such as brisk walking for half an hour three times a week, can lower blood pressure from three to fifteen points in a few months.[177] Swimming or bike riding are equally effective in improving cardiovascular health, but persons with existing hypertension should attempt a regimen entailing weightlifting or vigorous workouts only under the direction of a physician.

Folk Remedies

Apple Cider Vinegar Stir 1 or 2 teaspoons of vinegar—with or without an equal amount of honey—into a glass of water and sip with each meal.

Garlic One or two cloves of minced garlic (or garlic capsules) taken with two meals each day is a time-honored remedy for dilating blood vessels and reducing blood pressure. Calvin D. credits home-grown garlic for curing his hypertension after a neighbor introduced him to fresh, mildly flavored garlic bulbs with scallionlike tops. Besides adding the garlic to cooked dishes, he included slices of the half-inch bulbs in his noontime sandwich and tossed the minced tops with his dinner salad. Encouraged by a significant drop in his blood pressure, Calvin adopted his friend's "garlic-farming" method of planting cloves of dried garlic in flower beds and window boxes. By the time the second crop of green shoots appeared, Calvin's blood pressure was normal, and he continues to enjoy a lot of garlic to keep it that way.

Herbs Alfalfa, camomile, catnip, fennel, hawthorn berry, rosemary, sage, skullcap, and watermelon seed teas are considered specifics for lowering blood pressure.

Onions When eaten daily, onions are believed to be helpful antihypertensives.

Potato Broths The high magnesium-potassium content of potatoes lends credence to these two remedies. (1) Place the peelings from five well-washed potatoes in 2 cups water and boil for 15 minutes in a covered saucepan. Cool and strain, then drink 2 cups of the liquid each day. (2) Stir 2 cups chopped potato (scrubbed but not peeled) plus ½ cup *each* shredded carrots and chopped green beans into 3 cups of boiling water. Cover and simmer for 20 minutes. Strain and sip the liquid during the day.

Relaxation

Anxiety or anger causes blood pressure to soar as tension constricts arterial walls. Deliberate relaxation, through any of the methods described in the Introduction, help bring it back down. Even petting a cuddly pet, or watching flames flicker in a fireplace or fish swim in an aquarium can provide a transitory release from the continual pressure that contributes to hypertension.

Nerve Pressure and Massage

○ Once each day, for 3 minutes *each,* press and knead the area between the eyebrows; then massage the hollows in the back of the neck at the base of the skull, and the inside of the elbows.

○ For 30 seconds daily, stimulate any or all of the following points: Squeeze the vertical groove on the back of each ear above the earlobe; massage the thumbs and first two fingers, plus the webs between them, on both hands; press and massage 1½ inches directly below the navel, and just below the ball of the foot in line with the third toe.

Sources (see Bibliography)

2, 6, 13, 14, 17, 26, 42, 48, 49, 57, 58, 60, 63, 64, 72, 75, 78, 82, 86, 87, 98, 105, 108, 111, 112, 127, 130, 144, 150, 151, 164, 171, 177, 183, 186, 190, 205, 207, 229, 231, 237, 248, 260, 285, 293, 294, 300, 304, 306, 312, 313, 315

High Cholesterol

Chemically a lipid (fat), cholesterol is a soft, waxy substance present in all animal tissue. Essential to life, it is an important constituent of body cells, is used as insulation around nerve fibers, and is involved in the formation of digestive acids and certain hormones, as well as in the transport of fats. To supply these needs, the body (primarily the liver) utilizes saturated fats and refined carbohydrates to manufacture about 1,000 milligrams of cholesterol each day in addition to the dietary cholesterol consumed. To distribute cholesterol via the bloodstream, the liver combines it with proteins and triglycerides ("bad" fats derived directly from foods or made by the body) into molecular packets called lipoproteins. Low-density lipoprotein (LDL, "bad" cholesterol) carries cholesterol throughout the system and leaves unneeded cholesterol in the bloodstream, where it can accumulate on artery walls. High-density lipoprotein (HDL, "good" cholesterol) carries a smaller proportion of cholesterol than LDL, and as it moves through the blood, HDL picks up cholesterol that is either circulating or clinging to the arteries and transports it back to the liver for reprocessing or excretion.

Cholesterol Levels

The American Academy of Pediatrics suggests testing children only if there is a family history of heart disease. All adults are advised to have a cholesterol test as a precautionary measure, even though women who have not reached menopause rarely have heart attacks. Men should be retested every 5 years during their high-risk period between the ages of 40 and 60. Guidelines set by the National Institute of Health list a total serum cholesterol level below 200 milligrams of cholesterol per deciliter of blood (200 mg/dl) as safe; between 200 and 240 as borderline high cholesterol.[111] Recent research has shown that the proportionate amount of HDL is a more accurate indicator of the risk of heart disease or other cholesterol-related disorders such as gallstones, high blood pressure, impotence, and mental impairment. People with elevated total cholesterol levels may not be at risk if their HDL levels are high; individuals with a total under 200 may be at risk if the HDL level is low. Studies show that HDL levels above 70 protect against heart disease; those below 35 are a risk factor.[75, 300] LDL levels below 130 are desirable; those higher than 160 signal danger. For optimum cardiovascular protection, triglyceride levels should be 120 or lower; levels above 200 are considered dangerous. If test results are high, the National Cholesterol Education Program suggests averaging in one or two additional readings from different labs before starting strict dietary intervention or cholesterol-lowering drugs.

Cholesterol levels are influenced by heredity; diets rich in saturated fat, cholesterol, and refined carbohydrates; metabolic diseases such as diabetes; obesity (excess body weight stimulates the liver to produce more triglycerides and elevate cholesterol levels); smoking (smokers who quit have raised their HDL by 10 points in 1 month);[50] and lack of exercise (walking briskly for 30 minutes three times a week raises HDL and reduces triglycerides).[47] A few individuals are blessed with protective genes that adapt to high cholesterol and allow them to eat, drink, and smoke to excess and to evade exercise for 80 or 90 years with no ill effects. Conversely, a few others are burdened with defective genes that overproduce cholesterol and must have drug therapy to clear away the excess. For most normally active people, dietary alterations can control cholesterol levels.

Diet

Large meals stimulate the production of an enzyme that increases the liver's output of cholesterol; dividing the day's calories into frequently eaten small meals rather than the customary two or three can help lower cholesterol levels.[50] Cutting dietary consumption of cholesterol from the average of 500 milligrams a day to 100 milligrams per 1,000 calories—with an upper limit of 200 to 300 milligrams—is recommended by many experts.[294, 312] Plant foods do not contain cholesterol, but all foods of animal origin contain some. Those with the most are organ meats (two slices of liver sausage have 89 milligrams of cholesterol); egg yolks (one large yolk provides approximately 1 day's quota, even though its cholesterol content is now calculated as 213 milligrams, not the original 274); and milk products such as whole milk at 33 milligrams per cup, butter at 31 milligrams per tablespoon, and cheddar cheese at 30 milligrams per ounce.

Beverages can affect cholesterol levels. At least eight glasses of water or juices are needed daily to keep cholesterol-absorbing fiber flowing through the body. Herbalists suggest cayenne, chicory root, comfrey, fenugreek, hawthorn, mint, red clover, rose hip, skullcap, or turmeric teas (or capsules) to improve cholesterol levels. Studies reported by the American Heart Association in June 1991 show that boiled or percolated coffee increases the harmful LDLs, but that up to six cups daily of regular or decaffeinated coffee brewed with a paper filter have no effect on serum cholesterol. Having one or two alcoholic drinks every day raises the helpful HDLs while lowering LDLs,[254] but excess alcohol as well as sugar not utilized for energy is transformed into saturated fat. According to a report in *American Health* (December 1992), purple grape juice contains almost as much of the LDL-lowering substance as red wine.

Fats

Many authorities believe that the total amount of fat in the diet has a greater impact on blood cholesterol levels than does the amount of dietary cholesterol. Saturated fat (found primarily in animal products but also in coconut, palm, and cottonseed oils) encourages the liver to produce more LDLs and interferes with its ability to remove cholesterol from the blood. Monounsaturated fats (canola, olive, and peanut oils; avocados, nuts, and olives) maintain or elevate the levels of protective HDLs while decreasing the amount of cholesterol carried by the LDLs. Polyunsaturated oils (safflower, sunflower, corn) help lower total cholesterol. Hydrogenating vegetable oils for solid shortening or margarine transforms their health-promoting properties into a type of fat potentially more harmful than naturally saturated fat.[177]

The Pritikin diet, which allows only 10 percent of daily calories from fat, has lowered cholesterol levels by 25 percent in 1 month.[237] Other nutritionists have found that a less restrictive diet allowing one-third of calories from fat can lower total cholesterol and LDL levels even more effectively as long as a large proportion of the fats are monounsaturates.[293] The American Heart Association recommends a total fat intake of 30 percent of the diet with no more than 10 percent from saturated fat, the remainder from unsaturated sources. At 9 calories per gram of fat, 30 percent of the average woman's 2,000 daily calories equals 67 grams of fat; a man's 2,700 calories, 90 grams of fat.

A simple plan for reducing dietary fat calls for eating red meat three times a week (a 3-ounce portion of lean beef has 205 calories with 12 grams of fat—4.9 of them saturated), with fish, poultry, or protein-rich legumes on alternate days. Three ounces of baked salmon equals 140 calories and 5 grams of fat, including 2 grams of saturated fat; the same amount of turkey breast equals 3 grams of fat with 0.2 of them saturated; and cooked dried beans have only 1 gram of fat per cup. By reading labels and taking advantage of the fat-reduced and fat-free products available, a low-fat diet need not be deprivational.

Fiber

Water-soluble pectin (from fruits, vegetables, legumes, and nuts) and the soluble fiber present in corn and rice brans as well as in oat bran lowers LDLs and total cholesterol without reducing the levels of helpful HDLs. Wheat bran's insoluble fiber protects against colon cancer but does not affect cholesterol. Soluble fiber not only binds to excess cholesterol and carries it out of the system but is also believed to interfere with cholesterol synthesis in the liver.[48]

Augmenting a balanced 30-percent-fat diet with an extra 10 grams of soluble fiber can result in reducing cholesterol levels by as much as 19 percent in less than a month.[300] One serving of oat bran cereal contains 5 grams of fiber; a pear, 6 grams; an apple, 3; and a cup of cooked dry beans contains as much soluble fiber as two-thirds of a cup of oat bran.[47] Other good sources recommended for cholesterol reduction include apples, bananas, berries, broccoli, cabbage, carrots, cauliflower, corn, citrus fruits, dates, eggplant, figs, prunes, raisins, sweet potatoes, turnips, and zucchini. Garlic and onions also contain sulfur compounds that significantly affect the biosynthesis of cholesterol and triglycerides. Studies show that an onion a day increases HDLs by 30 percent while lowering LDLs and triglycerides.[150, 151] Other clinical studies reported in *Prevention* (January 1992) showed that taking 600 to 900 milligrams of garlic powder capsules every day for 3 or 4 months lowered cholesterol levels by 14 to 21 percent, triglycerides by 18 to 24 percent.

Supplements (see note on page xii)

Drastic changes in diet or supplements should not be initiated without medical approval, but because random nutrients may be swept up along with cholesterol as fiber clears out the system, a daily multivitamin-mineral is usually recommended.

Antioxidants These play a vital role in cholesterol control. Scientists believe cholesterol must be oxidized before it can cling to artery walls, and according to a study reported in *Atherosclerosis* (June 1990), vitamins C and E halt this oxidation within the body. Other studies have shown that 500 IUs of vitamin E daily can significantly increase HDL levels[293] and that 1,000 milligrams of vitamin C each day slowly reduces high cholesterol to normal levels without lowering the protective HDLs.[29] Some nutritionists recommend up to 5,000 milligrams of vitamin C daily to increase the cholesterol-lowering effectiveness of pectin.

B Vitamins These vitamins assist with fat metabolization. In addition to a B-complex tablet daily, individual supplements have been found to be beneficial. Smokers in particular are advised to take 100 milligrams of B6 daily to raise HDL levels.[312] Clinical studies demonstrated that taking 30 milligrams of B15 (pangamic acid) three times a day for 20 days reduced cholesterol levels for 90 percent of the people tested.[98] Lecithin, which contains high concentrations of choline and inositol, is believed to emulsify fats and cholesterol so they can be utilized by the body or flushed out of the system. One to six tablespoons of lecithin granules daily, or two or more 1,200 milligram capsules with each meal, is the suggested dosage. Under medical supervision, therapeutic amounts of B3 (niacin, not niacinamide) can be as effective as prescription drugs, for those who are not diabetic, by increasing HDLs while decreasing LDLs and triglycerides. Dr. Matt chose this natural method to correct his own dangerously high cholesterol. He began with 100 milligrams of niacin with two meals a day and gradually increased the dosage until he was taking 1,000 milligrams with each of three meals a day. Instead of using time-release niacin, which usually produces no skin flushing but is suspected of being potentially harmful to the liver, he lessened the skin-tingling reaction by taking an aspirin half an hour before each meal until his body adapted to the niacin. By combining this regimen with a low-fat, high-fiber diet, Dr. Matt soon had his cholesterol down to a safe level.

Minerals One study demonstrated that taking 1,000 milligrams of calcium carbonate daily for two months lowered overall cholesterol by 4.8 percent. Other studies have shown that taking 2,000 milligrams of calcium carbonate daily for one year reduced triglycerides and lowered cholesterol by 25 percent.[177, 294] At least 500 milligrams of magnesium is advised when taking calcium supplements. Chromium (from tablets or brewer's yeast) reduces total cholesterol and raises HDL levels. One study, reported in *Longevity* (June 1990), showed that daily ingestion of 200 micrograms of chromium picolinate produced positive changes in 6 weeks—half the time usually required for improvement with drug therapy.

Activated Charcoal A non-nutritional alternative that binds with cholesterol and carries it out of the system so efficiently that ¼ ounce of charcoal taken three times a day has lowered LDL levels 41 percent and elevated HDLs 8 percent. Charcoal can latch onto other substances as well as cholesterol, however, so should be taken an hour before or after meals, supplemented with a daily multiple, and taken only with medical approval if any medication has been prescribed.[151]

Psyllium A soluble fiber from the seed husks of plantain, it can be obtained in health food stores or from commercial bulk laxatives. When taken in conjunction with a low-fat diet, 1 teaspoon of psyllium plus 8 ounces of water three times a day has raised HDLs, lowered LDLs, and resulted in a 35 percent drop in total cholesterol after only 6 months.[112]

Sources (see Bibliography)

17, 28, 29, 40, 45, 46, 47, 48, 50, 75, 98, 99, 109, 111, 112, 130, 150, 151, 176, 177, 186, 237, 248, 254, 266, 268, 281, 283, 293, 294, 300, 303, 308, 312, 313

Hives (Urticaria)

Sometimes called nettle rash, because contact with nettle plants of the genus *Urtica* produces similar skin eruptions, hives (urticaria) occur as a form of allergic reaction. The itchy, inflamed welts or wheals appear when allergens or stress causes skin cells to release histamine, which makes fluid leak from capillaries into skin tissue. Giant hives (angioedema) is a rare condition that affects deeper layers of the skin on the eyelids, genitals, lips, mouth, and other parts of the body, producing swellings larger than the customary pea-to-walnut-size of urticaria. Giant hives require emergency medical care if breathing passages are obstructed.

Hives often result from reactions to foods such as berries or shellfish, or from drugs such as aspirin or penicillin, but they can be precipitated by anything to which an individual is sensitive. Cosmetic preparations, inhaled substances, insect bites, emotional upsets, physical overexertion, food additives or dyes, even the "fillers" in certain brands of vitamins are possible culprits. For persons allergic to cold or heat, sudden changes in climate, eating ice cream, swimming in cold water, or taking a steam bath can provoke a histamine release.

Solar urticaria (sun-induced hives) typically strikes after half an hour of exposure, but the usual time lag of hours or days for the appearance of other types of hives may require detective work for identification and future avoidance. Prime suspects are foods not normally eaten and recent changes in medication. In some cases, a combination of otherwise unnoticeable allergens can trigger an outbreak of hives. Rhea S. knew what the red-ringed bumps were when she was awakened by their excruciating itching, but she didn't know what she had eaten to deserve them. Then she remembered a childhood bout after gobbling raspberries while picking them for her grandmother, and another encounter following a teenage clambake. Rhea had not indulged in either of those foods but deduced that the previous day's strawberry pie at lunch had joined forces with her lobster dinner to set off the eruptions.

The itchy red welts normally disappear within a few hours or days—using over-the-counter antihistamines and natural remedies may shorten their duration and relieve the discomfort.

Supplements (see note on page xii)

Studies show that massive amounts of vitamin C can halt the harmful effects of all kinds of allergens immediately after they have entered the bloodstream. Suggested dosage is 1,000 to 2,000 milligrams every 4 hours for a total of 4,000 to 8,000 milligrams in 16 hours.[87] Taking vitamin C with bioflavonoids and milk (or up to 1,500 milligrams of calcium gluconate) helps suppress itching and lessens the likelihood of stomach irritation from the vitamin.

Tissue Salts Three tablets three times a day of 6X Kali. Phos., Mag. Phos., and Silicea. If the skin is dry and tending to scale, take Kali. Sulph. For hives that appear after heat exposure, take the same potency of Nat. Mur.

Folk Remedies

Drinking two cups of stinging-nettle tea is an old cure for adults who are under 65 and neither pregnant nor lactating. For temporary relief, aloe vera gel or bottled witch hazel can be smoothed over the wheals. If the hives are not an allergic response to cold, ice packs or cold compresses relieve the burning and itching sensations and shrink surface blood vessels to decrease the amount of irritating histamine being released.[16, 293]

Baths Soak for 20 minutes in cool water with one or more of the following skin soothers: ½ to 1 cup baking soda or cornstarch, ½ to 2 cups commercial colloidal oatmeal, 1 to 2 cups regular oatmeal or crushed camomile flowers tied in cheesecloth and squished in the water.

Pastes Cover the hives with milk of magnesia, or with a paste of baking soda or cream of tartar and water, or cornstarch and white vinegar. Rinse off and reapply when the coating dries.

Nerve Pressure and Massage

○ On each side, press and massage a point 1 inch toward the back from the middle of the muscle running between the neck and shoulder.

○ Using the left thumb, deeply massage the right palm directly below the fourth finger.

Stress Relief

If emotional stress is a suspected cause of the hives, it may help to sip nerve-calming herbal teas of camomile, catnip, passion flower, peppermint, red clover, or valerian—or to take a combination of hops, skullcap, and valerian in a capsule. Practicing the relaxation techniques described in the Introduction and visualizing the itchy eruptions being replaced with comfortably smooth skin may also be of benefit.

Sources (see Bibliography)

16, 29, 59, 64, 65, 75, 80, 86, 87, 109, 112, 135, 137, 148, 150, 151, 176, 177, 186, 201, 224, 254, 255, 256, 281, 283, 293, 294, 312

Hypoglycemia (Low Blood Sugar)

Functional hypoglycemia (FH) is a condition in which abnormally low blood sugar (glucose) forces the body to rob this essential fuel from the brain and muscles and utilize stored protein and fat to provide energy for life-sustaining functions.[254] Pancreatic oversecretion of insulin, abnormal carbohydrate and protein metabolism, and poor adrenal function contribute to FH.[17] Heredity is a susceptibility factor. Possible instigators include diets high in refined carbohydrates and sweets, meal skipping, and yo-yo dieting. Anger or anxiety, alcohol, tobacco, caffeine or other stimulants, and beta blockers or sulfa-containing medications can precipitate hypoglycemic attacks in some people.[29]

FH symptoms, which have a direct relationship to the frequency of meals and the type of food eaten, appear in astounding variety and can mimic many diseases: blurred vision, depression, dizziness, faintness, fatigue, headache, heart palpitations, indigestion, insomnia, irritability, memory loss and mental confusion, mood swings, muscle cramps or spasms, nervousness, night sweats, pain in various parts of the body, panic attacks, poor circulation, or poor physical coordination with staggering or trembling. These effects can be cumulative, producing perpetual malaise—in severe cases, bizarre behavior that suggests a mental disorder, or personality changes—and may lead to diabetes or other physical disorders. Functional hypoglycemia is believed to affect at least one-fourth of the American population;[191] to be a significant cause of childhood hyperactivity and learning disabilities as well as of adult alcoholism and auto accidents;[201] and to be responsible for much of the violent behavior of mental patients[251]—repeated studies have shown hypoglycemia to be present in over 80 percent of all criminal offenders tested.[98]

A 6-hour glucose tolerance test (GTT) is the most reliable method of diagnosis; having blood drawn while experiencing symptoms is an alternative. Even with these tests, FH is difficult to diagnose. Many cases are subclinical in that "borderline" levels of blood sugar may produce serious symptoms for some people. And since a hypoglycemic episode can be temporarily relieved with candy or a sugary drink in the same manner as for diabetes, that is often the suggested means of control. With FH, however, the relief is brief. Proteins and fiber-rich carbohydrates better serve a hypoglycemic because the sweet-triggered surge of insulin from an overreacting pancreas not only sweeps the new sugar out of the bloodstream but also removes much of the small amount of glucose that was present in the beginning—leaving the individual with even more pronounced symptoms.

During exercise or strenuous activity (which should be performed about an hour after eating) or when meals are delayed, a stabilizing snack like cheese and crackers or grapes and peanuts is usually more beneficial than candy for those with low blood sugar. Cindy B. was so determined to make it on her own with her first job away from home that she didn't tell her family about her fainting spells. She assumed they were her own fault for neglecting to bolster her "slightly low" blood sugar by eating a candy bar when she felt wobbly. But when she blacked out a few minutes after having eaten a piece of candy, Cindy called her dietitian-mother for advice. By following the high-protein, sugar-free diet that arrived by return mail, Cindy is no longer beset by either blackouts or the wobblies. Vivian V.'s symptoms were different—mental fuzziness and shaky hands—but the diagnosis and suggested treatment were the same as Cindy's. The chocolates worked for only a few minutes after ingestion, so 6 months later and 6 pounds heavier, Vivian sought a second opinion. The new test indicated FH and, after 2 weeks of sugar avoidance and between-meal high-protein snacks, Vivian was symptom-free.

Diet

Protein, fiber-rich carbohydrates, and enough fat to slow digestion are the cornerstones of a hypoglycemia-control diet. Ideally, some of all three should be consumed at each of at least six minimeals (or three major meals and three snacks) every day. Refined carbohydrates (white bread, white rice) are rapidly converted to the glucose that incites insulin production and lowers blood sugar,[201] so they, as well as sugars (corn syrup, molasses, sucrose, table sugar, etc.) should be avoided by most hypoglycemics. Since the pancreas is conditioned to react to sweet tastes and may be fooled by sugar substitutes, artificially sweetened desserts and drinks may need to be limited to one a day and consumed with meals. Research data indicate that garlic and onions, and the herbs cayenne, goldenseal, and pau d'arco can adversely affect blood sugar levels for hypoglycemics, so their use should be carefully monitored or avoided.

The therapeutic diet devised by Seale Harris, who identified hypoglycemia in 1924, allowed no starchy foods other than one slice of bread per meal.[1] More lenient diets are detailed in *Low Blood Sugar and You*,[123] and a vegetarian variation is offered in *How to Get Well*.[6] Most current guidelines advise ample amounts of complex carbohydrates and rely on meat as the principal source of protein. Meats (particularly beef and lamb) are the richest dietary sources of L-carnitine, an amino acid essential for the body's conversion of stored fat into energy. Vegetarians may need to take supplemental L-carnitine—dairy products and avocados contain small amounts of the amino acid; fruits, vegetables, and cereals provide little or none.[151] And, as reported in *Prevention* (September 1983), the American Diabetes Association considers functional hypoglycemia an early and treatable symptom of systemic L-carnitine deficiency.

Individual experimentation determines the most effective diet pattern for each hypoglycemic. Some people function comfortably with nothing more substantial than a glass of milk to bridge the blood sugar gap between regular meals. Others must have a glass of juice or milk upon arising, a minimeal every 2 or 3 hours during the day, and rouse for a snack in the middle of the night to prevent morning headache, nausea, or fatigue. To self-test for a week, stir a spoonful of brewer's yeast into tomato juice (or blend brewer's yeast, dry milk, or unsweetened protein powder with milk) for a prebreakfast drink each morning. Then divide the following foods among six meals and snacks with an ounce or two of protein plus some bread, milk, fruit, or vegetable with each one.

- ○ Twelve to 15 ounces meat, poultry, or seafood. If desired, 2 ounces of the meats may be replaced with 2 ounces of natural cheddar or Swiss cheese, two eggs, or ¼ cup peanut butter.

- ○ Two to 5 cups of any assortment of vegetables except beets, carrots, corn, dried legumes, parsnips, potatoes, pumpkin, or winter squash.

○ Three slices whole-grain bread. Once each day, a half-cup serving of one of the "forbidden" vegetables may be substituted for half a slice of the bread.

○ One to 3 tablespoons vegetable oil on salads or as a cooking ingredient.

○ Two servings of fruit—fresh, or unsweetened frozen or canned.

○ Two glasses milk.

Clear broths, herbs (especially basil, marjoram, oregano, saffron, and thyme), lemon juice and vinegar, unflavored gelatin, and moderate amounts of butter or margarine or mayonnaise are allowable embellishments. Decaffeinated coffee or tea, and caffeine-free herbal teas such as alfalfa, camomile, comfrey, dandelion, juniper berry, licorice root, peppermint, rose hips, and skullcap are considered acceptable beverages. If indulged in at all, alcohol should be limited to one or two drinks per day and, to prevent a precipitous drop in the blood sugar level, imbibed with food.

If improvement is apparent after the first week, the basic pattern can be continued while other favorites are added one at a time—eating a variety of foods helps avoid possible allergic reactions. One slice of bread can be traded for popcorn, whole-grain crackers, corn tortillas, brown rice, wheat pasta, or a bowl of oatmeal. Artificially sweetened soft drinks or desserts such as puddings or sponge cake may not present problems if accompanied by protein and complex carbohydrates.

Supplements (see note on page xii)

The stress reaction triggered each time blood sugar plummets increases the body's need for nutrients and can create deficiencies that further impair carbohydrate metabolization. In addition to a daily multivitamin-mineral, the following supplements have proven beneficial in many cases.

B Complex One comprehensive tablet daily to help metabolize carbohydrates and combat stress. Extra amounts of B_2 and pantothenic acid assist in the conversion of glucose and may decrease the craving for sugar—deficiencies of these two vitamins can prevent the liver from producing enzymes to inactivate insulin, thus causing blood sugar levels to plunge. Taking niacinamide with each of three daily meals has reduced tension and depression as well as other FH symptoms.[215, 317] People who cannot assimilate swallowed B_{12} may need to take sublingual tablets daily or have B_{12} injections every few weeks.[17, 98]

Calcium and Magnesium   800 to 1,500 milligrams of calcium plus 500 to 750 milligrams of magnesium in divided daily doses. Studies show that even with the two glasses of milk each day, the high-protein hypoglycemic diet results in a bodily loss of calcium, which can cause osteoporosis if not countered by supplements.[228] Magnesium is necessary for the proper uptake of calcium and is important in carbohydrate (sugar) metabolism. Under medical supervision, it may be beneficial to change the proportions of these two minerals to 1,600 milligrams of magnesium plus 800 milligrams of calcium.

Chromium   150 to 200 micrograms daily. There is growing evidence that lack of chromium—the active component of the glucose tolerance factor (GTF)—is a common cause of blood sugar disorders.[190] Augmenting chromium supplements with brewer's yeast (rich in chromium as well as B vitamins and protein) has been shown to increase the effectiveness.

Vitamin E   100 to 600 IU daily to improve circulation, energy, and sugar storage in the liver.

Potassium   An excess of ingested salt or the internal stress created by low blood sugar can cause a loss of potassium and trigger FH symptoms. Eating a few bites of banana, swallowing a pinch of potassium-containing salt substitute, or chewing a 99-milligram potassium tablet may abort an incipient blackout.[87] For hypoglycemic headaches, muscle cramps, or shakiness, some authorities recommend 200 milligrams of potassium daily in divided doses with meals, but continual supplementation should be medically supervised.

Zinc—10 to 50 milligrams daily. This mineral helps the body cope with carbohydrates, is important for the health of the pancreas, and is particularly effective when accompanied by 50 milligrams of manganese (many hypoglycemics are deficient in both of these minerals) and an equal amount of vitamin B6.[4, 98, 228]

Sources (see Bibliography)

1, 2, 4, 6, 14, 17, 29, 34, 35, 39, 41, 57, 75, 79, 87, 90, 94, 97, 98, 112, 122, 123, 136, 148, 151, 162, 167, 190, 191, 201, 215, 222, 224, 228, 234, 243, 251, 252, 254, 255, 283, 293, 300, 301, 316, 317, 320

Indigestion

Defined as imperfect digestion and medically termed dyspepsia, indigestion encompasses a varied selection of symptoms and causes. Stomach discomfort, bloating, belching (eructation)—sometimes accompanied by nausea and vomiting—most commonly result from eating too much or too fast; inadequate chewing; swallowing large amounts of air; or eating when constipated, physically fatigued, or emotionally upset. Biliousness, which leaves a bitter taste in the mouth, can occur when bile secreted by the gallbladder to help digest fats is brought up into the esophagus. Symptoms of gastritis (functional dyspepsia, inflammation of the stomach lining) may include abdominal cramps and diarrhea. Overindulging in alcohol, caffeine, or fatty or spicy foods; excessive smoking; and overuse of aspirin are potential irritants. Other instigators of indigestion can be food poisoning or reactions to specific foods or medications.

Symptoms usually disappear after the stomach has been allowed to rest for a few hours and the cause of the irritation is avoided. Recovery may be hastened by loosening tight clothing and lying down on the left side to allow gravity to help move the stomach contents along to the intestine. Stress worsens any condition and affects stomach activity to such an extent that food may linger as a partially digested lump or rush on through the gastrointestinal tract to cause diarrhea. A few minutes of deliberate relaxation (see Introduction) plus the affirmation "my stomach is relaxed and comfortable" is often beneficial. Antacids make the symptoms subside, but by neutralizing stomach acid, they prevent efficient digestion and interfere with the absorption of nutrients, and can interact with aspirin or prescription medications.[98, 108] Their continual use may produce side effects such as constipation, diarrhea, increased stomach acid secretion, or kidney stones.[109, 201] Recurrent dyspepsia warrants medical attention. In some instances, a lack of hydrochloric acid rather than overacidity is responsible for the condition and can be corrected with betaine or glutamic-acid hydrochloride supplements. In other cases, persistent indigestion may be a symptom of an underlying illness requiring treatment.

Diet

Eating at regular intervals three to five times a day and relaxing for a few minutes after meals aids digestion, but dining too close to bedtime may instigate indigestion—bodily functions slow during sleep and yet-to-be-used digestive acids can irritate the stomach or back up into the esophagus.[109] Getting too hungry allows gastric juices to accumulate and may trigger indigestion, especially for diabetics and hypoglycemics. If foods such as cabbage, cucumbers, onions, radishes, or turnips are indigestion instigators, an aftertaste usually identifies the culprit. Milk is a subtle suspect. Lactose intolerance, with its stomach-bloating gassiness, may develop after middle age due to the body's lessened production of the lactase required to digest the milk sugar lactose. Using lactase supplements or avoiding all dairy products except cultured ones like yogurt may resolve the difficulty. An overabundance of refined carbohydrates (which are digested more rapidly than other foods) can contribute to dyspepsia. Studies show that even substituting whole-wheat bread for white improves digestion in many cases,[147] but large amounts of soluble fiber (from oats, fruits, vegetables) may cause stomach bloating unless the intake of fiber is increased gradually.

Supplements (see note on page xii)

Taking acidophilus capsules with each meal helps control harmful intestinal bacteria that release gasses that can pass into the bloodstream to cause indigestion and nausea. Vitamins and minerals are necessary for proper digestion—a daily multiple may help chronic digestive difficulties—and additional supplements may be beneficial.

Vitamin A In the form of beta-carotene, for the stomach inflammation of gastritis, up to 25,000 IU twice daily for 5 days.

B Complex One comprehensive tablet daily plus 50 to 100 milligrams of B_1, B_6, niacinamide, and pantothenic acid may benefit all types of digestive problems.

Calcium and Magnesium These natural antacids are utilized in over-the-counter products. For after-mealtime distress: one 10-grain tablet of calcium carbonate can be chewed, or 500 milligrams of magnesium gluconate may be taken with milk. Chronic indigestion and nausea may be symptoms of magnesium deficiency.

Tissue Salts For occasional indigestion, take 3X Kali. Sulph. every 10 minutes for half an hour, then every 25 minutes for an hour or so.

○ For discomfort after eating fats or starches, take three tablets of 6X Kali. Mur. once each hour for 3 hours.

○ For bilious conditions or a bitter taste after eating, take 6X Nat. Sulph. at hourly intervals. If nausea is present, adding alternate doses of 6X Nat. Mur. and Silicea may be beneficial.

○ For gastritis, take 6X Ferr. Phos. and Kali. Mur. alternately each half hour, and if accompanied by nervous exhaustion, take 6X Kali. Phos. every 2 hours.

○ For indigestion with vomiting, take 6X Ferr. Phos. with sips of cold water every 30 minutes.

○ For chronic indigestion that is worse in the evening, take 12X Kali. Sulph. in the afternoon and again in the early evening.

Folk Remedies

Peppermint tea—used by ancient Egyptians and international folk healers—is now recognized as an effective stomach soother. Researchers have found that peppermint relaxes the muscular opening (sphincter) at the base of the esophagus so that trapped stomach gas can escape with a belch. Baking soda is more efficient as a burp inducer but should be used no more often than once a week; peppermint tea can be sipped three times a day.[51, 112] Anise tea is an antacid. Valerian root is recommended for "nervous stomach." Other widely used digestive teas include camomile, caraway, catnip, dill, fennel, fenugreek, and tarragon.

Digestion-improving liquids to be consumed before eating include mustard seed tea; tomato juice stirred with a spoonful of cod liver oil and an optional ¼ teaspoon of kelp granules; 2 teaspoons apple cider vinegar and 1 teaspoon honey in a glass of water; or the juice of a lemon in a cup of hot water. For chronic indigestion, stir ¼ cup *each* unprocessed bran and rolled oats in one quart of water, cover and let stand for a day, then strain and drink a cup of the liquid before each meal.

Fruits Slowly eating grated green apples is said to cool the burning sensations of gastritis and speed the healing process. For ordinary indigestion, sweeten shredded ripe apples with honey, or simmer apple parings in milk and sip a cup of the strained liquid until relief is felt. Potassium-rich bananas are recommended by folk practitioners. Blueberries or figs, sweetened with honey, and papaya or pineapple have scientific approval as digestive aids.[56, 150] An old remedy for chronic dyspepsia calls for chopping an unpeeled grapefruit into 2 cups of boiling water, letting the mixture stand overnight, then straining and drinking the liquid before breakfast.

Juices Blackberry juice (or blackberry wine), carrot, coconut, papaya, pear, and pineapple juices are believed to assist digestion. Because of their alkalinity, raw vegetable juices like celery and spinach and the liquid from sauerkraut are thought to be helpful for chronic dyspepsia.[311]

Milk Although a glass of milk may be as effective as commercial antacids for relieving "acid indigestion," it, too, may trigger acid rebound. Soured milks such as buttermilk, kefir, and yogurt are definite digestive aids. The Swiss prefer "Essig-Milch," made by stirring 1 tablespoon vinegar in ½ cup buttermilk.

Olive Oil A spoonful of olive oil every morning is a folk remedy for chronic gastritis; taking a spoonful before eating a spicy-hot meal may prevent an aftermath of stomach distress.

Vegetables Folk healers recommend thoroughly chewing a few bites of alfalfa sprouts or raw celery, parsley, potato, radish, or turnip. According to the *Book of Household Management*[20] published in 1861, the fruit of the tomato plant is a "sovereign remedy" for dyspepsia.

Water Sipping a cup of hot water before or after meals is credited with preventing or correcting indigestion. Evaline W. ate wisely and always had an excellent appetite but frequently suffered from a sour stomach. For 70 years, she relieved the discomforting episodes by "eating" hot water with a spoon. Eventually, however, the plain water seemed unpalatable. Adding ¼ teaspoon of potassium-containing salt substitute to the water not only solved that problem for Evaline but also made the remedy more effective—perhaps because potassium increases the internal contractions necessary for complete digestion.

Nerve Pressure and Massage

○ Press or massage the top of the head, about 1 inch in front of the center, press inward and upward at the base of the skull, then press inward on the corners of the mouth.

○ On the left hand, massage the palm between the thumb and index finger, then all four fingers.

○ Press or massage the outer side of the upper bone of each arm midway between elbow and shoulder, then a point about 2 inches toward the thumb from the elbow crease.

○ Press or massage 1 inch to the left of the center of the chest, then massage the area around both armpits and both kneecaps.

○ Massage and pull the middle toe on each foot for 1 minute, then massage the area between the ball of the foot and the center of the arch on both feet. If a tender spot is discovered, rub for 5 minutes twice a day to improve chronic indigestion.

See also **Food Poisoning, Heartburn, Nausea and Vomiting**

Sources (see Bibliography)

2, 5, 6, 10, 17, 20, 26, 42, 47, 51, 56, 57, 59, 64, 65, 72, 75, 83, 87, 98, 108, 109, 112, 116, 144, 147, 148, 150, 151, 166, 172, 177, 186, 189, 195, 201, 202, 203, 218, 225, 254, 255, 257, 265, 280, 283, 285, 294, 304, 305, 306, 311, 312, 313

Insomnia

Sleep-onset insomnia (difficulty in falling asleep) and sleep-maintenance insomnia (difficulty in staying asleep) may be either transient (lasting for less than 3 weeks) or chronic, long-term problems. Emotional upsets, excitement, a brief illness, and jet lag can cause short-term wakefulness or troubled sleep. Chronic insomnia may be due to anxiety; external sleep stoppers such as an uncomfortable mattress or too much light or noise; mental stress; nutritional deficiencies; poor sleep habits; physical disorders such as low blood sugar, sleep apnea (a breathing problem), or thyroid gland disturbances; or reactions to prescribed medications.

Individual minimum daily requirements for sleep are genetically determined, stabilize in early adulthood, and vary from less than 4 to more than 10 hours out of each 24. False insomnia can be self induced by attempting to force the body to sleep more than it should. A "good night's sleep" consists of four or five 60- to 90-minute cycles, each concluding with 10 to 20 minutes of rapid-eye-movement (REM) dream sleep after roller-coastering through four stages of light-to-deep non-REM sleep. All the stages are necessary for physical and mental well-being.

Habitual sleeplessness that does not respond to home remedies or professional treatment for underlying disorders may succumb to the behavioral modification strategies advised by experts at insomnia clinics. A 5-week study reported in the *Berkeley Wellness Letter* (July 1992) showed that insomniacs practicing relaxation exercises and these three facets of behavior training fell asleep faster and slept better than those who were treated with a sleeping drug. (1) Avoid caffeine, heavy meals, and strenuous exercise for 3 to 5 hours before bedtime. Limit alcohol (which can disrupt sleep patterns) and nicotine, which is a mild stimulant. Relax for an hour or so before retiring—listen to music, read, watch television, or take a warm bath. (2) Limit in-bed activities to sleeping and sex. If wakeful after 30 minutes, practice a relaxation technique (see Introduction) or get up and do something pleasantly monotonous until drowsy. (3) Arise at the same time every morning, regardless of the number of hours slept. Avoid daytime naps or limit them to 1 hour in the afternoon and then compensate by retiring an hour later at night.

Diet

Going to bed hungry can cause sleeping problems. For many people, eating an ounce or 2 of a low-fat, low-protein, sweet, starchy food an hour before bedtime is as effective as a sleeping pill—without the disruption of sleep rhythms or the adverse side effects of sleep drugs.[186, 319] Salty foods stimulate the adrenal glands so should be avoided before bedtime.

Although concentrated proteins are believed to increase the flow of alertness chemicals from the brain, bedtime snacks of crackers and cheese; half a meat, poultry, or tuna fish sandwich; or a glass of warm milk may encourage the release of sleep-inducing serotonin just as high-carbohydrate foods do. Increasing the consumption of foods rich in iron and copper (dried beans and fruits, red meat, nuts, shellfish, tofu) may improve the quality of sleep. When nervous tension creates sleeping difficulties, drinking carrot juice combined with apple, grape, papaya, pear, or pineapple juice may also be of help.

Supplements (see note on page xii)

Supplements differ from pharmaceutical drugs in that they lead to natural sleep and that the dosage can be decreased as nutritional deficiencies are corrected. In addition to a daily multivitamin-mineral, separate supplements may be beneficial.

B Complex One comprehensive tablet daily, plus 10 to 100 milligrams of B_6, 100 milligrams of pantothenic acid, 100 to 1,000 milligrams of niacinamide, and/or 500 to 1,000 milligrams of inositol, which has the tranquilizing effect of Librium and should not be taken on a regular basis.[98, 227]

Vitamin C 500 to 2,000 milligrams in divided daily doses to calm nerves and promote restful sleep.

Calcium and Magnesium Suggested dosages of these two minerals vary from 2,000 milligrams of calcium plus 250 milligrams of magnesium, or 1,000 milligrams of each, to 500 to 1,000 milligrams calcium plus 1,000 to 2,000 milligrams of magnesium. The most effective combination should be determined with the advice of each individual's physician, and the minerals taken in divided doses after meals and before bedtime.

Tissue Salts For occasional sleeplessness from nervous tension, take three tablets of 6X Ferr. Phos. an hour before retiring; 10 minutes later, take the same dosage of Kali. Phos. If needed, repeat in an hour. If wakefulness is accompanied by heart palpitations, take one tablet *each* 12X Calc. Fluor, Kali. Phos., and Nat. Mur. For insomnia accompanied by itching, take three tablets of 6X Nat. Phos. If necessary, repeat in an hour.

Exercise

A sedentary lifestyle contributes to insomnia by inhibiting the normal fluctuations in body temperature and metabolism. Even when a regular aerobic regimen is part of the daytime schedule, an after-dinner stroll or a routine of gentle bending and stretching exercises before bed can help relax tense muscles and facilitate the onset of sleep.[25]

Folk Remedies

In the first century A.D., the Greek physician Galen cured his insomnia by eating lettuce each evening. King George III reportedly relied on a bag of hops secured to his pillow to relieve the sleeplessness with which he was plagued. American folk healers suggest spraying the hops with alcohol to enhance their sedative effect.[313] Slowly eating a raw apple is another possible aid to restful slumber.

Alcohol An old German remedy calls for stirring a spoonful of honey into a cup of heated dark beer. American folk practitioners recommend sipping a glass or two of sweet wine, or steeping a teaspoon of dill seeds in ¾ cup of almost-boiling white wine for 30 minutes, then drinking the strained liquid while it is still warm.

Garlic Stir crushed garlic or garlic extract into chicken broth, warm water, or milk sweetened with honey.

Herbal Teas Those with soporific properties include anise, camomile, catnip, dill, hops, passion flower, peppermint, rosemary, skullcap, and valerian root. To ease muscle tension and promote sleep, steep 1 teaspoon *each* powdered hops flowers and valerian root in a cup of boiling water. Add ½ teaspoon of passion flower to relieve nervousness.

Honey A Vermont remedy is to blend 3 tablespoons of apple cider vinegar with a cup of honey, keep it in a jar by the bedside, and take 2 teaspoons whenever wakeful. One teaspoon to 1 tablespoon of honey may be stirred into herb teas, hot water, or warm milk. A European favorite is 2 tablespoons of honey mixed with ½ cup hot water and the juice of one lemon and one orange. A more potent variation calls for ¼ cup honey, 1 tablespoon apple cider vinegar, and 2 teaspoons bee pollen granules stirred into a cup of freshly boiled water. Colleen F. had such a full schedule and was so enthusiastic about teaching her seventh-grade class that she couldn't get to sleep at night. Neither could she teach while half awake. Not wanting to succumb to sleeping-pill dependency, Colleen combined folk remedies. At bedtime, she stirred 2 tablespoons of honey into a glass of warm milk, added a tablespoon of apple cider vinegar, and drank the mixture before it curdled. The results were fantastic. Colleen sleeps soundly and awakens refreshed and alert.

Onions Raw or cooked onions are thought to have great soporific power. Placing a cut raw onion beneath the pillow[150, 313] or in a jar to uncover and whiff when wakeful has relieved some cases of insomnia. Although not recommended for hypoglycemics, hardy souls eat raw onions before bed; the more timid prefer to down their onions cooked in chicken broth—with or without the addition of the juice of one lemon and a pat of butter.

Nerve Pressure and Massage

Once each day, press and massage one or two of these points for 30 seconds: above the bridge of the nose between the eyebrows; 1 inch behind each earlobe; the center of the nape of the neck, and the center of the chest; 1½ inches directly below the navel; 1½ inches toward the elbow from the inside of the wrist crease, in line with the little finger; or the indentation below the anklebone on the inside and outside of each foot. Or massage each foot for 3 minutes. Start with the toes, then massage the sole, the heel, the sides, the ankle, and the top of the foot.

Relaxation and Mental Imagery

Yogis believe that gazing at a lighted candle for 10 minutes before retiring will quiet the mind. Sounds soothe many people to sleep. Soft music, electric fans, or ticking clocks were used before the advent of "sleep-sound" recordings of rain, ocean waves, trickling brooks, and waterfalls. Slow, deep breathing can encourage drowsiness. Inhale through the mouth, exhale through the nose, repeat five times or until yawning. Or, take three deep breaths and stop breathing to the point of discomfort after the third exhalation. Repeat the cycle five or six times to derive a tranquilizing effect from the accumulation of carbon dioxide in the blood.[254, 261] Practicing any of the relaxation techniques described in the Introduction can help banish disturbing thoughts; focusing on "counting" can block their reentry. As an alternative to counting sheep, imagine entering an elevator on the hundredth floor and mentally recite the numbers on the indicator above the door as the elevator slowly descends. Or visualize a blackboard with the number "100" written on it inside a large circle. Mentally erase the number and write the next lower number, then write the words "deep sleep" beside the circle. Continue erasing, renumbering, and writing over the words as long as necessary.

Warm Baths

Soaking for 15 minutes in a tub of warm water is a standard cure for sleeplessness. Some researchers have found that slightly cool water (between 92 degrees and 97 degrees Fahrenheit) relaxes the blood vessels of the skin, soothes nerve endings, and has a pronounced sedative effect.[300] Dissolving a half cup of baking soda, epsom salts, or table salt in the water aids muscle relaxation. Herbalists suggest steeping ½ cup of any one or a combination of these soporific herbs in boiling water for 30 minutes and adding the strained tea to the tub: bergamot, camomile, hops, lavender, peppermint, pine needles, sage, thyme.

Sources (see Bibliography)

14, 16, 17, 25, 26, 37, 42, 47, 49, 51, 53, 57, 59, 63, 64, 75, 98, 111, 125, 135, 139, 143, 145, 147, 150, 151, 168, 172, 177, 180, 186, 201, 203, 204, 206, 218, 227, 240, 254, 255, 256, 261, 284, 285, 293, 294, 300, 302, 308, 312, 313, 319

Irritable Bowel Syndrome

Formerly referred to as mucous colitis, nervous bowel, or spastic colon, irritable bowel syndrome (IBS) is a common malady with an assortment of unpleasant symptoms: abdominal cramping, alternating episodes of diarrhea and constipation, bloating, flatulence, and sometimes, nausea, fatigue, and depression. Affecting three times more women than men, IBS is considered a functional abnormality, not a disease, because it is due to abnormal contraction and distension of bowel muscles. This irregular motility interferes with normal movement of food and waste material through the gastrointestinal tract, may stretch the intestinal walls to cause pain, and can produce excessive gas and mucus in the bowel. Although there may be a genetic predisposition toward IBS, the primary causes are believed to be emotional stress and food sensitivities. Symptoms may also be triggered by overuse of alcohol, coffee or tea, tobacco, or laxatives. By combining relaxation techniques with nutritional strategies, most sufferers are able to control the condition, but medical diagnosis should be obtained to rule out the possibility of complications or an accompanying illness.

Diet and Supplements (see note on page xii)

Eating small meals at frequent intervals, and eating them slowly, avoids overstimulating the digestive system and may help regulate abnormal bowel contractions.

Acidophilus Eating yogurt once or twice a week bolsters the friendly intestinal flora that help synthesize B vitamins and inhibit problem-creating putrefactive bacteria in the bowel. If IBS symptoms develop within a few months after antibiotic treatment, a yeast infection (Candida) may be the cause[201]—acidophilus yogurt (or capsules) helps restore the beneficial intestinal flora destroyed along with harmful microorganisms. Myrna G. suspected a yeast infection might be responsible for her symptoms of IBS because she had been hospitalized the previous month and had not taken acidophilus capsules during treatment with antibiotics as she had on other occasions. Eager to dispense with her discomfort, Myrna tried a nutritional assault against *Candida albicans* by eating no milk, sugar, or yeast breads, consuming ¼ cup of yogurt three times daily, and adding a folk remedy: Once a day for 2 weeks, she ate an avocado drizzled with a mixture of 2 teaspoons olive oil and 1 teaspoon apple cider vinegar. The experiment was a success; Myrna's symptoms subsided and have not recurred.

Beverages Folk healers prescribe 1 tablespoon of blackstrap molasses stirred into a cup of hot water. Herbalists suggest teas of cascara sagrada (to increase intestinal peristalsis), camomile, ginger root, or peppermint. The two alcoholic beverages most likely to aggravate an irritable bowel are beer and red wine.[250]

Essential Fatty Acids A deficiency of these acids (also called UFA, unsaturated fatty acids) is commonly associated with irritable bowel syndrome. Wheat germ, nut butters, and cold-pressed vegetable or seed oils are excellent sources. To assure absorption of the fatty acids and to prevent their oxidation within the body, many nutritionists suggest taking at least 10 IU of supplemental vitamin E for each tablespoon of oil used. Evening primrose oil, which should be taken only in capsules, is also a rich source of the essential fatty acids.[17]

Fiber A bland, soft diet benefits some IBS sufferers, particularly during bouts of diarrhea, but most people can reduce symptoms and the frequency of flareups by gradually increasing the amount of dietary fiber and drinking six to eight glasses of water each day. Whole grains, brans, vegetables, fruits, and pectin or psyllium supplements provide fiber, which expands with absorbed liquid to increase stool bulk and alleviate cramping, diarrhea, and constipation. In one study, 50 percent of the patients on a high-fiber diet reported improved bowel function and a reduction in pain, and 75 percent of those who had been passing mucus no longer did so. On a low-residue regimen, there was no change in mucus passing, and only 14 percent had any relief from IBS symptoms.[147]

Food Sensitivity Numerous studies show that food allergy or food sensitivity causes IBS flareups in one-half to two-thirds of the patients tested.[44] The most likely offenders are citrus fruits, corn, dairy products, eggs, nuts, potatoes, tomatoes, and wheat. Others are chocolate, fish, pork, and food additives or colorings. By eliminating suspects for 2 weeks then reintroducing the foods one at a time after symptoms have cleared, individual instigators may be identified. Lactase deficiency (a shortage of the enzyme needed to digest the lactose in milk and milk products) is a common cause of IBS symptoms. If using lactase supplements does not remedy the condition, a milk allergy may be the culprit—avoiding all dairy products except cultured ones like yogurt and kefir may provide relief. Refined carbohydrates and sugar (including the artificial sweetener sorbitol) can bring on this syndrome; as may an excess of fat, which can stimulate colonic contractions to cause diarrhea.[189] Limiting consumption of gas-producing foods and taking activated charcoal (see "Flatulence") helps prevent that part of the problem.

Tissue Salts Taking three tablets of 6X Mag. Phos. with a few sips of hot water may quickly relieve cramping and spasmodic pains. To improve a spastic colon, 2 tablets *each* of 3X Mag. Phos. and Kali. Phos. may be taken three times a day for a week.

Vitamin and Mineral Supplements Supplements compensate for malabsorption due to diarrhea and may help control IBS. Taken in addition to a multivitamin-mineral, a daily B-complex tablet plus 50 milligrams of pantothenic acid improves peristaltic action and helps combat stress reactions. Under the guidance of the attending physician, 800 to 1,500 milligrams of calcium plus 500 to 1,600 milligrams of magnesium to help soothe a spastic colon and calm the central nervous system.

Exercise and Stress Management

Performing a few bent-knee sit-ups may stop colon spasms and initiate a return to normal intestinal contractions. Emotional stress can instigate IBS by disrupting the coordination of bowel muscles; adhering to a program of physical activity helps prevent this effect. Exercise also improves bowel muscle tone, helps control discomfort by releasing painkilling hormones (endorphins) in the brain, and augments the stress-relieving relaxation techniques described in the Introduction.

Moist Heat

An old-fashioned sitz bath may alleviate abdominal pain. For a modernized version, fill the bathtub with hot (100 to 104 degrees Fahrenheit) water to the lower margin of the navel, then elevate both feet on the sides of the tub or hang them over the rim. Adding a tablespoon of apple cider vinegar, baking soda, epsom salts, or table salt to the water may increase the benefit. As an alternative, a cup of double-strength camomile, comfrey, lavender, or pekoe tea may be swished into the water.

Saturating a towel with hot water, salt water, or a strong epsom salts solution and applying it to the painful area is another option. The hot applications should be repeated for 2 or 3 hours or kept warm with a plastic-protected heating pad.

Nerve Pressure and Massage

Press and massage just in front of each ear at the top of the cheekbone; press above the thumb pad ½ inch toward the center of each palm; then massage both shinbones from just below the knee to mid-calf.

See also **Colitis and Diverticulosis**

Sources (see Bibliography)

10, 17, 44, 45, 47, 51, 59, 65, 75, 98, 101, 112, 147, 151, 164, 172, 177, 186, 189, 190, 201, 202, 203, 250, 254, 255, 262, 281, 286, 293, 294, 296, 300

Jet Lag

All living things operate according to a circadian rhythm, an inborn clock that determines when various bodily functions and the desire to eat, sleep, and wake occur. Transmeridianal fatigue, commonly called jet lag, is a modern ailment caused by passing through too many time zones too rapidly for the body's biological clock to make appropriate adjustments. It is easier to accept a gain than a loss in time because, as shown in clinical studies, the human "internal day" actually lasts 25 hours, not 24.[300] North/south trips usually evoke only normal weariness, but disrupting sleep/wake patterns by shortening the day with eastward flights or lengthening it by traveling westward more than two time zones often results in exhaustion, diminished alertness, disorientation, irritability, loss of appetite, sleepiness during the day, wakefulness at night, and perhaps, constipation or diarrhea.

Jet lag preventives and remedies can help reset the biological clock to significantly reduce the typical readjustment period of 1 day for each time zone crossed. Complete anti-jet-lag programs such as those developed by Charles F. Ehret[100] and Judith J. Wurtman[319] incorporate exercise, exposure to light, rest and sleep, along with foods and beverages, on a precise schedule determined by the direction and duration of each flight. Individualizing basic anti-jet-lag strategies may be equally effective.

Diet

Although some individuals are able to prevent jet lag by avoiding all food on the day of the flight and drinking only water and fruit or vegetable juices, "jetting diets" are based on eating proteins when it is time to stay awake; carbohydrates before time to sleep. Fatty foods and overeating also promote postmeal lethargy. Clear soups, nonstarchy vegetables, and unsweetened fresh fruits are considered "neutrals" in the sleep/wake game.

○ High-protein meals consisting mainly of lean meat, poultry, fish, eggs (when allowable), and low-fat dairy products stimulate neurotransmitters in the brain to provide mental alertness and energy for up to 5 hours.

○ High-carbohydrate meals composed principally of pasta, rice, starchy vegetables like potatoes, rolls, sweetened or dried fruits, and desserts boost energy for about an hour, then trigger the release of serotonin, a tranquilizing, sleep-inducing chemical.

Whether initiating a plan with high-protein breakfasts and lunches and high-carbohydrate dinners 3 days before the trip (Dr. Ehret advises "feasting" with hearty meals on days 1 and three, "fasting" with a 900-calorie limit on day 2) or waiting until departure day, it is important that each meal begin with a few ounces of the primary food. As explained in *Managing Your Mind and Mood Through Food*,[319] starting a high-carbohydrate dinner with a protein appetizer can block the production of serotonin; eating a breadstick before a high-protein lunch can diminish the flow of alertness chemicals.

Nibbling a carry-on, high-carbohydrate snack (gum drops or jelly beans) or a packet of high-protein beef jerky or dry-roasted peanuts can help evoke the required biological responses between meals. Drinking plenty of fluids fends off dehydration from the dry air in pressurized cabins. Inflight alcohol is forbidden with the U.S. Department of Energy's Anti-Jet-Lag Diet and limited to one drink per day with Dr. Ehret's, but one or two drinks are suggested as a sleep aid with other diets. To help regulate the body clock, most programs advise restricting caffeine-containing beverages to one cup in the afternoon for 3 days prior to departure. During the trip and the postflight adjustment period, they recommend having no caffeine other than one to three cups of black coffee or plain tea daily—with breakfast on westward journeys, at 6:00 P.M. on eastward junkets. Continuing the protein-for-alertness, carbohydrates-for-relaxation diet pattern for several days after arrival and adhering to normal mealtimes in the new time zone may hasten the body's adjustment. Herbalists suggest judicious use of herbal stimulants such as ginseng, gotu cola, and peppermint and sedatives such as hops, skullcap, and valerian to readjust sleep/wake cycles.

Supplements (see note on page xii)

Calcium, a natural tranquilizer available in chewable tablets, can help relax tense nerves during the flight and encourage sleep on the new schedule after arrival. Besides a daily multivitamin-mineral (two doses on flight day if more than five time zones are crossed), some nutritionally oriented doctors suggest additional supplements to assist the body in overcoming jet lag.

B Complex   One tablet each morning and evening.

Vitamin C with Bioflavonoids   Available in tablets or lozenges, 1,000 milligrams in divided doses.

Vitamin E   Preferably in the dry form, 100 to 400 IU twice daily.

Exercise

Physical activity a half-hour before destination-time breakfast helps bring the body back to optimal functioning. If stretching and walking up and down the aisle are not feasible, substitute deep breathing and seat exercises: Rotate both ankles, tense and relax one buttock at a time, press the palms of the hands together in front of the chest, press down on the thighs for a count of five, then pull up on the thighs without moving the hands.

After arrival, 10 to 15 minutes of moderately strenuous exercise helps reset the biological clock by raising the metabolism. Following a west-to-east trip, exercise should be performed early in the morning. In a time zone west of the home zone, late afternoon exercising postpones the desire for sleep.

Light

Research studies show that sunshine (or artificial light of equal brightness) can shift the body clock to an earlier hour if exposure is early in the day; to a later hour with late-afternoon exposure.[293, 300] Utilizing a brisk 10-minute walk in the sunlight for the before-breakfast or late-afternoon exercise maximizes the benefits.

Sleep

Switching to the sleep/wake cycle of the destination time zone as soon as possible helps resynchronize the biological clock. Wes H., who makes several business trips to Europe every year, plans to arrive the evening before his scheduled appointments, and follows an anti-jet-lag pattern. On a 13-hour flight from Phoenix to Frankfurt, for instance, he sets his watch to destination time after takeoff, inserts his earplugs, dons his dark glasses, and rests or sleeps from the 8:00 P.M. departure (5:00 A.M. in Germany) until four or five hours before arriving in Frankfurt at 6:00 P.M. Although it is 9:00 A.M. in Arizona, Wes has a leisurely dinner, including wine and dessert, reads or watches television for an hour or so, goes to bed by 11:00 P.M. (new time), and sleeps enough to be clear-headed the next morning. On short trips (two or three time-zone changes), Wes again uses earplugs and dark glasses to encourage relaxation during the flight and alertness upon arrival.

Night owls like Zelda G., who normally retires well after midnight and is not fully functional until midmorning, have additional adjustments to make. For 2 weeks prior to flying from San Diego, California, to visit her daughter in Atlantic City, New Jersey, Zelda gradually advances her inner clock by going to bed earlier each night and rising earlier each morning. During the flight and the week on the East Coast, she eats high-protein or high-carbohydrate foods as needed to encourage alertness or tranquility, and since she does not drink caffeine-containing beverages at home, she derives dramatically energizing benefits from a cup of coffee or tea early in the evening.

Daytime naps are not advised for travelers who are east of their home time zone. For the first few days after a westward flight, however, a 1-hour afternoon nap followed by 10 minutes of exercise, a cup of coffee, and a protein snack may allay jet-lag discomfort.[319]

Nerve Pressure and Massage

When it is time to relax, stimulating these acupressure points may help: Press and massage the depression at the base of the skull with a counterclockwise motion, then a spot on each shoulder about 2 inches out from the spine. Repeat each movement three times for 15 seconds each.[265]

Sources (see Bibliography)

48, 53, 56, 75, 86, 100, 151, 159, 176, 186, 206, 207, 234, 256, 265, 293, 300, 313, 319

Kidney Stones and Bladder Problems

Kidney stones (renal calculi) develop in the urine from crystals of mineral salts—60 to 80 percent consist of calcium oxalate and/or phosphate, 5 to 10 percent are uric-acid stones that usually occur in people with gout, up to 20 percent stem from urinary tract infections (UTIs).[75] Occasionally, stones form in the bladder as a result of obstructed urine flow or recurrent UTIs. Kidney stones, which afflict more men than women, may remain symptomless for years, then create excruciating pain when they migrate down the urinary tract, lodge in the ureter, or pass on into the bladder and cause dribbling or painful urination.

UTIs (also known as bladder infections and cystitis) are more common among women than men because the shorter female urethra (tube through which urine is excreted) leaves the bladder more accessible to contamination from bacteria such as *E. coli* that normally inhabit the intestines. Women prone to recurrent bladder infections are advised to wear cotton-crotch underwear, use sanitary pads rather than tampons, avoid using a diaphragm for birth control, and wipe from front to back after a bowel movement to avoid vaginal contamination with bacteria from the colon. Allergic reactions and yeast infections sometimes simulate UTI symptoms; other instigators are sexual contacts, infected urine sent from the kidney to the bladder, and, in males, an enlarged or infected prostate gland.

Heredity plays a leading role in the selection of stone formers and UTI sufferers, and both ailments tend to recur in susceptible people unless precautionary measures are practiced. All maladies of the urinary system should be diagnosed by a physician—particularly if there is blood in the urine or if fever is present. Although most kidney and bladder stones exit spontaneously, the intense pain may demand professional alleviation, and large stones may require prescriptive medication, fragmentation with sound waves or shock waves, or surgical removal. All "passed" stones should be chemically analyzed to determine proper treatment to prevent recurrence.

Cranberry Juice and Water

Scientific studies show that cranberry juice, the favorite folk remedy for kidney and bladder problems, not only acidifies the urine to discourage development of kidney stones and proliferation of harmful bacteria but also has even more beneficial properties. Recent research has found that cranberries contain antiadhesion compounds to keep bacteria from adhering to body tissues in the urinary tract and that drinking 3 to 6 ounces of cranberry juice cocktail a day may prevent recurrent UTIs.[186, 298] In clinical studies of patients with acute bladder infections, 70 percent showed moderate to excellent improvement after 3 weeks of taking a pint of cranberry juice as their only treatment.[29] Steeping a teaspoon of powdered goldenseal root in a cup of boiling cranberry juice daily may help destroy the harmful bacteria. If during an acute episode the juice further aggravates an irritated urinary tract, experts suggest drinking a glass of water mixed with ¼ to 1 teaspoon of baking soda two or three times a day.[132, 201]

The primary preventive and treatment for urinary ills, however, is drinking lots of water—eight to ten glasses per day. Well diluted urine discourages stone formation by flushing out seed crystals and assisting the passage of tiny stones, and the copious urine produced also washes out infection-causing bacteria. To irrigate the urinary tract and lessen the likelihood of infection, women are advised to drink a glass of water and urinate both before and after sexual intercourse.

Diet

Aside from the importance of fluid intake and the preventive value of acidifying the urine, the relationship of diet to urinary tract disorders is controversial. For some people, foods that prompt the release of histamines or that contain large amounts of amino acids may instigate or add to burning sensations during urination. Experimental food elimination may identify the culprits from a group that includes aged cheeses, alcohol, avocados, chocolate, coffee, fruits (except for berries, pears, and watermelon), pickled and spicy foods, tomatoes, and wines.[132]

Bladder, kidney, and ureter stones tend to recur—60 percent of patients treated for one stone develop another within 7 years.[75] Blood tests and the analysis of a passed stone determine the dietary approach most likely to forestall a recurrence. Since nutrients from all food groups are essential for total health, the following suggestions are for sensible limitation, not absolute avoidance.

Dairy Products Restriction of calcium-rich dairy products, antacids, and supplements may be recommended for individuals who overabsorb calcium or who have been consuming an overabundance of it. However, for people who ingest less than the 900 milligrams of calcium provided by three glasses of milk, who are not physically active, or who use excessive amounts of salt or sugar, calcium reduction may exacerbate stone formation because any of those factors can pull needed calcium from the bones into the blood and urine.[3, 147, 186, 300]

Oxalates Although the body synthesizes all but 2 percent of its oxalates, cutting back on oxalate-rich beans, beets, caffeine-containing beverages, chocolate, leafy greens, nuts (almonds, cashews, peanuts), peppers, tea, and wheat germ may be of benefit because oxalates are commonly a component of calcium-based stones.[147, 186, 234]

Protein Excessive amounts of animal protein put a strain on the kidneys and increase calcium loss in the body. For people with stones consisting predominantly of cysteine or uric acid, a daily total of only 6 ounces of cheese, fish, meat, and poultry is suggested—along with limitations on citrus fruits, grapes, and coffee.[186, 254]

Fiber Studies show that increasing the amount of dietary fiber to 18 grams by including 2 tablespoons of rice bran with each meal (or eating two corn bran or wheat bran muffins a day) sharply lowers the amount of calcium and oxalates in the urine and reduces the likelihood of kidney stone recurrence.[51, 186]

Supplements (see note on page xii)

A daily multivitamin-mineral is recommended to compensate for the requisite fluid intake that can flush water-soluble vitamins and minerals out of the system.

Vitamin A In the form of beta carotene, 25,000 IU daily to assist healing, maintain the health of the urinary tract lining, and discourage the development of kidney stones.

B Complex One comprehensive tablet daily. Clinical studies show that an additional 10 to 150 milligrams of B6 in divided doses reduces the amount of oxalic acid in the urine to discourage the formation of kidney stones.[47, 201]

Vitamin C 1,000 to 5,000 milligrams in divided daily doses to combat UTIs and acidify the urine to prevent recurrent infections. However, individuals who are disposed to form kidney stones should not take massive amounts of vitamin C without medical approval—for some people, more than 3 or 4 grams increases oxalate production. Uric-acid stone formers should use non-acidic forms such as calcium ascorbate.[17, 98, 151, 293]

Calcium and Magnesium 800 to 1,000 milligrams of calcium—not from phosphorus-rich bone meal, (because excess phosphorus leads to the formation of stones in some people) and not without a doctor's approval if stone prone—plus 500 to 750 milligrams of magnesium (up to 2,000 milligrams with medical approval) taken with meals. Although most kidney stones are formed with calcium, there is no evidence that their formation is related to calcium intake.[151] Magnesium regulates calcium flow between cells and bonds with oxalate to curtail the development of stones. Several studies show that combining magnesium and vitamin B6 supplementation can reduce stone recurrence from 68 to 90 percent.[151, 293]

Tissue Salts For UTIs with frequent urination and burning sensations, take three 6X tablets of Ferr. Phos. three times a day, or alternating doses of Ferr. Phos., Kali. Phos., and Nat. Mur. If urine emission is scanty, take 6X Silicea. For pain while passing kidney gravel, take three 6X tablets of Nat. Phos. and Nat. Sulph.

Folk Remedies

Drinking a glass of water containing 2 teaspoons *each* apple cider vinegar and raw honey with each meal is said to help prevent urinary tract infections. Eating three cloves of garlic a day (or taking the equivalent in capsules) is a remedy for cystitis. Imbibing four or five bottles of strong, dark beer, heated almost to simmering, is an old German remedy for getting rid of kidney stones in 2 days.

Herbal recommendations for kidney stones and bladder problems are catnip, cornsilk, parsley, red clover, uva ursi, and watermelon seed teas. Buchu, burdock, or a blend of burdock and catnip are believed to help dissolve and get rid of kidney stones. To soothe the burning sensation that accompanies cystitis, slippery elm tea or, according to *Natural Health* (October 1992), 4 teaspoons of marshmallow root steeped overnight in a quart of water can be sipped during the day.

Hot compresses or poultices may help relieve pain from kidney stones. Options include cloths squeezed out of hot water, or a quart of water in which an ounce of fresh ginger has been simmered for 5 minutes; or poultices made of wheat bran and hot water, or heated chopped onions and white wine.

Vegetable remedies for dissolving kidney stones include drinking ¼ cup pureed asparagus mixed with hot water twice a day, two cups daily of the water in which parsnips have been cooked, or a daily drink of ½ cup red wine whirred in the blender with two red radishes.

Nerve Pressure and Massage

For All Bladder and Kidney Problems   Press or massage each cheekbone just in front of the upper part of the ears, and the small depression about 1 inch below the top of the breastbone.

For Cystitis   Massage the center of each inner wrist, then the inner edge of each foot near the heel.

For Kidney Stones   Massage the center of the palms, then rub back and forth from the center of the palms to the inner wrists. Or massage the thumb, index, and middle finger of each hand. Or massage under the arch of each foot, then back and forth to the beginning of the heel pad.

Sources (see Bibliography)

2, 3, 5, 6, 10, 16, 17, 21, 26, 29, 37, 47, 49, 50, 51, 59, 60, 64, 65, 75, 98, 113, 132, 135, 143, 144, 147, 148, 150, 151, 164, 168, 171, 186, 201, 202, 223, 234, 254, 255, 293, 294, 298, 300, 304, 306

Leg and Foot Cramps

Painful, involuntary, contractions of leg and foot muscles can be instigated by a variety of factors: dehydration, fatigue, overexertion, nutritional deficiencies, or tight clothing that restricts circulation. A "charley horse" is usually caused by a blow to the leg or by a forceful stretch during physical activity—the term, which is applied to a "knotted" cramp or to any accidental lameness, originated at Ebbets Field in Brooklyn, where a lame horse named Charley dragged metal fencing around the infield between innings.

Intermittent claudication (leg pain brought on by walking and relieved by resting) feels like a cramp but is often accompanied by a sensation of heaviness, may be a symptom of atherosclerotic hardening of the arteries, and is contributed to by high blood pressure, high cholesterol, diabetes, and cigarette smoking. Repeated episodes of claudication, or of any cramping accompanied by numbness or coldness of a limb, should be medically evaluated to determine and correct the underlying cause.

Sleep-disturbing leg and foot cramps are sometimes interspersed with the muscle twitching and jerking called restless leg syndrome. Nocturnal leg problems may be resolved by environmental adjustments. Elevating either the foot or the head of the bed may prevent cramps caused by an accumulation of fluid in the lower extremities.[254] Tucking a pillow between the knees when sleeping on one side or under the knees when lying on the back helps prevent muscle-strain cramping. Loosening the bottom of the bed covers or placing a board or pillow at the foot of the bed removes cramp-triggering pressure on the toes. Wearing bed socks to keep the feet warm may help. New shoes were the solution for Rose B. Her nocturnal leg cramps began shortly after she retired from her position as an account executive and returned to her first love—art. Reveling in the freedom from heels and hose, Rose wore squishy-soled slippers all day while standing in front of the easel—and at night while she "walked off" leg cramps. Then she bought a pair of athletic shoes so comfortable that she wore them, instead of the scuffs, while painting. By the third night, Rose and her well-supported feet and legs were no longer disturbed by nighttime cramping.

Warm compresses or a heating pad may relax cramped muscles. For a calf cramp, grasping the toes and pulling them toward the knee with one hand while massaging upward from calf to knee usually brings quick relief; rubbing the area with cloth-covered ice may speed the process.

Diet and Supplements (see note on page xii)

Insufficient fluid intake (eight glasses of water per day are advised) can decrease blood volume and lead to circulatory problems that cause cramping. Muscle cramps that occur in conjunction with vigorous exercise may be prevented by eating a few bites of salty food and drinking at least half a glass of water before, every 20 minutes during, and immediately after the exertion. Eating generous amounts of potassium-rich bananas, beans, fresh vegetables, and whole grains is recommended; potassium supplements should be taken only with a physician's approval. A balanced diet plus a daily multivitamin-mineral usually satisfies muscular needs, but additional supplements may be required as compensation for blood sugar irregularities, dietary restrictions, or mineral deficiencies created by excessive perspiration or diuretic medications.

B Complex One comprehensive tablet daily, plus up to 50 milligrams of niacin three times a day to improve circulation, and 50 to 150 milligrams of B_6 to prevent nocturnal leg cramps. Additional amounts of B_1 and pantothenic acid may also be helpful.

Vitamin C with Bioflavonoids 1,000 to 3,000 milligrams in divided daily doses to decrease smooth-muscle contractions, improve circulation, and strengthen connective tissues. Taking vitamin C before, each hour during, and immediately after unaccustomed physical activity often prevents an aftermath of stiffness and cramping.

Calcium and Magnesium 800 to 1,500 milligrams of calcium plus 500 to 750 milligrams of magnesium in divided doses. Some researchers suggest 500 to 1,000 milligrams of calcium plus 1,000 to 2,000 milligrams of magnesium. Deficiencies of these two minerals are a common cause of nighttime leg and foot cramps. Calcium is essential for normal muscle contraction; magnesium helps regulate both calcium and potassium.[17, 49, 317]

Vitamin E   300 to 800 IU daily (beginning with the lower amount and increasing gradually) to improve circulation and claudication problems, and to relieve restless, cramping, nighttime legs.[98, 151, 301]

L-carnitine   For intermittent claudication, 900 to 1,600 milligrams daily. Several studies show that supplements of this amino acid can improve pain-free walking tolerance by up to 75 percent.[151]

Tissue Salts   For quick relief from restless legs and nocturnal cramps, dissolve three 6X tablets of Mag. Phos. under the tongue. For muscle cramps following exercise, 6X Calc. Fluor., Calc. Phos, and Mag. Phos. every 20 minutes for 2 hours. To prevent nighttime leg cramps, take three 6X tablets of Silicea plus calcium, magnesium, and vitamin B$_6$ supplements before retiring.[64, 65]

Zinc   50 milligrams daily to assist calcium absorption and the nerve-controlling action of B vitamins.

Exercise

Regular exercise improves muscle tone, assists calcium absorption, and lessens the tendency for cramping. Part of the treatment for intermittent claudication is walking until discomfort is noticed, resting while the pain subsides, then repeating the sequence. Easy exercises for stretching calf muscles to maintain flexibility and reduce cramps include standing at arm's length from a wall, and leaning forward with weight supported on both hands while legs are straight and heels are on the floor; or, while seated, stretching out the legs, extending the heels, and bending the toes toward the body.

Folk Remedies

Drinking a glass of water mixed with 2 teaspoons *each* apple cider vinegar and honey at mealtimes or walking in place for 3 minutes in 6 inches of cold water in a bathtub every night are favorite preventives. Quinine, an old remedy that modern studies have shown to be effective, is now available without prescription but medical approval is advised. For many cases, taking 200 to 300 milligrams of quinine sulfate every other night for a week or two has stopped nocturnal leg cramps for long periods.[151, 186, 254] If attacked by a midnight cramp, rubbing it with the bowl of a metal spoon is said to bring relief in 30 seconds. Herbalists suggest alfalfa, cayenne, horsetail, or red raspberry leaf for leg cramps. Ginkgo biloba extract increases blood circulation and, as demonstrated in European studies, provides significant improvement for patients with intermittent claudication.[151]

Nerve Pressure and Massage

For immediate relief at the onset of a leg or foot cramp, firmly pinch the skin between the nose and the center of the upper lip for 20 seconds. For knee pain while walking or running, press a point 3 inches above the knee and 3 inches toward the inside of the thigh; maintain firm pressure for 30 to 90 seconds. For leftover tenderness from a leg cramp, press and massage a point about 8 inches above the outside anklebone on the painful leg. Other cramp-relieving options are

○ Press and massage the base of both thumbs on the inside, across the inside of the wrists, and the backs of the hands above the wrist bone.

○ Press and massage an inch below the web between the big toe and the one next to it on the soles of both feet, side to side across the middle of the heel pads, and, on the right foot, the outer edge from 1 inch below the little toe to the center of the arch.

Sources (see Bibliography)

6, 14, 17, 26, 40, 47, 49, 59, 60, 64, 65, 98, 106, 108, 109, 111, 133, 148, 151, 159, 162, 172, 176, 177, 186, 202, 228, 244, 250, 254, 255, 256, 262, 265, 291, 293, 294, 300, 301, 308, 312, 313, 317

Low Blood Pressure (Hypotension)

Blood pressure readings below the average range of 110/70 to 140/90 are normal for some healthy people and are often considered a blessing. As explained in the January 11, 1992, issue of *British Medical Journal*, however, low blood pressure can become a problem when blood flow to the brain is reduced to the extent that dizziness or fainting spells are experienced. Hypotension is usually diagnosed when blood pressure is checked while lying down, then a twenty-point drop in the systolic pressure (upper figure) is registered when it is rechecked after 1 minute of standing.[293]

Chronic hypotension, which affects about 6 percent of the population, may be caused by anemia, diabetic nerve damage that disrupts blood pressure-controlling reflexes, internal bleeding, low blood sugar, malnutrition, an underactive thyroid, or a debilitating disease. Acute hypotension is the term for a sudden drop in blood pressure that results from injuries involving heavy blood loss or physiological shock such as a heart attack.

Postural (orthostatic) hypotension, the most common type, is evidenced by momentary dizzy spells when the position is abruptly changed. Rising slowly, sitting on the side of the bed before standing, and standing a moment before walking allows cardiovascular reflexes time to circulate blood to the brain. Elevating the head of the bed on 8- to 12-inch blocks also helps control hypotension.

Temporary episodes of lightheadedness can occur in connection with viral infections or influenza, and some cases of apparent hypotension may be reactions to antidepressants or antihypertensive medications. According to *Journal of the American Medical Association* (no. 4, 1991), the risk of heart attack increases if high blood pressure is forced down by drugs to a diastolic reading (the lower figure) of 85 or less. Continuing to take diuretics when they are no longer necessary can instigate all the symptoms of hypotension—headache, fatigue and weakness, lightheadedness and fainting—by reducing both blood pressure and blood volume from lack of fluid in the body. After medical evaluation and possible adjustment of medications, or treatment for underlying causes, home remedies may help alleviate the problem.

Diet

Nutritional deficiencies can cause the walls of the blood vessels to lose elasticity, become flabby, and expand. Since the volume of blood remains the same, blood pressure drops because pressure against the arterial walls is reduced, and fewer nutrients can penetrate into the tissues—thus producing fatigue, weakness, and lightheadedness. A high-protein diet that includes organ meats, potatoes baked in their skins, leafy green vegetables, soybeans or soy flour, and wheat germ helps restore elasticity to the arteries, stimulates the adrenal glands, and helps normalize blood pressure. (Desiccated liver powder or tablets may be used by those who do not enjoy eating liver or kidney.) Bell peppers, brewer's yeast, cabbage, citrus fruits, cucumbers, dates, onions, peas, raisins, sweet potatoes, tomatoes, and whole grains also are recommended. Eating small, frequent meals throughout the day equalizes blood sugar and helps avoid the hypotension that may occur after a heavy meal. To encourage nutrient absorption, as little liquid as possible should be taken with meals, but generous amounts should be imbibed between meals, and some salt should be included in the diet to maintain the body's fluid balance.

After a year on a salt-free diet, Gilda G. was tired all the time and experienced dizzy spells. A checkup showed that her formerly high blood pressure was well down in the normal range, and the doctor said she could stop taking her diuretic. Fearful that her blood pressure might shoot up without the medication, Gilda limited her liquids and continued using only a potassium-containing salt substitute for seasoning. A month later, too weak to walk and convinced she was suffering from a terminal disease, she checked into the hospital for a full battery of tests. Gilda's "fatal ailment" turned out to be sodium depletion compounded by dehydration. The prescription and successful cure? Drink six to eight glasses of liquid every day, throw out the salt substitute and use small amounts of granulated kelp or salt for seasoning, and, for 2 weeks, stir ¼ teaspoon of salt into 6 ounces of tomato juice and drink it between meals three times each day.

Supplements (see note on page xii)

In addition to a daily multivitamin-mineral tablet to help compensate for decreased nutrient assimilation, these individual supplements have been found helpful.

B Complex   One comprehensive, high-potency tablet daily.

Vitamin C   1,000 to 3,000 milligrams in divided doses during the day.

Vitamin E   100 IU a day, gradually increased to 600 IU.

Folk Remedies

Folk practitioners suggest one 6-ounce glass of beet juice plus one serving of beets 3 times a week for livening lagging blood pressure. Dandelion greens or dandelion tea, or ginger root or skullcap tea with a pinch of cayenne pepper are other favorites for raising blood pressure.

Nerve Pressure and Massage

Stimulating each of these points for 30 seconds once a day may be helpful in normalizing low blood pressure.

○ Press inward and upward under the center of the back of the skull, then hook the left index finger as far up as possible under the inside margin of the left rib cage and press inward and upward.

○ Press or massage 2 inches toward the front of the body from the center of the right underarm, then 1 inch below the tip of the breastbone.

Sources (see Bibliography)

15, 26, 72, 75, 78, 80, 81, 86, 87, 164, 173, 179, 226, 234, 257, 262, 268, 283, 293, 294, 300, 313, 317

Ménière's Disease

Characterized by a fluctuating, recurring group of unpleasant symptoms—ringing in the ear(s), unsteadiness, vertigo, nausea and vomiting, a sensation of fullness or pain in the ear(s), distortion of sound, and hearing loss—Ménière's disease results from excess fluid in the labyrinth (semicircular canals in the inner ear), which disturbs balance and hearing. Often affecting only one ear, episodes may last from a few minutes to a few hours, occur as rarely as once a year or as frequently as three times a day, and vary in intensity. During an acute attack, bed rest and a nonprescription motion sickness antihistamine is the generally recommended treatment.[148]

Medical evaluation is essential to make certain that an underlying disorder is not responsible. Diabetes, high cholesterol, hypoglycemia, low thyroid function, rheumatoid arthritis, and syphilis can produce symptoms that mimic Ménière's. Allergic reactions, eye or mental strain, poor circulation, impaired blood flow to the brain, the spasm of a blood vessel in the ear, or the consumption of alcohol or caffeine can precipitate an attack. Although stress is not a proven instigator of Ménière's disease, it can aggravate the symptoms. Practicing relaxation techniques (see Introduction) may alleviate the discomfort. Nicotine is a nervous-system stimulant that can induce the symptoms; stopping smoking has cleared some cases. Less than 10 percent of Ménière's patients require surgical intervention; the rest self-correct with time, home remedies (see "Hearing Loss," "Nausea," and "Tinnitus"), and dietary improvements.[254]

Diet

Clinical studies show that the majority of people with Ménière's disease are overweight and have abnormal carbohydrate metabolism, and that at least half have high blood fats. By adhering to a sodium-restricted, low-fat, low-sugar diet with a reduction of refined carbohydrates and by losing weight, some patients experience immediate relief; most report dramatic improvement within a month or two.[147]

Supplements (see note on page xii)

The first encounter with Ménière's symptoms frequently follows antibiotic treatment—which destroys helpful as well as harmful bacteria. Taking acidophilus capsules with each meal (or eating acidophilus yogurt) for a few weeks helps reestablish the body's synthesis of B vitamins. Possibly due to defective utilization, Ménière's patients have been found to be chronically deficient in B vitamins and other nutrients. Calcium and magnesium supplements may be helpful when the proper dosage is determined by the attending health care professional. Suggested amounts of these two minerals range from 1,500 milligrams of calcium plus 1,000 milligrams of magnesium, to 1,000 milligrams of magnesium plus 500 milligrams of calcium. Many cases have been cleared with adequate supplementation of needed nutrients.[17, 87, 98]

B Complex One comprehensive tablet daily, plus separate supplements of 10 to 25 milligrams *each* of B_1 and B_2, and 50 milligrams of B_6 four times a day for 2 weeks. Because of its vasodilating action, niacin is especially beneficial for Ménière's patients, but no more than 200 milligrams a day should be taken by anyone who is pregnant or suffering from gout or from a liver disorder. For others, taking 50 to 250 milligrams of niacin before each meal has corrected Ménière's in 2 to 4 weeks.[98] To reduce uncomfortable skin-flushing from niacin's beneficial dilation of the arteries, niacinamide (the synthetic form) may be substituted for half of the niacin.

Vitamin C with Bioflavonoids 1,500 to 5,000 milligrams in divided doses plus 400 IU of vitamin E each day to combat free-radical damage and promote efficient oxygenation.

Lecithin One tablespoon of granules daily (or two or three capsules with each meal) for brain function and cellular protection.

Manganese Five milligrams daily. A deficiency of this mineral may be responsible for Ménière's symptoms.

Folk Remedies

Drinking a mixture of 2 teaspoons apple cider vinegar and ¾ cup water with each of two daily meals is a folk cure for chronic Ménière's syndrome. Lessening of the symptoms is said to be evident after 2 weeks, with further improvement by the end of a month.[171] Butcher's broom, catnip, and ginger tea are other favored beverages. Recent studies in Europe show that twice-daily supplementation with 80 milligrams of ginkgo biloba (a medicinal herb used in Asia since 3000 B.C.) increases blood flow to the ears and significantly improves Ménière's disease in 30 days.[51]

Leila H. relies on a combination of old and new remedies to control her occasional bouts of Ménière's. She keeps bottles of 50-milligram B6, 100-milligram pantothenic acid, and ground ginger in her bathroom medicine cabinet for easy access. When she awakens with ringing ears and spinning surroundings, Leila makes a cup of "tea" by stirring a teaspoon of ginger into hot tap water, takes one of each of the vitamins with it, and goes back to bed for half an hour. If the symptoms persist, she repeats the treatment and, if necessary to quell any lingering nausea or wooziness, has a third cup of ginger tea an hour or so later.

Sources (see Bibliography)

2, 6, 17, 51, 75, 87, 98, 147, 148, 171, 186, 207, 234, 254, 255, 281, 283

Menopause

$\mathbf{M}$ost women experience menopause (also called the climacteric, or "going through the change") between the ages of 45 and 55, as ovarian function and menstrual periods gradually cease. The ovaries continue secreting small amounts of estrogen for several years while the adrenal and pituitary glands begin producing hormones to take over estrogen's duties other than those of preparing for pregnancy. For about 20 percent of women, menstrual irregularity and its eventual cessation are the only indications of the "change of life." During 6 months to several years of this hormonal transition, however, the majority of women experience at least some of the traditional symptoms: hot flashes, mood swings, night sweats, and sleeping difficulties.[75, 147, 300]

Fluctuating hormone levels dilate blood vessels, disturb the body's thermostat, and are responsible for the hot flashes that occur with varying frequency and severity in more than half of menopausal women. A typical hot flash comes and goes in 30 minutes, with a 3-minute peak of an 8-degree rise in skin temperature.[293] Dressing for hot flash episodes calls for breathable fabrics worn in layers that can be peeled off and quickly replaced if a chill follows the profuse perspiration. Sucking ice chips helps chill out a facial flush. Body-cooling methods include taking a cool shower, soaking the feet in cold water, standing next to an open-door refrigerator-freezer, or hovering over the frozen-food bin in a supermarket.

Menopause is a "rite of passage," not a medical condition requiring drugs, but a physician should be consulted if mental or physical symptoms are severe. Hormone replacement therapy (HRT) may be prescribed to control menopausal problems and protect against the accelerated bone loss that can lead to osteoporosis—which affects 25 percent of postmenopausal women.[231] Although combining progesterone with estrogen in HRT diminishes the possibility of negative side effects (breast cancer or cancer of the uterus, elevated blood pressure, gallstones, migraine headaches), many women prefer to avoid potential risks by utilizing self-help measures to master menopause.[51, 254]

Diet

Eating four to six small meals throughout the day helps regulate body temperature—large meals may trigger hot flashes—and stabilizes blood sugar levels to help control emotional upheavals and other menopausal symptoms. Limiting sweets and stressing fruits, vegetables, and whole grains may be beneficial. Sugar and refined carbohydrates require adrenal action for their conversion into energy for bodily functions, thus diminishing the adrenal gland's ability to produce estrogenic replacements.[96]

Peas, soybeans, and other legumes are rich in natural estrogens to help replace the dwindling supply. Low-fat milk products, broccoli, dark leafy greens (especially collard, kale, and turnip greens), and canned fish such as salmon and sardines eaten with the bones are good sources of calcium to help retard bone loss. Drinking generous amounts of liquids helps regulate the body's thermostat, but alcoholic or caffeine-containing beverages should be limited—both interfere with calcium absorption, and their consumption sparks hot flashes for some women.

Supplements (see note on page xii)

Menopause and the resulting inactivity of the reproductive system slow the metabolic rate and reduce caloric requirements for maintaining ideal weight by as much as 45 percent, yet nutrient needs increase rather than decrease.[253] Eating less to avoid unwanted pounds makes a daily multivitamin-mineral, plus other supplements, important for supporting normal bodily functions and preventing bone loss.

B Complex One comprehensive tablet one to three times a day. Folic acid, B_6, B_{12}, niacin, PABA, and pantothenic acid enhance the effect of existing estrogen and stimulate the production of estrogenic hormones to reduce hot flashes and relieve nervous disorders. Taking an additional 50 milligrams of B_6 three times a day reduces fluid retention; 50 milligrams of pantothenic acid with each meal helps combat stress and improve adrenal function.[14, 17, 96]

Vitamin C and Bioflavonoids 1,000 to 5,000 milligrams of vitamin C and 800 milligrams of bioflavonoids in divided daily doses. Vitamin

C stimulates the body's production of estrogen; bioflavonoids contain natural plant estrogen. Together they help suppress hot flashes, night sweats, and mood changes.[6, 184]

Calcium and Magnesium   1,000 to 2,000 milligrams of calcium and 500 to 1,000 milligrams of magnesium in divided daily doses. With medical approval, reversing the proportions of these two minerals may be beneficial. Lack of calcium reduces the output of already decreasing sex hormones; lack of estrogen diminishes the body's ability to absorb calcium; magnesium (plus vitamin D from a daily supplement) is essential for calcium absorption. Without sufficient calcium, menopausal symptoms of depression, headaches, insomnia, and irritability are magnified and the bones are demineralized to provide calcium for such life-sustaining functions as muscle contraction and nerve conduction. Several long-term studies show that supplementation with these minerals results in reduction of discomfort during menopause and increases rather than decreases bone mass.[51, 98]

Vitamin E   400 to 800 IU daily (with the upper amount under medical supervision) not only potentiates estrogen production to reduce hot flashes, night sweats, insomnia, dizziness, and shortness of breath for many women but also lowers the incidence of breast cancer.[98, 106, 190]

Selenium   100 to 200 micrograms daily amplifies the action of vitamin E and is linked to normal hormone balance.[17]

Tissue Salts   6X potency, dissolved under the tongue. For hot flashes, three tablets of Ferr. Phos. every 10 minutes until relieved; for alternating hot and cold sensations or headache, use Kali. Sulph. For nervousness, three tablets of Kali. Phos. each day until relieved.

Exercise

Deep-breathing exercises may exorcise hot flashes: Inhale and exhale for 5 seconds each; repeat 10 times. Weight-bearing exercise (walking, dancing, low-impact aerobics) for at least 20 minutes three times a week not only burns excess calories and relieves tension but also increases bone mass by improving calcium absorption. Research studies show that for people unable to walk, even standing for some time each day helps offset the bone loss accelerated by bed rest.[105]

Folk Remedies

To relieve hot flashes, folk healers suggest using chervil, chives, garlic, raw honey, horseradish, nutmeg, shallots, and tarragon as seasonings, teas, or in capsules. Oatstraw tincture (20 drops in water three times a day after meals) has prevented night sweats for many women.[312] For general symptoms as well as hot flashes, herbalists recommend herbs that either provide natural estrogen or stimulate the body's production of estrogenic hormones: alfalfa, angelica (dong quai, tastes like celery—one or two capsules may be opened and sprinkled on food three times a day), black cohosh, blessed thistle, blue cohosh, cramp bark (squaw vine), damiana, gotu kola, licorice root, red raspberry leaf, sarsaparilla, unicorn root, and yarrow.

For some women, natural estrogen is more successful than hormone replacement therapy. One herbal combination that has resolved some menopausal problems is prepared by steeping 1 tablespoon powdered red clover flowers and 2 teaspoons *each* bruised anise and fennel seeds in a cup of boiling water for 15 minutes, then straining and drinking up to 3 cups a day.[16] Nadine P., who had never had severe headaches before undergoing HRT for her hot flashes, appreciated the relief the treatment provided but forsook hormonal therapy in favor of home remedies after the migrainelike headaches incapacitated her for several days every week. Under the guidance of a naturopathic practitioner, she took a capsule of black cohosh with each meal and 400 IU of vitamin E twice a day. The headaches disappeared in less than 3 weeks, and her hot flashes were controlled as effectively as they had been with the hormones.

Nerve Pressure and Massage

To relieve hot flashes, massage the inside of both wrists from side to side. To stimulate estrogenic hormone production, massage the thumbs of both hands, the undercenter of each big toe, and the outside of each foot just under the anklebone.

Relaxation and Mental Imagery

The mood swings, depression, and other symptoms attributed to menopause are sometimes the result of stressful personal and family changes during this period, not a reaction to estrogen depletion. Emotional stress can exaggerate or prolong all menopausal discomforts by overworking the adrenal glands so they cannot secrete the hormones needed to replace ovarian estrogen. Practicing relaxation techniques (see Introduction) often offsets stress reactions. In one study, half of the participants reported that daily periods of deliberate relaxation reduced the frequency, intensity, and duration of their hot flashes.[186] With practice, it may be possible to halt a hot flash by relaxing with closed eyes and imagining wading in a mountain stream, splashing the cold water over arms and face, and feeling the coolness of a pine-scented breeze.

Sources (see Bibliography)

6, 14, 16, 17, 26, 28, 29, 37, 46, 47, 51, 56, 59, 60, 64, 75, 77, 96, 97, 98, 105, 112, 144, 147, 150, 173, 176, 177, 184, 186, 190, 202, 217, 231, 252, 253, 254, 255, 256, 281, 293, 294, 298, 300, 312, 313

Menstrual Cramps (Dysmenorrhea)

At the beginning of each menstrual period, the uterus secrets hormonelike substances called prostaglandins to assist contraction of uterine muscles and expulsion of menstrual fluid. An excess of prostaglandins forces muscles to tighten more than necessary, creating spasmodic cramps that can be as intense as labor pains. Relaxing tense muscles with the relaxation techniques described in the Introduction may be helpful. For women who are not aspirin sensitive, the preferred painkiller is nonprescription ibuprofen, which contains prostaglandin inhibitors—studies have found it to be three times more effective than acetaminophen or aspirin for menstrual cramps.[294, 300] If birth control is desired, oral contraceptives relieve menstrual pain by preventing ovulation and the production of prostaglandins. Experimentation with the home remedies women have relied upon for centuries usually controls dysmenorrhea, but persistently painful periods warrant a gynecological examination to rule out an underlying disorder of the reproductive system.

Diet

Initiating dietary adjustments the week before a period can reduce menstrual bloating and cramping and provide iron to compensate for the monthly blood loss. Animal fats should be avoided; they contain a substance that stimulates the secretion of cramp-producing prostaglandins. Limiting salt intake cuts down on water retention; eating high-fiber foods prevents the constipation that can intensify menstrual pain. Nutritionists recommend a low-fat diet emphasizing fruits, legumes, vegetables (especially leafy greens), and whole grains.

Supplements (see note on page xii)

Minerals and Vitamins The radical changes in female hormones cause blood calcium levels to decrease prior to and during menstruation. In one study, taking 1,000 milligrams of calcium carbonate daily reduced menstrual discomfort for 72 percent of the women.[186] If cramps do occur, taking one or two dolomite tablets (calcium and magnesium) every hour often brings relief—500 milligrams of magnesium a day (with medical approval, up to 1,800 milligrams) may also be beneficial.

Crampiness that is not relieved with calcium may respond to a daily B-complex tablet plus additional B6 and 50 milligrams of niacin with each meal. Accompanying the B vitamins with 300 milligrams of vitamin C with bioflavonoids brought relief to 90 percent of the 220 cramp sufferers in an Australian study.[57] In other cases, taking evening primrose oil or 400 IU of vitamin E each day prevented dysmenorrhea.[201, 312]

Tissue Salts Hourly doses of the tissue salts Calc. Fluor. and Mag. Phos. in the 6X potency often relieve painful menstruation. An additional dose of three tablets of Mag. Phos. or Kali. Phos. dissolved in hot water may be taken to remedy spasmodic pains. For dysmenorrhea with profuse loss of blood, three 6X tablets of Ferr. Phos. every 2 hours are suggested.

Exercise

A daily exercise routine may reduce monthly cramping. For Brenda L., performing this postural exercise each night between menstrual periods for 2 months abolished the dysmenorrhea that had forced her to stay in bed at least 1 day while menstruating: Stand with feet parallel to a wall, about 6 inches away from it. Place the forearm and hand nearest the wall flat against it at shoulder level, then bring the hip in to touch the wall three times. Repeat with the opposite side. Exercising vigorously on the days preceding a period sometimes diminishes discomfort after the bleeding starts—Nikki. S. credits her misery-free menses to playing tennis or racquetball the day her period is scheduled to begin.

Gentle stretching exercises often relieve cramps in progress.

○ Stand with feet 24 inches apart, arms extended, and knees relaxed. Slowly bend to touch the left toes with the left hand. Straighten up and breathe deeply, then touch the right foot with the right hand. Repeat the sequence three times.

○ Lie on the back with knees bent and feet flat on the floor. Place a large paperback book on the abdomen. Inhale to raise the book, hold for 5 seconds, then tighten stomach muscles and exhale slowly to lower the book. Or, from the same position, raise the knees to the chest and pull them closer with the arms for 5 seconds, then release the legs and slowly lower them to the floor.

Folk Remedies

Spirited panaceas for the monthly miseries range from straight gin or whiskey, or gin in which juniper berries have been steeped, to Ozark stew—a mixture of corn whiskey, ginger, and a modicum of boiling water. Medicinal quantities are advised. Aunt Ruby still smiles over her "lost weekend" at college. Attacked by cramps on a Saturday morning, she tried to duplicate her mother's blackberry brandy and hot water remedy by half-filling a large tumbler with brandy, adding some cranberry juice, and topping it with tap water. "When my roommate returned on Sunday and woke me," she recalls, "the cramps had vanished. Of course," Aunt Ruby adds, "I did get the correct formula from Mom: 2 tablespoons of the brandy in a cup of hot water!"

Herbalists suggest drinking a cup of cramp bark (squaw vine) or red raspberry leaf tea each morning and evening for several days before the start of a period to prevent dysmenorrhea. Herbal teas used to relieve menstrual cramps include black cohosh, camomile, caraway seed, catnip, comfrey, ginger, ginseng, licorice root, mint, and sarsaparilla. Adding a teaspoon of powdered meadowsweet to each cup of raspberry leaf tea provides the painkilling benefits of aspirin.[16]

Hot and Cold Remedies

The application of heat to either the lower back or the abdomen helps relax tense muscles. Before the advent of heating pads, hot salt, a mustard poultice, or towels squeezed out of hot water and sprinkled with turpentine were recommended. Alternating abdominal warmth with a 10-minute ice pack on the lower back once each hour may bring relief. Drinking hot lemonade or herbal tea during a 20-minute soak in a warm bath swished with enhancers such as a cup of baking soda, salt, or 2 cups of strained, double-strength camomile tea may increase blood flow and relieve cramping.

Nerve Pressure and Massage

○ With a tongue depressor or popsicle stick, press three-fourths of the way back on the tongue.

○ On both hands, exert pressure on the tips of the thumbs and first and second fingers, press and massage the fleshy mound formed on the top of the hand between the thumb and index finger when the two are pushed together, then massage both sides of the wrists.

○ Press or massage 1 inch above and to both sides of the navel.

○ On each foot, squeeze the web between the big toe and the one next to it, massage the center of the sole of the foot, then press and massage the hollows beneath the inner and outer anklebones.

Sources (see Bibliography)

6, 16, 26, 37, 57, 59, 60, 61, 64, 65, 75, 92, 98, 109, 111, 112, 116, 135, 147, 148, 151, 164, 176, 186, 201, 202, 203, 227, 252, 254, 255, 256, 265, 278, 281, 293, 294, 298, 300, 312, 313

Migraine and Cluster Headaches

Migraines may be humanity's oldest malady. The name is derived from the word the Greek physician Galen used to describe the disorder in 200 A.D.; 6,000-year-old Sumarian writings refer to their ravages, and prehistoric skeletons bear testimony to a crude form of trephination—holes chiseled in skulls to allow the escape of pain-creating demons. Once referred to as sick headaches, migraines now fall under the vascular heading; are subdivided as common, classic, or cluster headaches; and, according to statistics reported in *American Health* (November 1991), increased in incidence by 60 percent during the 1980s.

In common migraine, the throbbing pain develops gradually from distended veins around the brain, usually attacks only one side of the head, may be accompanied by nausea, vomiting, and sensitivity to light, lasts for hours or days, and recurs at varying intervals. In classic migraine, the miseries of common migraine are preceded by 15 to 90 minutes of an "aura" caused by blood vessel constriction around the brain. During an aura, symptoms can include distorted perception, flashes or zigzags of light, temporary loss of sight or hearing, numbness in an arm or leg, and hallucinations. Some of the religious visions of the Middle Ages are attributed to the visual effects of migraine aura; Lewis Carroll immortalized his in *Alice in Wonderland*. Cluster headaches, a relatively rare migraine variant, attack without warning, cause intense pain (usually behind one eye) for about an hour, recur several times a day for weeks, then disappear for months before returning in another cluster.

A number of factors, singly or in combination, can cause migraines. Predisposition may be inherited. If both parents have migraines, there is a 70 percent chance of developing the syndrome; if only one parent is

302

affected, the likelihood is lowered to 50 percent.[111, 300] Ninety percent of cluster headache victims are men—typically, hard-driving perfectionists who drink and smoke heavily. Female hormone fluctuations due to menstrual cycles, oral contraceptives, or estrogen supplements help account for the fact that seven out of ten migraine sufferers are women.[293, 294]

Almost anything can bring on an attack in a susceptible person. The trigger may be stress-related (anger, anxiety, excitement, exhaustion, or changes in routine or weather), diet-related (sensitivity to certain foods, beverages, or medications), or sensory-related (bright or flickering light, loud noise, perfume or intense odors).

Migraine management involves prevention as well as pain relief. Practicing relaxation techniques (see Introduction) can reduce reactions to stress. Keeping a "headache diary" helps identify diet- or sensory-related triggers so they can be avoided. As reported in *Longevity* (December 1990), a study in which 22,000 doctors participated showed that taking one aspirin every other day reduces the incidence of migraine recurrence by 20 percent. Several recent studies by British researchers demonstrated that the herb feverfew can reduce the number and severity of migraine attacks by between 24 and 44 percent when a 100-milligram capsule of the freeze-dried herb is taken daily.[45, 113, 151]

Aspirin, acetaminophen, or ibuprofen may be helpful when taken at the onset of migraine pain, but their prolonged use can damage the stomach, liver, or kidneys.[300] Oxygen, now available in tiny tanks, is another option. Breathing pure oxygen for 5 minutes will often relieve a cluster headache, and its regular use may reduce the incidence of migraine attacks. Medical diagnosis and assistance should be sought if self-help therapies do not control headaches that interfere with work and regular activities. Although almost all drugs can have undesirable side effects, prescription medications are available to prevent migraines as well as to block their severe pain.

Diet

Snacking on wholesome foods between three light meals each day helps stabilize the blood sugar swings that can precipitate migraines. Some doctors summarily dismiss the relationship of diet to migraine headache; other experts have found that half of all migraines are triggered by food sensitivities or high fat, salt, or sugar intake.[147, 312] Any edible can be the culprit. The most common villains are aged cheeses, chocolate, citrus fruits, cured meats, eggs, fermented foods such as relishes and yogurt, freshly baked yeast breads, milk and milk products, wheat, and food additives such as MSG (monosodium glutamate) and the nitrates in cold cuts and hot dogs. For some people, eating ice cream without allowing it to melt in the mouth can trigger a migraine; or alcohol's distention of cerebral blood vessels can set one off. Studies show that although red wine causes attacks in nine out of eleven people subject to migraines, taking two aspirins before drinking the wine may prevent a reaction. Beer and champagne affect some susceptible individuals, but vodka has been shown to have no effect unless imbibed during a lull between cluster headaches.[254]

Supplements (see note on page xii)

For migraine-susceptible people, many nutritional experts recommend a daily multivitamin-mineral plus individual supplements.[14, 17, 98]

B complex One comprehensive tablet daily to help maintain normal vascular control. Additional niacin (50 milligrams with each of three meals a day) dilates blood vessels and increases blood flow to the brain.

Vitamin C with Bioflavonoids Including 200 milligrams of rutin, 3,000 to 6,000 milligrams in divided daily doses to assist the production of antistress hormones and counteract substances that may instigate migraines.

Calcium and Magnesium 1,000 to 2,000 milligrams of calcium and 500 to 1,000 milligrams of magnesium (with medical approval, 1,000 to 2,000 milligrams of magnesium and 500 to 1,000 milligrams of calcium) in divided doses throughout the day to soothe nerves and help control muscle contraction.

Tissue Salts At the onset of a migraine, take three tablets of 6X Nat. Mur.; repeat in four hours, if needed. For throbbing pain, take the same amount of Ferr. Phos. every 30 minutes for up to 2 hours.

Folk Remedies

For some people, covering both nose and mouth with a paper bag and then inhaling and exhaling several times brings relief. Folk healers suggest binding watermelon rind or a ripe banana peel over the forehead—perhaps because of the cooling effect. Other old-fashioned migraine relievers include eating fifteen almonds or a bowl of strawberries, drinking a cup (or taking a capsule) of meadowsweet or white willow bark tea, or ¼ teaspoon grated nutmeg in a cup of water.

Apple Cider Vinegar Taking 2 teaspoons of vinegar in a glass of water with each meal is said to reduce the frequency of migraines. When the pain has started, inhaling the fumes from a jar of strong mustard, or taking seventy-five breaths of the vapors from a half-and-half mixture of boiling vinegar and water has brought headache relief in as little as 5 minutes.[159, 172]

Cold and Hot Applications Cold cloths, ice, or gel-filled packs help constrict swollen blood vessels and reduce the sensitivity of painful nerve endings. Warming the hands and/or feet with hot water or a heating pad helps relieve pressure in the head by causing the blood to rush to the extremities. Adding lemon juice or dry mustard to a hand or foot bath is said to increase the benefits. (Headache clinics have found that patients who vividly visualize their hands near a fire are more successful in diverting blood from the brain than those who physically heat their hands.)[51] When utilized at the beginning of a migraine aura, the heat and high-pitched hum of a stand-type hair dryer may prevent a headache from developing.

Coffee Drinking a cup or two of strong black coffee (with or without the juice of half a lemon) at the onset of pain may abort a migraine by constricting cerebral blood vessels.

Herbs Sipping a cup of camomile or catnip tea daily is said to prevent migraines. Besides its established virtue as a migraine preventive when one capsule a day is taken, feverfew combined with thyme is a pain eradicator—the recommended dosage is three capsules of each at two-hour intervals.[46, 176] Other herbs advised for the treatment of migraine headaches are ginkgo biloba extract, peppermint, rosemary, and wormwood; or a combination of fenugreek, thyme, and wood betony.

Nerve Pressure and Massage

○ Extend the tongue ½ inch and hold it between the teeth for 10 minutes.

○ Place the thumbs behind the earlobes, then squeeze and massage the bottom of the lobes with the fingers.

○ Using the thumb of the opposite hand, firmly press and massage the center of each palm; then each thumb, concentrating on tender points—usually between the second joint and the tip.

Dr. Tad R.'s frequent migraines were more than miserable; they were a menace to his psychiatric practice. When a friend suggested he try foot reflexology, Tad was willing to experiment. The visitor began by massaging the ball of Tad's foot, worked his way up to the pad behind the nail on Tad's big toe, and smiled when Tad winced with pain. They had located the pressure point. Continued gentle rubbing gradually lessened the pain in the toe, and surprisingly, the pain in Tad's head began to diminish. Even more amazing, by massaging his toe at the first indication of an approaching headache, Dr. Tad remains free of migraines.

Relaxation and Mental Imagery

Visualization and self-suggestion can enhance the benefits of relaxing in a darkened room with a cold pack on the forehead. For some migraine sufferers, imagining themselves in a peaceful, pain-free time and place is sufficient. Others prefer an anatomical vision of distended arteries shrinking to ease the pressure. A few migraine sufferers fare better with the fanciful image of lifting off the top of the skull to remove the hammer-wielding gremlin banging around in the brain.

Sources (see Bibliography)

14, 16, 17, 26, 29, 45, 46, 49, 50, 51, 56, 58, 59, 60, 61, 64, 65, 75, 98, 102, 108, 111, 112, 113, 144, 147, 150, 151, 158, 159, 164, 172, 176, 186, 201, 202, 212, 213, 235, 236, 238, 244, 254, 255, 256, 281, 293, 294, 297, 300, 312, 313

Morning Sickness

A lthough it may occur at any time of day or evening, the nausea experienced by about three-fourths of all pregnant women is commonly called morning sickness. Apparently caused by hormonal changes activating the vomiting center in the brain, morning sickness usually begins during the first 6 weeks of pregnancy and subsides after the fourth month. The intensity and duration, which differs with each individual, ranges from a few brief episodes of nausea to months of all-day queasiness and frequent vomiting. Experts theorize that morning sickness may be nature's method of guarding the fetus from ingested toxins that might instigate birth defects—studies have shown that miscarriage is three times more likely among expectant mothers who do not experience nausea during their first trimester—but severe or protracted nausea and vomiting warrants medical attention. [111, 293]

With the approval of their obstetricians, many women have resolved the discomfort of morning sickness by experimenting with home remedies. Self-help measures such as remaining upright during the day by sitting or standing (and not bending over) helps keep stomach acids from backing up and avoids added pressure on the abdomen, which can aggravate nausea.

Diet

A developing fetus is constantly nourished by glucose drawn from the mother's bloodstream. Having frequent small meals plus a bedtime snack and eating a few bites before arising replenishes the supply of glucose and prevents the nausea that can result from low blood sugar levels. Nibbling half-a-dozen raw almonds often calms waves of nausea occurring during the day. Avoiding fried or fatty foods and adapting the diet to individual food aversions also helps. The most common culprits are highly flavored foods and those with strong odors such as brussels sprouts, chili peppers, fish, garlic, and onions. Increased milk consumption may be responsible for stomach upsets due to difficulty in digesting the milk sugar lactose. Cultured milk products (yogurt, kefir), soybean tofu, or, with the doctor's approval, lactase or calcium supplements can be used.

Drinking small amounts of liquid at frequent intervals helps neutralize the extra stomach acid produced during pregnancy and, if the fluids are clear broths or fruit juices, helps maintain normal blood sugar. Orange juice is excellent; papaya juice halts queasiness for some expectant mothers; folklore has it that sipping a mixture of two-thirds sparkling water to one-third Concord grape juice will not only provide temporary relief from morning sickness but will also guarantee long hair for the infant. Alcoholic beverages should be abjured; most obstetricians advise restricting caffeine to one or two cups of coffee per day.

Supplements

During pregnancy, supplements as well as over-the-counter drugs should be taken only with the consent of the attending physician.

Unless preformed vitamin A is ordered by the obstetrician, beta carotene is advised because the body converts it to vitamin A only as needed.[147, 150] B vitamins, particularly B_1 (25 to 100 milligrams) plus 50 to 200 milligrams of B_6 in divided daily doses (especially when accompanied by vitamin C) often relieve the nausea suffered by expectant mothers.[2, 176] Diana H. overcame her family history of nauseous pregnancies by following her Aunt Ruth's advice. The obstetrician was doubtful about the benefits of supplements in addition to the prenatal formula she was already taking but agreed that they would do no harm. Within three days, the extra B_1, B_6, and vitamin C, plus 15 milligrams of zinc, lessened Diana's nausea—and also left her free of the swollen ankles that had been caused by fluid retention.

Folk Remedies

Eating saltines in bed before arising may prevent early morning nausea. Drinking ½ cup of warm water mixed with ⅓ cup papaya or pear juice and ⅛ teaspoon of cinnamon has also proven effective.[313] Daytime options for quelling queasiness include munching a few bites of alfalfa sprouts or raw celery, potato, or turnip; or sipping the liquid from 2 tablespoons of oats boiled for 30 minutes in a pint of water.

Ginger is the primary herbal remedy for morning sickness. A cup of ginger tea or two capsules of powdered ginger before breakfast has resolved the problem in many cases. Other beneficial herbs include alfalfa, camomile, catnip, cloves, fennel, hops, mint, red raspberry leaf, and sage. According to a report in the August 1992 issue of *Natural Health*, the herbs to be avoided during pregnancy are angelica (dong quai), coltsfoot, comfrey, ephedra, feverfew, ginseng, goldenseal, licorice root, tansy, and yarrow. Some health practitioners recommend black cohosh or blue cohosh as a uterine tonic late in pregnancy, but these herbs should not be used until a month before the due date, and then only under professional guidance.

Nerve Pressure and Massage

Reflexologists offer several options for stimulating acupressure points to relieve the nausea of pregnancy.

○ Without exerting any pressure, use the teeth of a comb or the fingernails of the opposite hand to lightly scratch the inside of the thumb and index finger of the left hand and the first three fingers of the right hand, then the back of each hand from fingers to wrist.

○ Using the thumb or a fingertip, firmly press and massage each inner forearm 2 inches toward the elbow from the center of the wrist.

Sources (see Bibliography)

2, 17, 26, 42, 49, 59, 75, 98, 109, 111, 147, 150, 151, 154, 176, 186, 201, 202, 218, 226, 228, 244, 254, 255, 256, 265, 281, 293, 300, 312, 313

Motion Sickness

Constant movement, compounded by conflicting signals from the body's balance system (eyes, inner ears, sensors in muscles and joints), produces motion sickness. On a ship, for instance, the eyes record movement, the inner ears detect rolling motion, yet the body is stationary. Preventive measures and natural remedies may prevent, or at least ameliorate, the clamminess, dizziness, nausea, and vomiting symptomatic of motion sickness. Experts advise focusing on the horizon or on a fixed, distant object instead of looking at swirling waves or "passing" roadside shrubbery. Facing forward is helpful. Traveling in darkness diminishes the potential for motion sickness. Positional arrangements also make a difference.

In an Airplane Motion is less pronounced in an aisle seat over a wing, preferably on the right side where there is less swaying because most flight patterns call for left turns.

In a Car Ride in the front seat and, unless driving (drivers are seldom subject to motion sickness), lean back against a stable headrest to minimize inner-ear reaction to movement. Looking down or reading while riding can produce motion sickness because of the apparent movement outside the windows.[293]

At Sea Reserve an amidship cabin near the waterline where motion is minimal and, as much as possible, stay topside in the middle of the deck.

Diet

Dining lightly before a journey, and eating small amounts at frequent intervals while traveling is the recommended pattern. An empty stomach readily succumbs to queasiness. Overindulgence in food or alcohol may trigger motion sickness symptoms. Sucking on a mouth-puckering lemon or nibbling olives at the first hint of nausea are old remedies that have scientific justification. Motion sickness engenders superfluous saliva, which trickles down to the stomach and contributes to nausea. Lemons and olives contain mouth-drying agents that diminish the queasiness. Drinking a small glass of papaya or pineapple juice, or munching soda crackers may also be helpful.

Swallowing additional liquid is a modern folk cure that prevented Virginia T.'s first flight from becoming a disaster. By the time they had been airborne for half an hour, sensations of butterflies fluttering in her stomach could no longer be attributed to happy excitement—she was nauseous. Noticing her distress, the flight attendant handed Virginia a paper cup of cool water and said, "Lean back, breathe deeply, try to relax, and take a sip of this every few minutes." After the queasiness faded away, the stewardess explained that sipping water helped adjust pressure on the balancing organs in the ears. On her return flight, Virginia avoided discomfort by requesting a cup of water when she boarded the plane and started the sipping before takeoff.

Supplements (see note on page xii)

Taking a daily B-complex supplement for 2 weeks before traveling may prevent motion sickness for those who are marginally deficient in these vitamins. Possibly due to this combination's antihistamine action, taking 500 milligrams of vitamin C, 100 milligrams of pantothenic acid, and 50 milligrams of B_6 before a trip, then repeating the dosage 30 minutes later and again in four hours thwarts motion sickness for some individuals. An additional 50 milligrams of B_6 has successfully quelled nausea in some after-the-fact cases.[98] The tissue salts Kali. Phos. and Nat. Phos. act as a preventive when two 12X tablets of each are dissolved under the tongue before starting and every 2 hours during travel. For acute motion sickness, the same dosage may be taken at 30-minute intervals.

Folk Remedies

Tightening a wide belt or towel around the waist for 30 minutes, placing an ice-cold container of anything behind the left ear, chewing one or two whole cloves, or drinking strong green tea may help calm a stomach upset by motion sickness. Herbalists suggest anise, basil, camomile, caraway seed, clove, marjoram, mint, or savory tea. Sipping ginger ale over crushed ice has long been a favorite shipboard remedy for *mal de mer*. Ginger's reputation as an antidote for motion sickness has been validated by recent studies showing it to be more effective than Dramamine.[49, 51, 186] And since ginger works in the gastrointestinal tract rather than in the brain, it does not cause the side effects of drowsiness and blurred vision produced by motion sickness drugs. For best results, two 500 milligram capsules of ginger should be taken a few minutes before departure. If preferred, ½ teaspoon of powdered ginger can be dissolved in a cup of hot water or other beverage, or crystallized ginger may be chewed. Repeat doses may be taken each hour, if needed, or every 4 hours for prevention.

Nerve Pressure and Massage

- Press or massage the mastoid bone behind each ear, just below the earlobes where the jawbones end, and the hollow at the base of the skull.

- Press or massage 1 inch below the bottom of the breastbone and 2 inches above the navel.

- Massage the last two fingers on both hands for 5 minutes per hand. If no relief is felt, massage (or lightly scratch with the fingernails) the thumbs and first three fingers, including the webs between, on each hand.

- Press and massage each inner arm 2 inches toward the elbow from the base of the thumb.

- Massage both kneecaps for 3 minutes, or press and massage the shinbones from 3 inches above the anklebones.

Sources (see Bibliography)

2, 6, 10, 26, 49, 50, 51, 56, 57, 59, 63, 64, 75, 87, 98, 111, 135, 164, 176, 186, 193, 195, 201, 202, 203, 213, 226, 254, 265, 282, 286, 284, 285, 293, 294, 300, 312, 313

Mouth and Tongue Problems

Mouth discomfort may be an early warning sign of nutritional deficiencies (see note on page xii) or may be caused by a variety of factors such as allergy, gingivitis or pyorrhea (see "Periodontal Disease"), poor oral hygiene, or improperly fitted dentures. Soothing mouth rinses include aloe vera juice and herbal teas brewed with angelica root, anise seeds, camomile, catnip, cloves, comfrey, lemon balm, marshmallow, or white oak bark. To inhibit bacteria, a half-and-half mixture of hydrogen peroxide and water can be swished in the mouth for 30 seconds once every other day.[293]

Burning Sensations Taking a B-complex tablet plus 50 to 100 milligrams of B_6 daily may correct the problem. Additional B_2 is helpful in some cases. Burning or stinging gums (often associated with dentures) may respond to increased amounts of fruit, vegetables, and protein in the diet, plus 2,000 milligrams of vitamin C taken in divided daily doses. For a fiery mouth caused by hot pepper, slowly drink a glass of milk—holding each swallow in the mouth for several seconds. According to the *Berkeley Wellness Letter* (April 1992), the casein in milk neutralizes capsaicin, the burning component in hot pepper. Folk practitioners suggest eating a slice of cold cheese, chewing a mouthful of white bread, or rinsing the mouth with a mixture of ½ cup cold water and 1 teaspoon lemon juice.

Coated Tongue If not due to debauch or dehydration, a coated tongue may result from the destruction of beneficial intestinal bacteria by antibiotic treatment. The condition usually clears when a B-complex supplement plus *Lactobacillus acidophilus* yogurt (or acidophilus

313

capsules) accompany each meal. A hairy tongue—yellow, brown, or black "hair" growing out of the tongue—may be due to similar causes or to poor oral hygiene. Preventive measures include taking acidophilus along with antibiotics and brushing the tongue each time the teeth are brushed. Remedies include scraping the tongue once a day with a tongue scraper or small spoon to remove bacteria and fermenting food trapped in its crevices, rinsing the mouth with hydrogen peroxide, and avoiding irritants like alcohol and tobacco.

Cracks in the Corners of the Mouth Also called angular cheilosis, these most frequently occur from a deficiency of vitamin B_2. Taking a daily multivitamin-mineral plus a 50-milligram B-complex tablet with each meal is recommended because a lack of other B vitamins and of iron is implicated in a high percentage of cases.[190]

Dry Mouth This problem may be a side effect of drugs such as antidepressants, antihistamines, blood pressure medications, diuretics, or tranquilizers. Many diabetics and hypoglycemics suffer from dry mouth engendered by blood sugar imbalance. Drinking fluids at frequent intervals (apple juice or warm tea stimulates salivary flow), and taking 25,000 IU of beta carotene plus a B-complex tablet daily may be beneficial. Immediate relief may be obtained by chewing sugarless gum, gargling with honey and water, or by gently chewing the tongue or running the tongue over the teeth for 20 seconds. Chronic dry mouth (xerostomia) should be medically evaluated to rule out infections or Sjogren's disease (an autoimmune disorder involving dry mouth, dry eyes, and painful joints).

Inflammation of the Mouth Also known as stomatitis, this condition includes cold sores (see "Canker Sores") and Vincent's disease—sometimes called "trench mouth" because of its prevalence in World War I—and often occurs during times of stress. Predisposing factors include poor oral hygiene and irritation from alcohol or tobacco. The inflammation often disappears when 25,000 IU of beta carotene, a high-potency B-complex tablet, and at least 1,000 milligrams of vitamin C are taken each day. Including orange or tomato juice and brewer's yeast in the diet is advised. Practicing relaxation techniques (see Introduction) and rinsing the mouth every half hour with a solution of 1 teaspoon baking soda or ½ teaspoon salt in a glass of water, a two-to-one mixture of hydrogen peroxide and water, or strawberry leaf tea (with or without a pinch of alum) may be beneficial. If home remedies are not effective, Vincent's disease should have professional care to prevent its spread into the gum margins and the lining of the cheeks.

Loss of Sense of Taste   This may be due to aging, allergies, infections, certain medications, nasal polyps, nerve damage, or deficiencies of B vitamins and zinc. Taste buds on the tongue detect the four basic sensations of bitter, salty, sour, and sweet—food odors that pass through the back of the throat identify the nuances of flavors. Taking a B-complex tablet plus 50 milligrams of zinc daily for a few weeks, then reducing the zinc dosage to 15 milligrams for maintenance, may normalize sensory acuity.

Sore Mouth and Gums   These problems may be due to allergic reactions to specific brands of toothpaste or mouthwash. Overly vigorous brushing or toothpick poking can cause gum tenderness and "pink toothbrush" unrelated to gingivitis. Plaque (a conglomeration of bacteria and food debris) can accumulate on the gums to cause discomfort for denture wearers if the gums are not gently brushed and the mouth rinsed every day while the dentures are removed. Bolstering the diet with 1,000 milligrams of calcium and 500 milligrams of magnesium daily (some researchers advise reversing these proportions) may help prevent jawbone shrinkage and dentures from becoming uncomfortable. To hasten healing and relieve the pain of sore spots from seeds or food particles caught under dentures, coat the gums and the inside of the dentures with vitamin E from a snipped capsule. An alternative cure worked for Grant. W. after the peanuts he munched left two excruciatingly painful spots under his lower denture. He took 25,000 IU of beta carotene, let a chewable vitamin C dissolve in his mouth, followed it with a zinc lozenge, and continued alternating the C and zinc until he had swallowed a half-dozen of each. By the next morning, Grant could wear his denture without discomfort.

Folk medicine relies on herbs to relieve mouth soreness and hasten healing. Sore gums can be rubbed with aloe vera gel, tincture of myrrh, a drop of oil of cloves or tea tree oil; or with powdered catnip, goldenseal, or myrrh. To apply powdered herbs to sores on mouth tissue, medical anthropologist John Heinerman[150] suggests sprinkling the herb on a tiny piece of bread spread with peanut butter. Mouthwash can be made from ½ cup water plus ¼ teaspoon *each* baking soda and goldenseal; ½ cup water with ¼ teaspoon tincture of myrrh; or by brewing double-strength tea from chaparral, goldenseal, myrrh, sage, or thyme. To increase the tea's germ-fighting benefits, soak the dry herbs in 80-proof vodka for a week, strain, then dilute with an equal amount of distilled water.

Sore and/or Swollen Tongue Also called glossitis, this can be caused be allergic reactions, ill-fitting dentures, heavy smoking, or overindulgence in alcohol or spicy foods, but usually it indicates a deficiency of B vitamins. A painfully red tongue may be a sign of insufficient B2 or niacin; a smooth, shiny one, an undersupply of B12 or folic acid; and a sore, enlarged tongue may result from lack of B1, B2, B6, or pantothenic acid. If taking a 50-milligram B-complex tablet three times a day does not remedy the problem, a physician should be consulted. A persistently painful tongue may be an indication of disorders in other parts of the body.

First-Aid Tip If a self-inflicted bite produces profuse bleeding, press a wet tea bag against the tongue so that the tannin it contains can promote blood coagulation.[29]

White Patches on the Tongue or the Mouth Lining Also called leukoplakia or thrush, these patches commonly follow radiation treatment or long-term antibiotic therapy but may result from pipe smoking or the rubbing of a rough tooth, or develop in the elderly due to the thickening of tissues. The painless patches often disappear when a B-complex tablet and acidophilus capsules are taken with each meal. Folk remedies for thrush (a fungal yeast infection) include rinsing the mouth with aloe vera juice or a mixture of 2 tablespoons *each* apple cider vinegar and water plus a pinch of cayenne pepper; or with tea brewed from goldenseal, myrrh, red raspberry, or white oak bark. Swishing diluted garlic oil in the mouth or wiping the white spots with cloth dipped in a solution of borax mixed with glycerin, honey, or water are other options.

Sources (see Bibliography)

29, 41, 42, 53, 75, 77, 87, 98, 111, 113, 129, 150, 151, 173, 176, 177, 190, 202, 206, 234, 254, 255, 256, 281, 286, 293, 312, 313

Nausea and Vomiting

Nausea can be initiated by sights (blood, road kill), smells (rancid grease, rotten fish), sounds (graphic descriptions of surgery or pus-filled wounds), or by a combination of all three—like being in close proximity to someone in the throes of throwing up. Other potential instigators range from allergic reactions, anxiety, dietary indiscretions, and motion sickness to low blood sugar or any of over twenty-five physical conditions or diseases. Nausea progresses to vomiting when interactive signals from the digestive tract inform the brain that harmful substances are present, and the mind's "vomiting center" issues the command. Retching (dry heaves) can result when the brain's vomiting orders continue after the stomach is empty. A doctor should be consulted if vomiting occurs within 48 hours after a head injury, if vomit is black or bloody, if nothing can be kept down for 24 hours, or if nausea and vomiting persist for more than a few days.

Whatever the cause of the nauseous condition, slow, deep breathing and deliberate relaxation (see Introduction) accompanied by an affirmation such as "my stomach is calming; I will feel fine in a few minutes" may quell the queasiness. Home remedies can be utilized to curb the churning, prevent dehydration, and hasten recovery.

Diet

Eating a small amount of dry toast or crackers often clears nausea, especially when it has been instigated by excessive exercise. Including protein with the snack may help a hypoglycemic. A few bites of candy or swallows of orange juice may resolve the problem for a diabetic. If the cause of the nausea is something recently consumed, vomiting may be a quick cure. Repeated vomiting, however, expels fluid from ingested foods and beverages before it can be absorbed and can dehydrate the body unless the fluid is replaced.

Sucking on ice chips is fine, but after an episode of vomiting, plain cold water or more than a tablespoon of any chilled liquid has been found to trigger an encore performance in some cases. Sips of warm broth or room-temperature fruit juices, cola, ginger ale, or other soft drinks may help de-nauseate while replenishing lost fluid and minerals. A report in *Berkeley Wellness Letter* (July 1991) advises allowing carbonated beverages to sit until flat because the carbonation may bloat an uneasy stomach and provoke vomiting. For severe symptoms, a package of unsweetened soft-drink mix can be blended with 2 tablespoons sugar, 1 tablespoon salt, and 2 teaspoons baking soda in 4 cups of water.[264] Before food can be faced, a teaspoon of sweetened orange juice or honey every 15 to 30 minutes may be tolerated. Shredded raw apple mixed with honey may be retained by those who are unable to keep anything else down. When eating seems feasible, bland, low-fat foods (chicken breast, rice or noodle soup with crackers, gelatin desserts) help ease the return to normalcy.

Supplements (see note on page xii)

Research studies have found that taking two 500-milligram capsules of ginger prevents postoperative nausea as effectively as antiemetic drugs.[49] In one hospital study, taking two garlic capsules after meals relieved chronic nausea for 75 percent of the patients.[2] Frequent episodes of nausea and vomiting in people with deficiencies of magnesium and vitamin B6 have been corrected with a daily B-complex supplement plus 500 milligrams of magnesium.[98] Tissue salts may remedy ordinary bouts: Take three doses 20 minutes apart of two tablets *each* 6X Kali. Phos. and Nat. Phos. If the nausea is instigated by recently ingested food, add two tablets of 6X Nat. Sulph.

Folk Remedies

Holding half a peeled, raw onion under each armpit is said to control incessant vomiting. Eating a minced chicken gizzard cooked with two chopped lemons reportedly alleviates both nausea and vomiting. Sniffing the ink on a black-and-white newspaper eliminates nauseousness for some people. Megan and Stuart A. discovered that the effectiveness of any remedy is an individual matter. On two occasions Megan had soothed a rebellious stomach by slowly chewing ¼-inch pieces of raw celery and celery leaves one at a time. However, when her husband tried this "sure cure" it aggravated his nausea. Stuart's successful solution was an old folk medicine prescription: Stir 1 teaspoon *each* apple cider vinegar and salt in a glass of water. Take a teaspoonful each 5 minutes until the nausea begins to subside, then take one swallow each 15 minutes for the next hour.

Alternative "Sipping Solutions" Plain hot water; hot broth with some cayenne pepper in it; and herbal teas prepared from basil, camomile, comfrey, ground cinnamon or cloves, ginger, licorice root, mace, nutmeg, peppermint, or yarrow. A potent blend of equal amounts of allspice, cinnamon, cloves, and ginger in boiling water is said to stop violent vomiting. Warm peppermint tea with a little brandy is believed to calm the stomach after an episode of vomiting. Cold, carbonated beverages are no longer advised, but bubbly champagne or ginger ale over cracked ice is a favorite folk remedy. Cold water with a teaspoon of baking soda in each cup is also highly recommended.

Chewable Denauseators Cinnamon sticks steeped in red wine; one or two whole cloves; ½ teaspoon dry, grated grapefruit peel; or fresh mint or sage leaves.

Cold or Hot Packs Applying an ice pack against the back of the neck sometimes settles churning internals. A hot pack made by saturating a wash cloth with cinnamon tea or vinegar—or a poultice of crushed mint leaves wrapped in moistened cloth—may negate nausea when placed over the bare stomach and kept warm with a heating pad set on low.

Nerve Pressure and Massage

○ On each hand, massage the thumb and first and second fingers, then firmly massage the webs between the thumbs and index fingers.

○ Press and massage the inside of each arm 2 inches toward the elbow from the center of the wrist.

○ Press or massage 1 inch to the left of the center of the chest for 10 seconds, release for 10 seconds, and repeat three times.

○ Firmly press and massage the area between the ball of the foot and the beginning of the arch on both feet, or the area between the second and third toes on each foot.

Sources (see Bibliography)

2, 6, 10, 26, 37, 41, 49, 51, 59, 60, 64, 65, 78, 87, 98, 123, 135, 144, 148, 150, 166, 172, 176, 186, 187, 193, 201, 202, 203, 226, 252, 254, 255, 262, 264, 265, 284, 293, 294, 304, 312, 313

Nosebleeds

The most common site of nasal hemorrhaging is the nose partition (septum) in the forward part of the nose, where relatively large blood vessels lie just beneath a thin mucous membrane. These anterior nosebleeds (epistaxis) can occur when the membrane is disturbed by a bump or blow, the interior of a nostril is scratched with a finger or other object, or when the nose is forcefully blown while it is irritated from a cold or sinusitis. Spontaneous bleeding can be set off by sudden changes in atmospheric pressure or by the extremely low humidity in overheated rooms, arid climates, or airplane cabins. Nutritional deficiencies are sometimes responsible for nosebleeds without apparent cause, and people with high blood pressure who take aspirin or other blood-thinning drugs may experience frequent nosebleeds.[300]

Posterior nosebleeds, which flow from the rear of the nose down the back of the throat no matter what position the person is in, primarily affect the elderly but may occur as the result of an injury. This type of nosebleed is potentially serious and warrants medical attention. A physician should also be contacted if spontaneous nosebleeds recur frequently, if a nosebleed follows a blow to the skull, if a broken nose is suspected, and for any nosebleed that continues to bleed after 20 to 30 minutes of home ministrations.

First-Aid Tips Gently blow the nose to remove any clotted blood. With thumb and index finger, pinch the fleshy part of the nose above the nostrils for 5 to 15 minutes while sitting quietly and leaning forward to keep the blood from draining back into the throat. Slowly release pressure, and if bleeding continues, squeeze the nose closed for another 5 or 10 minutes. Holding cloth-wrapped ice or a cold compress against the nose and face may constrict blood vessels to slow the bleeding.

If the nosebleed is not the result of an injury that might have fractured the nose, inserting a twist of gauze or clean cloth (not absorbent cotton or facial tissue, which might adhere to the clot) before the second compression session may help seal the ruptured blood vessel—leaving one end of each plug exposed eases removal half an hour after the bleeding ceases. Remaining upright and refraining from blowing the nose for several hours, as well as limiting vigorous activities for a few days, avoids dislodging the newly formed clot. During the week or 10 days required to completely heal the rupture, applying a coating of petroleum jelly or vitamin E from a snipped capsule several times a day helps keep membranes moist and speeds healing. If nosebleeds on airline trips are a problem, either substance may be applied before departure.

Diet and Supplements (see note on page xii)

Many cases of recurrent nosebleeds can be corrected with dietary adjustments and daily supplements. Eating generous amounts of broccoli, cabbage, and dark leafy greens provides vitamin K, which is essential for normal blood clotting. If blood-thinning medications are suspected of contributing to the problem, foods such as almonds, apricots, bell peppers, berries, cherries, coffee, cucumbers, grapes, peaches, plums, tea, and tomatoes, which are high in salicylate (an aspirinlike substance) should be avoided or used sparingly. In some cases, eliminating sugary sweets stops recurrent nosebleeds; other cases respond to daily supplementation with a high-potency B-complex tablet.

Increasing the daily intake of vitamin C plus bioflavonoids to 500 to 5,000 milligrams in divided doses, and eating citrus fruits with their white inner skin, strengthens the walls of the blood vessels so there is less chance of spontaneous nosebleeds. Alice T. blamed the dry desert air for the frequent nosebleeds and subsequent cauterization suffered during her first year at an Arizona university. After repeated nosebleeds and a day in bed with noseplugs during her summer vacation on the East Coast, however, Alice accepted the advice of a friend. When the next nosebleed struck, she took two 2-milligram tablets of copper, then two more for each of the next 3 days. Results were miraculous, and by taking a daily multivitamin-mineral containing copper (essential for the formation of collagen and elastin), Alice has remained free of nosebleeds regardless of her geographical location.

Tissue salts may help halt a nosebleed in progress. Take three 6X tablets *each* Ferr. Phos. and Kali. Phos. at 10-minute intervals until the bleeding stops. If the blood is dark and clotted, substitute three tablets of 6X Kali. Mur.[64, 65]

Folk Remedies

To quell nasal hemorrhages, ancient nostrums called for applying crushed raw garlic to the insteps of the feet; cabbage leaves or sliced onions to the back of the neck; or pressing down on a fold of cloth, brown paper, or a fresh green leaf placed under the upper lip. Persons beset by frequent nosebleeds were instructed to tie a string around the little finger just below the nail or wear a bright silk ribbon around the throat with or without an iron key dangling between the shoulder blades. American folk practitioners suggest taking 1 or 2 teaspoons of apple cider vinegar in a glass of water three times a day, or eating chickweed (*Stellaric media*, an actual weed) as a salad or cooked vegetable to forestall recurrent nosebleeds. Drinking a cup of yarrow tea (also known as soldier's woundwort) daily is believed to reduce clotting time and keep nosebleeds away. Snuffing bistort, golden-seal, or white oak bark tea up the nose, or applying a daily coating of aloe vera gel or carbolated petroleum jelly is said to toughen nasal membranes.

During the 1800s, folk healers recommended "stoppering" a bleeding nostril with bacon grease (or fat pork cut to fit), or nasal plugs of cloth saturated with mineral oil or vinegar (a gentle cauterizing agent). To draw blood away from the head while the nose is either plugged or compressed, one or both arms can be raised over the head; the feet or hands immersed in hot water; a cup of cayenne tea sipped; or the neck, nose and temples sponged with vinegar.

Sources (see Bibliography)

17, 21, 28, 42, 64, 65, 75, 92, 111, 116, 135, 148, 151, 171, 176, 186, 202, 203, 216, 255, 256, 257, 262, 264, 281, 283, 284, 293, 294, 300, 311, 312, 313, 322

Periodontal Disease

Plaque is the villain in the story of periodontal disease. A transparent, sticky film of food debris and bacteria that adheres to teeth, especially along the gumline, plaque hardens into a yellowish substance called tartar (dental calculus) unless it is cleaned off daily. An accumulation of tartar irritates the gums to cause gingivitis—a mild form of periodontal disease with swollen, inflamed gums that bleed easily. If the tartar is not professionally removed, gingivitis can escalate into pyorrhea (periodontitis). The gums recede, leaving pockets of infection that gradually erode supportive bone and tissue, teeth loosen and may be lost. Contributing factors are improper brushing, diabetes, glandular or blood disorders, medications such as antibiotics and anticoagulants, osteoporosis, poor dietary habits, and nutritional deficiencies. With proper care during its early stages, periodontal disease can be reversed. Puffy, spongy gums can shrink and grow firm, wobbly teeth become more stable.

Dental Hygiene

Both prevention and treatment of periodontal problems require periodic tartar-removal sessions in a dental office, plus twice-a-day brushing and at least once-a-day flossing to dislodge plaque before it hardens. Bedtime brushing is particularly important to prevent bacteria and food particles from wreaking their havoc during sleeping hours. Holding a soft-bristled toothbrush at a 45-degree angle against gums and teeth and wiggling it in small circles cleans the gumline as well as spaces between the teeth. The areas adjoining a bridge with an artificial tooth require special care to prevent periodontal disease from destroying the teeth supporting the bridge.

Diet

Eating a bite or two of aged cheddar or Swiss cheese after a meal or chewing sugarless gum for 10 minutes neutralizes some of the plaque-forming acids.[111, 293, 312] Concluding each meal with a few bites of crunchy raw fruits or vegetables and/or a mouth rinse of water removes food debris—eating a quarter of a raw apple has been found to be 30 percent more effective than an immediate brushing.[195]

A varied diet emphasizing green vegetables, fresh fruits, lean meats, and whole grains supplies nutrients for dental health and provides the exercise needed to stimulate blood flow to the teeth and gums. Bacteria thrive on sugar and starchy foods; fat makes food particles cling to the teeth—doughnuts, potato chips, and raisins are among the worst offenders. Suggested snack foods include air-popped popcorn and raw vegetables. Although low-fat dairy products and vegetables contain vitamin K (essential for bone maintenance as well as for preventing bleeding), the major portion of the body's vitamin K is synthesized by intestinal flora. Eating *Lactobacillus acidophilus* yogurt (or taking acidophilus capsules) can replenish the vitamin-K-producing bacteria destroyed by treatment with certain antibiotics or other medications.[151] As explained in *American Health* (February 1993), smoking or using smokeless tobacco reduces blood circulation to the gums and may interfere with healing.

Supplements (see note on page xii)

In addition to a daily multivitamin-mineral, these individual supplements prove helpful in many cases.

Vitamin A In the form of beta carotene, 50,000 IU for 1 month, then 25,000 IU daily.

B Complex One comprehensive tablet with meals. Taking extra folic acid and niacin has stopped bleeding gums for some individuals.[206]

Vitamin C with Bioflavonoids 1,000 to 5,000 milligrams in divided doses daily. Even subtle deficiencies of vitamin C can cause "pink toothbrush." Bioflavonoids, first isolated as a remedy for bleeding gums that were not corrected by vitamin C, strengthen and preserve the capillaries while C firms and tightens gums and teeth.[49, 151, 255]

Vitamin E 100 to 400 IU, gradually increased to 800 IU. To speed improvement, the capsules may be punctured and rubbed on the gums before swallowing.[17]

Calcium and Magnesium 1,000 to 1,500 milligrams of calcium plus 500 to 750 milligrams of magnesium daily (some researchers suggest taking twice as much magnesium as calcium) in divided doses to prevent or reverse jawbone shrinkage and help correct pyorrhea.

Zinc 15 to 50 milligrams daily to improve vitamin absorption and encourage healing.[98]

Tissue Salts For bleeding gums, take three tablets of 6X Kali. Phos. daily. If the gums are painful on slight pressure, add the same dosage of 6X Silicea.[65]

Folk Remedies

To heal and strengthen the gums, folk healers advise rubbing them with aloe vera gel, figs cooked in milk, or tincture of myrrh. "Healing" dentifrices include baking soda, equal parts of baking soda or cream of tartar and salt, a paste of baking soda and hydrogen peroxide, or powdered goldenseal. To relieve gum pain, rinse the mouth once an hour with a solution of ½ teaspoon salt in ½ cup water. A half-and-half mixture of water and 3 percent hydrogen peroxide is suggested as a three-times-a-day mouthwash to inhibit bacteria.

Apple Cider Vinegar Each night and morning, stir a teaspoon of vinegar in a cup of water; use a little as mouthwash and drink the remainder—or drink a glass of the same blend with each meal.

Herbs Teas may be sipped as a beverage or brewed double-strength for a mouth rinse. As reported in *Longevity* (March 1991), research scientists have found that the tannin in pekoe tea can reduce plaque-producing bacteria by 85 to 90 percent. Astringent teas (agrimony, eyebright, sage, sandalwood, white oak) are advised for bleeding gums. For antiseptic qualities as well as astringency, use goldenseal, myrrh, or thyme. Camomile, comfrey, marshmallow, white oak bark, or yellow dock can be used to reduce gum inflammation and pain. Steeping ¼ teaspoon *each* dried anise, mint, and rosemary in ¾ cup boiling water for 10 minutes then using the strained liquid as a mouthwash every hour is believed to correct bleeding gums.

Friction Massage

To help preserve a tight collar of gingival tissue around the teeth and guard against periodontal disease, massage the gums with a modern gum-stimulator, or rub them with old-fashioned remedies of table salt, coarse cloth, or the white portion of a slice of lemon peel.

Sources (see Bibliography)

3, 6, 13, 17, 41, 42, 49, 50, 53, 65, 72, 87, 98, 99, 108, 109, 111, 147, 150, 151, 173, 176, 177, 186, 190, 195, 199, 202, 206, 217, 228, 255, 256, 262, 283, 286, 293, 294, 300, 301, 308, 312, 313

Poison Ivy, Oak, and Sumac

U rushiol (the substance in the foliage, stems, and roots of poison ivy, oak, and sumac that causes a blistering rash) is considered an allergen, not a poison. The first contact seldom produces a reaction; rather, it merely sensitizes the individual. A second or third encounter then triggers this form of allergic contact dermatitis in 85 percent of the population.[46] Contacts need not be direct. Invisible, odorless, and incredibly potent, urushiol can be brought home on the fur of pets, be spread from person to person, and can be deposited on anything that is touched before the irritant is removed. Even more insidious is the durability of this allergen. Smoke from burning plants or dead roots may cause lung problems as well as skin rash. As explained in *Berkeley Wellness Letter* (August 1991), enough urushiol can endure on shoes, shovels, or other objects to instigate the blistery rash a year later. The reaction of reddened, burning, itching skin can begin within a few hours or delay for a week after the exposure. As the rash develops, oozing blisters form on swollen skin, then gradually heal. Medical help should be obtained if the rash lingers longer than 2 or 3 weeks, involves the eyes, mouth, or genitals, or if a fever occurs.

First-Aid Tip Removing urushiol from the skin within 15 minutes of contact forestalls or at least lessens the reaction. Water from a canteen, garden hose, or stream inactivates urushiol.[46] Some experts recommend three soap-and-water latherings and rinsings;[17, 111] others believe washing with rubbing alcohol is more effective—either before or between water rinses;[294] herbalists suggest using cold flaxseed or mugwort tea.[312] Gasoline or nail polish remover can be utilized in emergencies but should be rinsed off to avoid skin irritation. Clothing should be removed and laundered as soon as possible. Rosemary K. was having a wonderful time at a family picnic until her husband noticed that the wildflowers she was gathering were surrounded by poison ivy. He dumped a thermos of water over her legs and rushed her home where she could douse with rubbing alcohol and take a shower. Rosemary's extremities were fine, but 2 days later, she developed a blistery behind. Although she had not been sitting on the plants, recalling her actions following the poison-ivy encounter revealed the correlation—she had piled her clothes on a chair before showering, then sat on the garments while dressing in clean clothing.

"Second Aid" Decontaminate everything that might have touched the plants or been touched by anything harboring the urushiol—backpacks, car-door handles, even steering wheels. Ammonia or solvents like paint thinner will get the irritant off of bike tires, golf clubs, tools, and other products used outdoors. One cup of hydrogen peroxide can be added to each 5 gallons of water for washing shoes, tents, or dogs;[186] chlorine bleach can be included when laundering suitable fabrics.

Supplements (see note on page xii)

Augmenting the cleansing by taking 1,000 to 2,000 milligrams of vitamin C plus 50 milligrams of B$_6$ and 100 to 300 milligrams of pantothenic acid immediately following exposure, then repeating the dose twice at 4 hour intervals may prevent a rash from appearing. Applying a paste of powdered vitamin C mixed with water is said to clear up poison ivy or oak within 24 hours when adequate amounts of oral vitamin C are taken in divided doses during the day.[98]

To hasten healing, nutritionists recommend daily supplements of 25,000 IU of beta carotene and 80 milligrams of zinc. Swabbing the blisters with a mixture of crushed zinc tablets and water often relieves itching. Applying vitamin E squeezed from capsules aids healing, reduces pain, and helps prevent scarring.[98] If applied to the red area before blisters erupt, a solution of the tissue salt Nat. Mur. and water may reduce the reaction. Once the rash is apparent, taking three tablets *each* of 6X Nat. Mur. and Kali. Sulph. every few hours may be helpful.

Folk Remedies

Remedies for poison ivy's itchy, blistery miseries predate the identification of urushiol and its classification as an allergen. Over 2,000 years after oriental physicians advised applying crushed crab to the blisters, folk practitioners suggested sponging the sores with the water in which crab had been boiled.[313] Slitting the stems of jewelweed or milkweed and drizzling the juice over the rash is said to stop the itching as effectively as prescription cortisone preparations; dabbing pulverized chalk mixed with water (or liquid white shoe polish) on oozing eruptions is as drying as calamine lotion.[293] When the rash first appears, rubbing it with lemon or orange slices has provided immediate relief.[2] Smoothing the fleshy rind of watermelon or the inside of a banana peel over the affected area has brought same-day improvement for some individuals.[150]

Liquids Sponge over the rash or apply as compresses: aloe vera gel; alum water; apple cider vinegar; 1 tablespoon of baking soda, epsom salts, or table salt in a quart of water; buttermilk or fresh milk (mixed with vinegar and salt or with ½ teaspoon baking soda, if desired); diluted lemon juice; green tomato juice; witch hazel; or the fluid strained from cooked oatmeal. Black walnut extract can be swabbed on the sores to inhibit itching.[256]

Herbs Burdock, rose hips, or yellow dock can be sipped as a beverage or sponged over the sores. Goldenseal has been found to speed healing and relieve itching when taken orally in capsules (no more than ½ teaspoon per day) and another ½ teaspoonful dissolved in 1 cup hot water for topical application after cooling; or when a paste of powdered goldenseal, vitamin E oil, and a bit of honey is applied.[42, 57] Crushed fresh catnip or plantain leaves can be rubbed over the rash, or dried plantain or mullein may be moistened for use as a poultice. Powdered slippery elm mixed with hot liquid from cooked okra, then cooled and applied every few hours may relieve itching. To assuage both pain and itching, folk healers suggest cold compresses of mugwort or peppermint tea, or a half-and-half blend of strong white oak bark tea and lime water.[17, 149]

Hot Water A 5-minute application of hot water briefly intensifies the itching but is said to stop the itch for several hours.[16]

Pastes Baking soda or cornstarch and water can be rinsed off when dry, then reapplied. Tofu or cooked oatmeal can be bound in place; crushed raw garlic or ground green-bean pods can be encased in gauze as a poultice to relieve itching and promote healing.

Sources (see Bibliography)

2, 16, 17, 21, 29, 42, 46, 49, 57, 64, 65, 72, 75, 86, 87, 92, 98, 109, 111, 144, 148, 149, 150, 176, 179, 186, 202, 255, 256, 281, 293, 294, 300, 311, 312, 313, 316, 322

Premenstrual Syndrome (PMS)

Since its recognition as a "real" disorder rather than an all-in-the-head female problem, over 150 symptoms in addition to premenstrual tension have been attributed to PMS and are experienced to some degree by 90 percent of women at some time during their reproductive years.[77] Emotional symptoms include anger, anxiety, depression, irritability, and unprovoked hostility. Physical aggravations include abdominal discomfort, acne, bloating and weight gain, breast swelling and soreness, constipation, dizziness, food cravings, headaches, and lack of muscular coordination. The body's anticipation of pregnancy is largely responsible for these unpleasantries. During the second half of the menstrual cycle, estrogen levels rise, the lining of the uterus thickens, and extra breast cells form to enlarge milk ducts. The hormones controlling the menses also affect the nervous system, making susceptibility to stress another PMS symptom.

While no single method of treatment is effective for all symptoms, or for all PMS sufferers, practicing relaxation techniques (see Introduction) and experimenting with self-help remedies often overcome the biochemical causes of premenstrual problems. Wearing a support bra and applying ice packs may alleviate breast discomfort. Warm baths, enhanced with 1 cup of salt or soda, or with relaxant herbs such as camomile, lavender, oatstraw, sage, or thyme; or ginger poultices or hot-water bottles applied to the abdomen may relieve muscular tension and discomfort. Persistent or severe symptoms, however, warrant professional evaluation and treatment.

Diet

Dietary changes during the week or two before each period often relieve or abolish PMS. Food cravings—usually for sweets and salty foods—may be a biologically protective mechanism intended to prepare for pregnancy or menstrual fluid loss but should be controlled because excess salt or sugar causes water retention, which exacerbates bloating and breast swelling. Stabilizing blood sugar levels by eating small, frequent meals helps prevent fatigue, headaches, and wide emotional swings. Restricting caffeine (from coffee, tea, colas, chocolate, or medications) reduces breast discomfort as well as anxiety and irritability.[108, 186]

Alcohol, animal fats, and the lactose in milk products can elevate already high estrogen levels and may contribute to overproduction of preperiod breast cells and other discomforts. Nutritional consultants suggest substituting poultry, fish, and legumes for red meats and limiting dairy products to two servings per day.[17, 293] Emphasizing high-fiber fruits, vegetables, and whole grains helps the body clear out excess estrogen and prevents constipation—which can worsen PMS problems. Besides drinking at least a quart of water each day, drinking a cup or two of any of these herbal teas (or taking the equivalent in capsules) may relieve premenstrual symptoms: angelica (dong quai), blessed thistle, camomile, comfrey, cramp bark (squaw vine), garlic, juniper berry, raspberry leaf, sarsaparilla, Siberian ginseng, spearmint, yarrow, or yellow dock. As reported in *Natural Health* (October 1992), PMS problems may be lessened by taking capsules of black cohosh, dandelion root, false unicorn root, or skullcap daily for 10 days before the anticipated onset of menstruation and until 3 days after its cessation.

Supplements (see note on page xii)

Many experts recommend dietary supplementation to relieve PMS. Although some improvement may be noticeable within a few days, two or three menstrual cycles are needed to achieve maximum benefits. Taking a multivitamin-mineral guards against borderline deficiencies that may be magnified by preperiod biochemical changes. Cravings for chocolate, for instance, may result from the body's need for magnesium or for the amino acids it contains.

Amino Acids L-carnitine (2,000 milligrams daily) acts as a diuretic to help with bloating. L-lysine (500 milligrams daily for 5 days preceding a period) is helpful for hypoglycemics and for those who frequently suffer from herpes. DL-phenylalanine (400 milligrams daily) provides amazing relief for some PMS sufferers. L-tyrosine (500 milligrams before each of three meals a day) helps relieve premenstrual anxiety, depression, and forgetfulness.[17, 109, 151]

Vitamin A In the form of beta carotene, 25,000 IU daily may help relieve PMS symptoms.[98]

B Complex One comprehensive tablet daily. Clinical tests show that an additional 50 to 100 milligrams of B_6, taken every morning and evening for 2 weeks prior to each period, reduces or eliminates acne, backache, breast discomfort, depression, fluid retention and weight gain, headaches, mood swings, nervous tension, and sugar cravings, for most PMS sufferers—especially when used in conjunction with calcium and magnesium. Extra amounts of B_1, choline (a constituent of lecithin), folic acid, niacin, B_{12}, and/or pantothenic acid may also be helpful.[75, 147, 151, 190, 201]

Vitamin C with Bioflavonoids 1,000 to 3,000 milligrams in divided daily doses helps relieve breast discomfort, stress reactions, and general symptoms of PMS.

Calcium and Magnesium 1,000 to 1,500 milligrams of calcium and 500 to 1,000 milligrams of magnesium, or 1,000 to 2,000 milligrams of magnesium and 500 to 1,000 milligrams of calcium in divided daily doses during the latter half of each menstrual cycle. The most beneficial dosage should be determined by the health professional. A deficiency of either of these minerals may be at least partially responsible for premenstrual symptoms, and supplementation has provided significant relief for many PMS sufferers.

Vitamin E 400 IU daily. Recent studies show that this amount reduces abdominal bloating, anxiety, breast tenderness, cravings for sweets, depression, and fatigue.[46, 281]

Gamma-linoleic Acid (GLA) Two capsules of evening primrose oil (or the equivalent in black currant seed oil) three times daily. Several studies show that this essential fatty acid reduces depression, irritability, and other PMS symptoms.[17, 190, 201]

Tissue Salts Three 6X tablets of Nat. Mur., dissolved under the tongue three or four times a day may relieve preperiod depression, lassitude, and morning headaches.[65]

Zinc 15 to 50 milligrams daily may be helpful for PMS symptoms. In conjunction with B_6, niacin, vitamin C, calcium, and magnesium, zinc helps regulate prolactin, the breast tissue activator.[111, 151]

Exercise

Increasing physical activity during the 2 weeks prior to a period may help combat PMS by relieving mental and muscular tension, reducing fluid retention, and increasing the production of endorphins—the pain-blocking, pleasure-promoting hormones responsible for the euphoria of "runners' high."

Nerve Pressure and Massage

○ To dissipate the mood swings of PMS, apply 30 seconds of pressure and massage between the eyebrows directly above the nose, and beside the nails on the thumb side of both middle fingers.[265]

○ To relieve premenstrual discomfort, press the hollow just below the collarbone (in line with the nipple) for 10 seconds, release, and repeat three times on both sides.[57]

Sources (see Bibliography)

6, 14, 16, 17, 28, 29, 46, 49, 51, 53, 57, 61, 65, 75, 77, 98, 108, 109, 111, 112, 147, 151, 176, 186, 190, 201, 252, 254, 265, 281, 293, 294, 300, 312, 319

Psoriasis

A dysfunction of the skin-renewal process, the silvery-scaled plaques of psoriasis result when the rate at which old cells are shed remains the same but new cells force their way to the skin's surface ten times faster than normal, then pile up to form the sometimes itchy and reddened patches. Arms, legs, lower back, and scalp are the most common sites, but any part of the body may be affected. In severe cases (which require professional care), the plaques may spread, fingernails may become pitted, and, in approximately one-third of psoriatic sufferers, a form of arthritis develops with pain and swelling in several joints.[255]

Medically considered a chronic condition of unknown origin, psoriasis may linger interminably or may clear and remain in remission for months or years. Heredity is a factor—one out of three psoriatics have a family history of the disorder.[51] Some cases may be due to faulty metabolism (particularly of fats) or to hormone imbalance; others may be precipitated by almost anything. Key triggers and aggravators include emotional stress, infections, reactions to medications prescribed for heart disease or other ailments, and skin damage from irritation or dryness. Psoriasis is so capricious that what is effective for one person or for one episode may not work for the next. Professional diagnosis is always wise, but the relief proffered by most current medical therapies is fraught with potentially serious side effects.[186, 281] Home remedies often prove equally effective in minimizing discomfort and reducing the frequency of flareups.

Diet and Supplements (see note on page xii)

A low-sugar diet stressing fruits, vegetables, fish (especially salmon and mackerel), and whole grain breads and cereals is usually recommended. If Candida overgrowth is involved, a yeast-free diet may be indicated.[192] In other cases, a gluten-free diet (no barley, oats, rye, or wheat) brings good results. Some nutritionists advise against the use of citrus juices. Fresh apple, beet, carrot, cranberry, cucumber, and grape juices are considered especially helpful. Saturated fats (animal or hydrogenated) should be avoided, but 1 or 2 tablespoons of unsaturated oil should be included daily.

Dairy products, eggs, meat, and poultry contain arachidonic acid, a natural inflammatory substance that has been found to cause psoriatic lesions to turn red and swell.[17, 109] Primrose oil (one capsule three times a day) or fish oil (EPA) helps counteract arachidonic acid. Therapeutic use of fish oil should be under medical supervision—fish oil is high in fat-soluble vitamins A and D that can be toxic in high amounts. Numerous studies show that taking EPA capsules daily (or substituting fish oil for 2 or 3 ounces of fats in the diet) for several months significantly reduces the itching and size of psoriatic patches for up to 61 percent of the patients tested.[51, 147, 151, 294] Taking three capsules daily of cod liver oil *and* of linseed oil (from a health food store) has completely cleared some cases of chronic psoriasis in 5 months. If no improvement is evidenced within 2 months, however, this remedy should be forsaken in favor of a different one.[42] Including 3 or 4 tablespoons of lecithin granules (or the equivalent in capsules) in the diet each day for 2 months then reducing the dosage by one-half, has effected relief in a number of instances.[98, 157] Other cases have responded to two or three lecithin capsules with each meal plus topical applications of lecithin squeezed from capsules.[42]

Sprinkling kelp granules on foods provides additional minerals. Taking three tablets of the tissue salt Kali. Sulph. in the 6X potency three times daily, has alleviated psoriasis in some instances—adding the same dosage of Calc. Phos. has brought improvement to others. Studies indicate that, in addition to a daily multivitamin-mineral, individual supplements may be beneficial.[190]

> **Vitamin A** In the form of beta carotene, 30,000 to 50,000 IU daily for 1 month, then 25,000 IU for 3 months. If the psoriasis has not cleared, the sequence may be repeated, or with medical approval a higher dosage of beta carotene or the emulsion form of vitamin A may be used.

> **B Complex** One comprehensive tablet once or twice daily, plus extra B_6 and B_{12}.

Vitamin C with Bioflavonoids 500 to 5,000 milligrams in divided daily doses.

Calcium and Magnesium 500 milligrams of each daily. Some researchers advise an additional 500 milligrams of magnesium.

Vitamin E 300 to 800 IU daily. When combined with topical applications of vitamin E oil, some longstanding cases have been completely cleared in 6 weeks.[301]

Zinc—50 to 75 milligrams daily. In one study, oral zinc sulfate brought improvement to patients suffering from psoriatic arthritis as well as psoriatic skin lesions.[151]

Folk Remedies

Scientists have found that aloe vera gel, the oldest of all anti-itch skin soothers and healers, contains a substance of specific benefit to psoriasis sufferers.[29] For a temporary itch reliever, an ice pack or a plastic bag filled with ice cubes can be held against the affected area.

Comfortably warm baths—enhanced with a cup of apple cider vinegar or 2 teaspoons of powdered ginger, if desired—reduce psoriasis by flattening plaques and cutting down scaling.[17, 293] Rubbing the patches with avocado oil several times each day may help remove the scales. Other helpful applications include the liquid strained from cooked oatmeal or okra, or ¼ cup of almond oil blended with the juice from one lemon and one lime.

Herbalists suggest drinking a cup of burdock tea before breakfast and dinner, or a cup daily of comfrey, dandelion, goldenseal, sarsaparilla, or yellow dock, then sponging another cup of the tea over the scaly spots. Poultices made from chaparral, chickweed, mullein, sassafras, or slippery elm can be applied to affected areas.

Sea Water and Sunshine

Ocean swimming is a time-honored remedy for psoriasis. Studies conducted at spas near the Israeli Dead Sea show that 85 to 95 percent of psoriatics who combine daily sea bathing with sun exposure are either completely cleared of symptoms or symptoms are greatly improved within a month.[108] As a substitute for the mineral-laden sea, 1 to 4 pounds of sea salt from a health food store can be dissolved in the bath water; or bottled sea water can be applied to the scaly patches several times a day with a cotton ball.[6, 17]

Besides producing vitamin D in the skin, sunlight's ultraviolet rays fight psoriasis by slowing down the rapid proliferation of skin cells. Exposure should be moderate to prevent the possibility of sunburning (which can cause psoriatic patches on previously unaffected areas), and sunscreen should be applied to the clear skin to avoid increasing the risk of skin cancer.[293] Ultraviolet lamps and infrared heat lamps are of benefit in some cases but are not as efficient as the sun's ultraviolet rays.[75, 294]

Stress Management

Recent studies show that emotional stress can cause psoriatic patches to erupt on 50 to 62 percent of people subject to the disorder.[112, 201] Practicing relaxation techniques (see Introduction) during periods of remission may defuse stress before it can initiate a flareup. When psoriasis is active, combining other remedies with relaxation and mental images of clear skin replacing the scaly rash often reduces discomfort and speeds healing.[137, 186]

Sources (see Bibliography)

6, 17, 29, 42, 50, 51, 64, 65, 75, 98, 108, 109, 112, 137, 144, 147, 150, 151, 157, 176, 177, 186, 190, 192, 195, 201, 233, 254, 255, 256, 275, 281, 283, 293, 294, 301, 303, 312, 313

Rosacea and Facial Redness

osacea (formerly called acne rosacea because the flushed-red skin on nose, cheeks, and chin may be accompanied by small acnelike pimples), telangiectases or spider veins (cousins of varicose veins that wander over faces, often radiating from a central point in spidery-looking splotches), and cherry angiomas (red spots resulting from minuscule tumors in dilated blood vessels) affect 85 percent of Americans over 50.[112] Although fewer males than females experience rosacea, many of the afflicted men develop a proliferation of tiny tumors and thickened tissue to create the bulbous purplish red nose associated with chronic alcoholism—which could account for the term "grog blossoms" being applied to all red-faced problems in colonial times.

Hormonal fluctuations may be at least partially responsible for the occurrences of rosacea in pregnant or menopausal women. Triggered or worsened by emotional stress, extreme heat or cold, medications such as vasodilators that enlarge blood vessels, spicy foods, and caffeine as well as alcohol, these facial discolorations may require professional treatment but usually respond favorably to a regimen of internal and external nurturing. Rosacea can recur, however, when encouraged by a combination of instigators.

"Oh, no! Not again!" Noreen L. whispered to the mirror when she recognized the redness on her nose and cheeks as rosacea. "My skin's been fine for 5 years, why now?... Maybe the stress of the trip and caring for the twins, and Rena, and the new baby... Maybe lounging in the sun by the pool yesterday... Maybe that exotic Thai food, or last night's wonderful Italian dinner and red wine... Of course the rosacea showed up today! At least I know what to do, and what not to," she thought as she put her cosmetics in the suitcase instead of on her face, toasted a slice of white bread to accompany a poached egg for breakfast, and purchased a bottle of B vitamins on the way to the airport for her return flight home.

Diet and Supplements (see note on page xii)

The standard treatment calls for a bland diet and the elimination of alcoholic or caffeine-containing beverages. Not everyone need be as strict as Noreen, who must forego seasonings, acid foods, and whole grains for at least a month to clear her skin. Some individuals find that drinking a glass of papaya-pineapple-orange juice or tomato-cucumber-radish juice daily helps balance the distribution of skin-lubricating sebum.[305] Orthomolecular physicians and nutritionally oriented dermatologists attribute these permanent flushes and conspicuous veins to dietary deficiencies and have reported consistent success when a B-complex tablet plus 1 or 2 tablespoons of brewer's yeast and 25 milligrams of B2 are taken daily. Improvement may be speeded by adding 10,000 to 25,000 IU of beta carotene (nontoxic vitamin A), 1,000 milligrams of vitamin C in divided doses with 400 to 800 milligrams of bioflavonoids, 100 to 400 IU of vitamin E, and a multivitamin-mineral tablet containing at least 15 milligrams of zinc.

External Treatment

Exterior care as well as internal nourishment should be bland: mild exercise without excessive perspiration, adequate rest and relaxation, and gentle cleansing. Exposure to heat from the sun, an open fireplace or oven door, or from facial steaming can burst dilated capillaries close to the skin's surface. Icy chilling, tingly toners or after-shave lotions, and harsh soaps or scrubs are equally hazardous.

Folk Remedies

○ After cleansing, splash on a final rinse of the water in which potatoes have been boiled; or use a mixture of ½ cup water and 1 tablespoon of apple cider vinegar.

○ Smooth cod liver oil over the discolorations.

○ For 5 minutes each evening, massage olive oil (or baby oil) outward from nose to ears with circular movements of the fingers.[283]

Sources (see Bibliography)

3, 17, 42, 53, 74, 75, 77, 86, 98, 112, 190, 203, 207, 218, 233, 234, 281, 283, 304, 305

Shingles (Herpes Zoster)

Medically termed herpes zoster, shingles is a viral infection of the nerves caused by the same varicella virus responsible for chickenpox. Most of these viral organisms are destroyed during a childhood attack of chickenpox, but the survivors hide in spinal nerves, where they lie dormant for decades. They can reactivate after emotional stress, a cold or other illness, or when the process of aging lowers resistance and weakens the immune system. The virus, which usually is harbored in only one nerve root, creates an eruption of rashlike sores closely resembling chickenpox on the skin area served by those nerves. There may be several days of localized skin sensitivity or pain before the red bumps appear; itching and burning sensations for 2 weeks to 2 months as the sores blister, burst, crust over, and heal; and in about one-third of the cases, residual pain (postherpetic neuralgia) that lingers for weeks or years.

Although shingles itself is not generally considered a communicable disease, exposure to the rash (which contains active virus particles) may cause small children to develop chickenpox; and pregnant women, adults who have never had chickenpox, and persons with impaired immune systems are advised to avoid direct contact.[80] Medical assistance should be obtained if the outbreak is near the eyes or ears, or if the symptoms are severe. Mild to moderate cases may be controlled with over-the-counter painkillers and self-help remedies. For postherpetic neuralgia, a nonprescription cream containing capsaicin from hot red peppers provides relief for 75 percent of sufferers by anesthetizing the skin's surface.[151, 254]

Supplements (see note on page xii)

In addition to a daily multivitamin-mineral, individual supplements may be beneficial.

Vitamin A   In the form of beta carotene, 25,000 IU twice a day for 2 weeks, then once daily to promote healing and potentiate the immune system. With medical approval, higher dosages of the emulsion form of vitamin A may be beneficial during the first 2 weeks. [17]

B Complex   One comprehensive tablet each morning and evening. All the B vitamins are essential for proper functioning of the nervous system. Taking an additional 5 to 100 milligrams of B_1, B_6, and pantothenic acid with a teaspoon of brewer's yeast in half a cup of milk each 2 or 3 hours until the symptoms begin to subside, then once or twice a day, speeds recovery and helps prevent a painful aftermath. [86, 87] Under medical supervision, injections of B_{12} have provided relief from excruciating pain in as little as 2 hours. [233] Mary Ellen R. was controlling her itching with an ointment the doctor prescribed, but the pain continued and new blisters kept popping up. When she heard that supplemental B vitamins had worked wonders for a friend's shingles, Mary Ellen immediately checked with her doctor and began taking 1,000 micrograms of B_{12} plus 50 milligrams of B_1 each morning. Within a few days, the burning pain lessened and the rash was receding rather than spreading.

Vitamin C with Bioflavonoids   1,000 to 4,000 milligrams in divided doses throughout the day to aid in destroying the virus, help prevent postherpetic neuralgia, and boost the immune system. Dosages should be continued for several days after the symptoms disappear, then gradually reduced.

Calcium and Magnesium   1,000 to 1,500 milligrams of calcium and 500 to 750 milligrams of magnesium in divided daily doses (some researchers advise 1,000 to 2,000 milligrams of magnesium and 500 to 1,000 milligrams of calcium), plus vitamin D (400 IU daily for 1 week, then reduced to 100 IU) to assist healing and protect sensitive nerve endings.

Vitamin E   400 to 800 IU daily to assist the immune system, protect cell membranes from viral attack, and help prevent the nerve damage responsible for residual pain. Direct applications of the oil from snipped capsules may relieve discomfort and help avoid any scarring.

L-lysine   500 milligrams twice daily. Studies show that when taken at the onset of shingles, this amino acid helps inhibit viral action to reduce the severity and duration of symptoms. [17, 293]

Tissue Salts In the 6X potency: Ferr. Phos., two tablets three times a day for the pain preceding shingles; Calc. Phos., Ferr. Phos., and Kali. Phos., two tablets of *each* twice each day after the rash erupts. Kali. Mur. and Nat. Mur. can be taken in alternation three times a day to help speed healing. Either Ferr. Phos. or Nat. Mur. may be dissolved in water and sponged over the blisters to alleviate pain.

Zinc 10 to 50 milligrams daily to promote healing of the skin lesions.

Folk Remedies

A variety of remedies are suggested for symptomatic relief from pain and itching. Aloe vera gel, raw honey, or fresh leek juice may be smoothed over the rash several times a day. Hydrogen peroxide can be used on infected blisters. Apple cider vinegar; cool goldenseal, mugwort, or peppermint tea; or a solution of baking soda and water may be sponged over the sores or applied as a cold compress. A 20-minute soak in a tub of tepid water enhanced with a cup of colloidal oatmeal or cornstarch helps soothe the way to slumber at bedtime. For pain that lingers after the blisters have healed, contemporary folk remedies call for applying a mixture of 2 tablespoons of hand lotion and a crushed aspirin tablet, or vigorously rubbing the area with cloth-wrapped ice cubes.

Sources (see Bibliography)

2, 6, 17, 42, 50, 64, 65, 75, 80, 86, 87, 98, 112, 135, 148, 149, 150, 151, 176, 177, 186, 189, 233, 254, 255, 267, 281, 283, 293, 312, 313, 316

Snakebite, Spider Bite, and Sea Scrapes

A ny penetration of the skin by poisonous creatures warrants medical attention. Even nonvenomous bites and scrapes can trigger infections or allergic reactions, and may require a tetanus injection. Herbalists recommend immediately drinking an antispasmodic tea (asafetida, sarsaparilla, skullcap) to reduce tension and help localize the venom.[149] To lessen the possibility of severe reactions and to alleviate painful symptoms, holistic practitioners advise therapeutic doses of these three supplements (see note on page xii).

Vitamin C 1,000 to 2,000 milligrams immediately; repeated each hour but in reduced amounts if diarrhea develops. (Vitamin C powder dissolved in water is speedily assimilated and can be sipped when swallowing is difficult.) If the injury is from a poisonous snake, spider, or sea dweller, a first dose of at least 4,000 milligrams is recommended as a detoxifying agent. When this dosage was repeated several times, all symptoms reportedly cleared in as little as 38 hours.[98]

Calcium Gluconate 500 milligrams every 6 hours to relieve pain and abdominal cramping from snake or spider venom, and to prevent stomach upset from massive amounts of vitamin C. Accompanying each dose of calcium with 1,000 milligrams of magnesium gluconate or orotate may be beneficial.

Pantothenic Acid 500 milligrams each 8 hours for 2 days to augment vitamin C's detoxifying, antiallergy properties.

Snakebite

There are two species of poisonous snakes in the United States. Pit vipers (rattlesnakes, copperheads or highland moccasins, cottonmouths or water moccasins) are found in every state except Alaska. The coral snake (a member of the cobra family found in southern states from the East Coast to Texas) "chews" instead of creating fang punctures. Prevention is the ideal remedy for snakebite. When in wilderness areas, tuck long pants into footgear at least ankle high, be cautious when turning over rocks or fallen logs, camp in an open space, and wear thick gloves when gathering firewood.

Most bites are by nondangerous species, and even poisonous snakes do not always inject venom. The severity of the reaction depends on how much venom is injected; the age, size, and allergic proclivity of the human; what part of the body is bitten; and how soon medical help is obtained—an antivenin is effective only if administered within 12 hours after the bite.[281] A snakebite victim should not attempt to drive. Besides the customary pain and swelling, symptoms can include nausea, weakness, and loss of consciousness.

First-Aid Tip If bitten, stay calm, and after getting out of range (a snake can bite more than once), move as little as possible. To slow blood circulation through the bitten area, keep it immobile and level with or lower than the heart. If soap and water are available, cleanse the wound and cover it with a clean bandage. Applying a paste of water and the contents of several activated charcoal capsules, then taking ten of the capsules;[312] or immediately swallowing five papaya tablets with sips of water in which papain-containing meat tenderizer has been dissolved may neutralize some of the venom.[150] Do not apply ice—chilling may damage tissue and drive the venom deeper. If the bite is on an arm or hand, remove rings and bracelets before any swelling commences. Seek medical assistance immediately. If the snake has been killed, it can be taken along, but no time should be squandered by searching for it.

If medical help is more than 30 minutes away and if the bite is on an arm or leg, a tourniquet should be applied between the wound and the heart during the first 5 minutes after the bite. The constricting band should be 2 to 4 inches above the wound and loose enough to allow a finger to be inserted between it and the skin and for a pulse to be felt below the bite site—this pulse should be checked every few minutes and the tourniquet loosened when necessary. If the swelling reaches the tourniquet, it should be left in place and a second constricting band applied a few inches higher.[322]

According to the August 1991 issue of *Berkeley Wellness Letter*, cutting a snakebite to suction out the venom should be attempted only when medical care is several hours away and when the bite is on an arm or leg; then it should be done as soon as the tourniquet is in place. Without a snakebite kit containing a poison-extracting suction pump, the emergency procedure is

1. Sterilize a sharp knife or razor blade in alcohol or with a flame. Make cuts ⅛ of an inch deep through each fang mark, cutting down the length of the limb, not across it.

2. Suck out venom and blood, spit it out, and continue the suction for 30 to 60 minutes—snake venom is not a stomach poison but the mouth should be rinsed.[148] Then wash the wound and bandage it.

While awaiting medical help, small sips of water containing powdered vitamin C may be beneficial, but food and alcoholic beverages should be avoided. Whiskey is not snakebite medicine.

Spider Bite

All spiders are poisonous—they inject venom to paralyze their prey— but only a few species are harmful to humans. In the United States, the most dangerous are the female black widow and the brown recluse. Both may be encountered indoors or out, and bites from either have been known to be fatal; medical evaluation for possible antivenin therapy is essential.

The black widow, a glossy black spider with a red hourglass marking on the underside of her quarter-inch body, injects a neurotoxin similar to rattlesnake venom. The bite produces brief pain; then, about 30 minutes later, abdominal cramps and muscle spasms, breathing difficulty, and occasionally, paralysis may develop. The brown recluse (also called a fiddleback or fiddler spider) is approximately the same size with a dark brown violin-shaped marking on the top front portion of its body. Its bite is relatively painless, but within a few hours or days, there may be pain, fever, chills, nausea and cramps, and the wound may blister, ulcerate, and enlarge.

First-Aid Tip Wash the bite and disinfect it with alcohol or hydrogen peroxide to prevent secondary infection. Rub an aspirin over the moist area to neutralize some of the poison, then apply an ice pack to slow the spread of venom while awaiting professional care. If medical help will be delayed more than half an hour, and if the bite is on an arm or leg, apply a tourniquet as for a snakebite. If the dead spider is available, bottle it for positive identification.

Sea Scrapes

Poisonous marine creatures are a hazard to waders, swimmers, snorkelers, and scuba divers. Aesthetically appealing coral is composed of coral skeletons and is inhabited by coral polyps equipped with the same toxic cells as jellyfish. When touched, coral can cause painful abrasions and may discharge small barbs along with a dose of poison. Sea urchins are shallow-water as well as ocean-floor denizens whose spines instigate pain and infection. Stingrays get their name from the barbed, toxic spines located at the base of their long, threadlike tails. All such wounds should be medically evaluated as soon as possible. Barbed spines may require professional removal; symptoms of intense pain, nausea, and possible shock could necessitate life-support procedures.

First-Aid Tip Flush the site with saltwater, then splash with alcohol, ammonia, vinegar, or alum or meat tenderizer dissolved in salt water to inactivate some of the toxins. Remove small spines or coral fragments with tweezers or cloth-covered fingers, then immerse the injured part in hot water for at least 30 minutes to neutralize more of the poison. If medical assistance cannot be obtained within half an hour and if the injury is on an arm or leg, apply a tourniquet between the wound and the heart as for snakebite.

Home Remedies to Augment Professional Care

To draw out venom, folk healers use tobacco poultices or apply powdered mustard mixed with garlic juice or wine vinegar when medical help is not available.[203] Wild plantain is said to serve the same purpose for rattlesnake or black widow bites—juice from the leaves should be squeezed onto the wound while the victim chews additional plantain leaves.

> **Herbal Remedies** For venomous encounters remedies include drinking a cup of echinacea, sarsaparilla or yellow dock tea (or taking two capsules) every hour until symptoms are relieved and applying a poultice of moistened black cohosh, blue cohosh, comfrey, slippery elm, or white oak bark.
>
> **Pain Relief** A poultice of alum powder beaten with egg white, a prepared-ahead salve made by simmering equal amounts of tar and

tobacco until thick, or Trisha P.'s sweet solution may be effective. When the 3-year-old ventured beyond the patio to admire a butterfly, one bare foot was bitten by something she could identify only as "bug." To quiet the anguished howls, Trisha's mother poured peroxide over the swelling red spot, swished a cup of sugar into a pan of water, and immersed the little foot. The pain and tears subsided before Trisha and her mother reached the doctor's office, and, whether Trisha had been bitten by a vicious ant or a garden-variety spider, no further treatment was required.

Swelling, Itching and/or Pain Alleviate by taking three or four daily doses of the tissue salts Kali. Mur., Kali. Phos., and Silicea, and applying a paste made by mixing them with water; or with applications of aloe vera, ammonia, eucalyptus oil, lemon juice, vinegar, or vitamin E oil.

See also **Bites**

Sources (see Bibliography)

17, 20, 41, 42, 57, 64, 69, 72, 75, 80, 85, 87, 92, 98, 104, 111, 135, 144, 148, 149, 150, 159, 169, 176, 196, 202, 203, 216, 252, 264, 281, 282, 283, 284, 285, 293, 300, 311, 312, 322

Sore Throat and Laryngitis

Inflammation of the wall of the throat (pharyngitis) or of the vocal cords (laryngitis) commonly accompanies a cold or the flu but can result from allergic reactions; chronic coughing; emotional stress; excessive smoking; inhaling chemical fumes, dust, or smoke; overindulgence in hard liquor; overly dry air; overuse of the voice; or from swallowing extremely hot food or beverages. Most sore throats run their course in a few days or weeks. Two or three days of complete voice rest is advised for laryngitis—whispering puts more strain on the vocal cords than normal speech does. Throat and voice problems that linger, swallowing difficulty, or soreness with white spots in the throat should receive medical evaluation and, possibly, antibiotic treatment for a bacterial infection such as strep throat.

Breathing through the nose with the mouth closed helps prevent throat dryness and deflects airborne irritants. A study reported in the *Berkeley Wellness Letter* (January 1992) indicates that dry air impedes the effectiveness of nasal cilia in keeping the respiratory tract clear of viruses and bacteria. Portable humidifiers help maintain the ideal 30 to 50 percent level of moisture in the air. Inhaling steam for 5 minutes at a time several times a day soothes throat irritation. Adding a teaspoon of tincture of benzoin (or menthol or eucalyptus oil) to a pan of boiling water increases the benefits of the inhaled vapors.

Diet and Supplements (see note on page xii)

Chewing whole cloves (no more than four per day) or eating onions cooked in molasses are folk remedies for a sore throat accompanied by hoarseness. Fresh pineapple and its juice contain an enzyme (bromelin) that is believed to speed recovery by destroying dead tissue in the throat without affecting healthy tissue; fresh grapefruit may also be helpful. Increasing fluid intake lubricates the vocal cords to relieve hoarseness and ease discomfort. Iced beverages can aggravate the problem; hot soups and liquids slow viral reproduction by raising the temperature of the throat. Orange or tomato juice, or warm lemonade made with honey and fresh lemon acidifies the throat to help destroy invading viruses. Herbalists suggest sipping honey-sweetened tea: bayberry root bark, catnip, comfrey, ginger, licorice root, or mullein. Slippery elm tea, with or without the addition of ¼ teaspoon goldenseal, may be combined with an equal amount of cow's milk or soy milk for super soothing. Holistic doctors advise dietary supplements to shorten the duration of a sore throat.

Vitamin A In the form of beta carotene, 75,000 IU daily for 1 week, reduced to 50,000 IU for 1 week, then 25,000 IU daily—to aid healing and strengthen the immune system.

Vitamin C 1,000 to 5,000 milligrams in divided daily doses. Hourly gargling with 500 milligrams of powdered vitamin C stirred in a glass of water, plus taking a 250 milligram tablet of vitamin C each hour, has cleared sore throats by the second day.[301]

Zinc One zinc gluconate lozenge dissolved in the mouth every 2 hours until pain is relieved—not over 12 in 24 hours and for no longer than 1 week.[118]

Garlic Two 15-grain capsules with each meal for its natural antiseptic, antibiotic properties.[17, 293]

Tissue Salts For an inflamed throat with hoarseness or loss of voice, dissolve three 6X Ferr. Phos. tablets under the tongue each hour until pain is ameliorated; then three tablets every 3 waking hours until inflammation subsides. For a sore, aching throat with pain on swallowing, take three 6X Calc. Phos. on the same schedule.[65]

Compresses and Poultices

A cold compress may help relieve pain and inflammation—covering it with plastic to keep it airtight for 4 to 8 hours increases the benefits. Hot-water packs or cloth squeezed out of double-strength camomile tea should be renewed when cool or be repeated four times a day. Poultices of ripe banana or ½ cup tofu blended with 2 tablespoons wheat flour and 1 teaspoon grated fresh ginger can be spread on a strip of cloth, placed next to the throat, then wrapped with a covering cloth and replaced every 2 hours.

Gargles

Gargling provides temporary relief for a raw, scratchy throat, helps shrink swollen tissue, and may be repeated every 20 to 30 minutes.

Stir-and-Use Solutions Half-and-half mixtures of water and aloe vera gel, apple cider vinegar, lemon juice, or pekoe tea. One-fourth cup brewer's yeast and 1 tablespoon honey may be stirred into 1 cup of water. Or ¼ cup *each* honey, cider vinegar, and water can be combined. Or the water in which figs have been cooked may be used as a gargle.

Cooked Gargles These are old-fashioned favorites. Simmer 1 tablespoon dried currants in 1 cup water for 10 minutes, add ½ teaspoon cinnamon, cover and let stand for 30 minutes, then strain. Or boil 2 tablespoons dried, grated pomegranate rind in 3 cups water until reduced to 2 cups; strain when cool. Strong white oak bark tea is another option. For a gargle with character, steep 2 teaspoons *each* cayenne pepper and dried sage in 1 cup boiling water; then stir in 2 teaspoons *each* honey, salt, and vinegar before straining.

Salt and Baking Soda Singly or combined (¼ to ½ teaspoon per half-cup of warm water), these are preferred by many folk practitioners. Stage performers rely on baking soda when threatened with laryngitis. Rhonda P. had recovered from her cold and was excited about her first appearance with the Little Theater group. More nervous than she realized, however, her vocal cords reacted by tightening up just before show time. "I know my lines but I can't say them," she squeaked to the director "I'm losing my voice." He stirred half a teaspoon of soda in a paper cup of water and told her to gargle; take 10 slow, deep breaths; and gargle again. Amazingly, Rhonda's throat relaxed, her voice returned to normal, and she was able to perform on cue.

Liquid Remedies

To relieve throat irritation, folk healers recommend a variety of fluids to be sipped or taken by the spoonful at frequent intervals. Coconut milk, prune juice, or the juice of one lemon heated with ¾ cup water and a tablespoon of honey has soothed many sore throats. Other options are honey-sweetened liquid from ¼ pound miller's bran simmered in a pint of water for 30 minutes; double-strength sage tea, with or without honey and a teaspoon of lime juice; or strong slippery elm tea with the juice of half a lemon.

Syrups

Sugar or honey is the basic ingredient of syrups to be taken by the spoonful. Combinations include equal amounts of brown sugar and brandy; a half-and-half blend of honey and bee pollen; equal parts of egg white, honey, and lemon juice; ¼ cup hot lemon juice stirred with ½ cup honey and 1 tablespoon glycerin; or honey in which peeled garlic cloves have been steeped for several days.

Nerve Pressure and Massage

O Pull down on the top margin of the breastbone for 10 seconds, release for 10 seconds, and repeat three times.

O Press and massage the lower part of each thumb and the web attaching it to the hand; then press the bottom portion of each thumbnail on the side closest to the index finger. With the right thumbnail, press the bottom outside corner of the left thumbnail for 7 seconds. Release and repeat three times, then apply the same sequence to the right thumbnail.

O Massage each big toe and the web between it and the next toe.

Sources (see Bibliography)

2, 17, 20, 21, 26, 49, 51, 57, 58, 65, 69, 75, 84, 87, 92, 98, 110, 111, 116, 117, 118, 135, 144, 148, 150, 151, 159, 164, 171, 172, 186, 202, 203, 250, 254, 264, 265, 281, 293, 294, 300, 301, 302, 304, 308, 312, 313

Sprains and Strains

S trains, also called muscle pulls, are injuries in which muscle fibers are stretched and sometimes partially torn through overexertion. Shoulder strain, for instance, can result from painting a ceiling; back strain from improperly lifting a heavy object. Sprains occur when the fibrous bands (ligaments) connecting the bones in a joint are torn, as in a twisted ankle or sprained wrist. Muscles, tendons, and blood vessels may also be damaged during a sprain, thus adding a strain and a bruise to the accompanying pain and swelling. Sprains and strains are treated according to the degree of injury. First- and second-degree injuries are subject to home remedies; third-degree injuries warrant immediate medical evaluation. Fractures can be detected only by X-rays; being able to walk on a sprained ankle does not preclude the possibility of a fracture.

- ○ **First degree** is a mild injury evidencing minimal pain and little loss of movement.
- ○ **Second degree** is a moderate injury that produces sharp pain with motion, swelling, and possible discoloration.
- ○ **Third degree** is a severe injury with extreme pain, swelling, and spasmodic muscle contraction.

First-Aid Treatment

RICE, an acronym for "rest, ice, compression, and elevation," is the accepted treatment for sprains and strains.

Rest The injured area should be kept immobile. If a weight-bearing body part is involved, walking should be attempted only with crutches for 1 week for a mild sprain, 2 weeks for a moderate one.

Ice Applying ice on a 20-minutes-on/20-minutes-off schedule for an hour or so serves as a local anesthetic and slows blood flow and seepage from damaged blood vessels to reduce swelling. Placing a damp cloth over the injury protects against frostbitten skin. The ice treatment, or cold compresses, should be repeated four or five times a day for at least 24 hours; for several days if needed. (See Introduction for homemade, flexible, reusable ice packs that will conform to a joint.)

Compression Wrapping an elastic bandage around an injured joint helps slow the accumulation of fluids in the tissues. The bandage should be snug but not tight enough to cut off circulation and should be loosened then rewrapped at least once an hour. By using an elastic bandage to hold an ice pack in place, compression and chilling can be accomplished simultaneously.

Elevation If the injured body part is kept raised, gravity helps control inflammation and swelling by moving blood and fluids away from the sprain. Elevating extremities is especially important. A twisted ankle should be raised above waist level as much of the time as possible for the first 24 hours; a sprained wrist should be placed in a sling adjusted so that the fingers are several inches higher than the elbow.

Milly M. and her friend Barb discovered that necessity can be the mother of improvisation as well as invention, and that for-fashion-only suspenders can be functional. The weekend campout with their husbands had been fun, but they were not overly enthusiastic about fishing so opted for sleeping late on Sunday while the men made a final effort to increase the supply of take-home, iced-down fish in the picnic cooler. The ladies had dressed and were rolling up the sleeping bags when Milly slipped and twisted her ankle. By the time the men got back to camp, RICE was in progress in a thoroughly modern manner. Milly was reclining on an open sleeping bag, her foot was propped on a rolled-up sleeping bag, and surrounding her swelling ankle were two plastic-wrapped frosty fish firmly held in place with Barb's stretchy, bright-red suspenders.

Supplements (see note on page xii)

If tissue salts are available when the injury first occurs, one 6X tablet *each* Calc. Fluor., Calc. Phos., and Mag. Phos. taken every 20 minutes for 2 hours may lessen the pain and binding of muscles. Following each dose with a drink of hot liquid increases the effectiveness. Alternating cold compresses of Ferr. Phos. and Kali. Mur. tablets dissolved in cold water may help alleviate both swelling and discomfort.

Taking 250 to 1,000 milligrams of vitamin C (and/or a capsule of the herb horsetail) with each meal can aid the repair of connective tissue. Other daily supplements to augment the healing process are a multivitamin-mineral plus 15,000 IU of beta carotene, a B-complex tablet containing 50 milligrams of B6, 100 to 600 IU of vitamin E, 50 milligrams of zinc, and 1,000 to 2,000 milligrams of calcium plus 500 to 1,000 milligrams of magnesium (some researchers suggest 1,000 milligrams of calcium plus 2,000 milligrams of magnesium) taken in divided doses.

Heat Therapy

The appropriate time to begin heat treatments varies from 24 hours to 7 days, depending on the degree of injury. Without medical evaluation, the best guide is to wait until the swelling starts to subside.[165] As soon as the damaged blood vessels are repaired, heat can be utilized to increase blood flow and promote healing by irrigating the tissues with nutrients and removing waste products. An acute muscle tear or a bruised area should not be massaged for at least 72 hours after the injury,[291] but after that length of time, interspersing hot compresses and gentle massage with applications of cold may reduce stiffness and speed recovery.

Pain Relief

If a painkilling pill is needed the first day, ibuprofen or acetaminophen is advised—aspirin inhibits the blood clotting necessary for repair of damaged blood vessels and could contribute to swelling. For pain relief after the first day or two, however, aspirin or ibuprofen is recommended to help reduce inflammation—acetaminophen lacks this capability.[186]

Liniments and rub-on balms produce a feeling of warmth and reduce pain by stimulating the nerves and increasing blood flow. Topical pain relievers should not be covered with a heating pad or hot compress that could dangerously increase their absorption and injure the skin.[112]

Folk Remedies

For the deep-seated congestion of sprains, folk healers recommend both soothing and stimulating applications.

Casts of a Sort Beat an egg white with salt and spread it over the sprain or, if the skin is not broken or irritated, apply strips of newspaper soaked in vinegar and then overwrap with airtight material.

Compresses Towels wrung out of hot burdock or catnip tea, hot milk, or warm vinegar can be applied several times daily. Or the injury can be bathed in hot water, then fomented with a solution of 2 tablespoons salt in 1 cup *each* alcohol, vinegar, and water.

Liniments As soon as possible after a sprain occurs, shake one egg white with 1 teaspoon *each* turpentine and vinegar in a jar, then apply to the area. For later use, simmer 1 tablespoon cayenne pepper in 2 cups cider vinegar for 10 minutes and use while warm. Or heat 2 tablespoons of petroleum jelly and blend in a teaspoon of cayenne. Or combine one egg white with 1 tablespoon *each* honey and salt, beat until stiff, let stand for an hour, then spread the liquid it produces over the sprain and cover with a bandage. To relieve the pain of strained muscles, mix one beaten egg yolk with 1 tablespoon eucalyptus oil or turpentine and 1 tablespoon vinegar, then massage into the painful area.

Poultices Binding orange peel (with the white side next to the skin) over a sprain is said to reduce swelling. A variety of substances can be spread on gauze and bandaged over a sprain: ground caraway seeds cooked to a paste in water; grated raw carrots; cider vinegar mixed to a paste with breadcrumbs, unprocessed bran, or oatmeal; comfrey tea leaves softened in hot water or steeped in alcohol; the white of an egg blended with 2 tablespoons ground ginger and ½ teaspoon salt; grated raw onion mixed with granulated sugar; a paste of ground turmeric and water; or a mixture of ground black pepper and hot vinegar that should be removed and rinsed off after 3 hours.

Nerve Pressure

To help relieve the pain of a sprain anywhere in the body, press just below each outside anklebone (unless one of the ankles is injured) for 10 seconds, release for 10 seconds, and repeat three times for a total of 30 seconds pressure.

Sources (see Bibliography)

17, 42, 46, 47, 64, 65, 69, 75, 92, 112, 135, 144, 148, 150, 159, 164, 165, 168, 176, 186, 187, 202, 256, 264, 281, 282, 283, 291, 294, 299, 300, 312, 313, 322

Stings

Unless a person is allergic or supersensitive, stings from soaring, scuttling, or swimming creatures usually are unpleasant but not life-threatening encounters.

Supplemental Tips (see note on page xii). Immediately after being stung by anything, take 1,000 to 2,000 milligrams of vitamin C; repeat in an hour or so if discomfort lingers. Vitamin C helps detoxify venom; 10,000 milligrams during the first hour is suggested for people with known sensitivity to stings.[17] Massive amounts of vitamin C have been found nontoxic; taking it with calcium (up to 1,000 milligrams— some experts suggest including up to 2,000 milligrams of magnesium—per day) lessens pain and decreases the likelihood of stomach irritation. Adding 500 milligrams of pantothenic acid provides antiallergenic benefits. Tissue salts suggested for potentially severe stings are 6X Kali. Phos., Nat. Mur. and Silicea taken every 10 minutes for 1 hour. If swelling develops, substitute Kali. Mur. for Nat. Mur. and take three or four doses each day.

Bees, Hornets, Wasps, and Yellow Jackets

Honeybees are kamikazes—their barbed stingers pull out of their bodies, causing the bees to die. Bumblebees, wasps, hornets, and yellow jackets have smooth stingers that can sting repeatedly. Although Egyptian hieroglyphics indicate that King Menses perished from the sting of a hornet in 2641 B.C., only one person in two-hundred experiences severe symptoms of throat swelling, breathing difficulty, vomiting, and possible anaphylactic shock.[75]

First-Aid Tip If an allergic reaction is suspected, or if the sting is in the eye, mouth, or throat, cover the area with an ice pack and keep it elevated while enroute to the nearest doctor; apply a tourniquet between the heart and the sting if it is on an arm or leg—check to make sure a pulse is present below the tourniquet and loosen it for a few seconds each 5 minutes.

For known cases of insect allergy, immunotherapy (desensitization shots) or a prescribed emergency kit containing epinephrine or adrenalin in preloaded syringes is recommended. For most stinging situations, however, sensible precautions and home remedies suffice. To avoid being stung:

○ Establish an internal insect repellent. The daily consumption of large amounts of garlic, 2 tablespoons of brewer's yeast, or 60 milligrams of zinc makes people unappealing targets.[293] Taking 100 milligrams of B_1 (half that amount for a child) before and each 3 or 4 hours during exposure is said to produce a skin odor repellent to bees.

○ Forego any scent (perfume, after-shave, hair spray, even deodorant) that might entice a bee into relating a human body with a nectar-bearing plant.

○ Dress in plain, light-colored, long-sleeved shirts and long pants, and wear shoes—bees in the grass are more easily disturbed than those in the air, and sometimes confuse people with flowers.

○ Do not aggravate a bee by swatting at it. If approached by an insect dive bomber, walk away—do not run. Seek sanctuary indoors, dodge between buildings, or head for the woods to discourage pursuit, or if threatened by a horde, dive into any available water.

First-Aid Tips and Treatments

Smashing a stinging creature is not advisable. The blow may cause more venom to be injected and, if the insect is a yellow jacket, release a chemical that signals for a full-scale attack by its nest mates. If the stinger is still in the skin, immediately scrape under it with a knife, credit card, or fingernail, and flip it out—the stinger can continue to pump venom for 2 or 3 minutes and attempting to pull it out will squeeze more poison into the system. Wash and disinfect the sting, especially if it is from a carnivorous wasp that may have had its feet in contaminated material.

Cold Chilling the area keeps the venom localized and has an anesthetic effect. An ice pack can be used every 2 hours if needed for pain control.

Soaking a stung hand or foot in a basin filled with water, ice cubes, and half a cup of baking soda is usually effective. For swelling, dissolve 1 tablespoon epsom salts in hot water and use in place of the baking soda. For swelling around the eyes, cover with cloths squeezed out of a mixture of 1 teaspoon baking soda and 1 cup ice water. An ice bag or cold compress can be placed over any of the paste or poultice remedies.

Heat A heating pad or hot compress can be applied, or a hair dryer can be aimed at the sting to deactivate one of the inflammation-causing chemicals.

Aspirin Moisten the site and rub with an aspirin tablet to neutralize several of the inflammatory agents in bee venom.

Liquids and Lotions Dab for 5 minutes or cover with cloth saturated in any of these liquids: aloe vera gel, rubbing alcohol, household ammonia, baking soda and water (plus salt, if desired), castor oil or vitamin E oil, cinnamon tea (eat the sticks from which the tea was brewed), lemon juice, or vinegar.

Pastes and Poultices Meat tenderizer is a modern folk remedy for neutralizing venomous stings. Sprinkle papain-containing tenderizer on a moistened gauze pad, or make a paste with water, then apply for 30 minutes. Activated charcoal (crushed tablets or opened capsules) combined with water, applied to the sting and covered to keep moist, draws out the poison and reduces both pain and swelling. A water-based paste of vitamin C powder helps alleviate pain and itching, as does a paste of the tissue salts Kali. Mur., Kali. Phos., Nat. Mur., or Silicea. Rubbing toothpaste on the sting may make it feel better because of menthol's cooling effect. Older remedies are honey, mud, or moistened tobacco; or a paste of baking soda and/or salt mixed with water, witch hazel, or vinegar. Herbalists prescribe poultices of damp tea leaves (or opened capsules) of black cohosh, camomile, comfrey, pekoe, slippery elm, or white oak bark.

Vegetables Crushed cabbage leaves or leek blades, mashed garlic (or the oil from capsules), freshly grated horseradish wrapped in cheesecloth, onion juice, or grated or sliced raw potatoes have been used to relieve the pain of stings. Raw onion is another option that worked for Casey K. Attired in his Hawaiian shirt, he was having a wonderful time in his grandmother's backyard until the bee stung.

She quickly scraped out the stinger, gave him an ice cube to hold over the spot to deaden the pain, and took him with her to the kitchen while she sliced an onion and secured it over the swelling site. By the time Casey's parents arrived to pick him up, the only evidence was his tear-streaked face—which he explained by declaring, "The onion made me cry."

Beverages—Herbal remedies call for 1 cup (or two capsules) of black cohosh, echinacea, or yellow dock tea each hour until symptoms are relieved.[176] Alcoholic drinks are ill advised because they intensify the effects of the venom by dilating blood vessels and speeding up circulation. Regular coffee, tea, or caffeinated soft drinks may help counteract bee sting discomforts.

Scorpions

Two to four inches in length, with clawlike pincers, a scorpion presents a crablike appearance but possesses a flexible tail that arches over its back to administer poison with a sharp stinger. Scorpions dwell in warm regions, are nocturnal creatures that lurk in dark crevices or under rocks during the day, and attack if disturbed. In scorpion-infested areas, clothes and footwear should be shaken out before being put on.

Most scorpion stings are no more dangerous than a bee sting and can be treated with the same remedies—only two of the forty species in the United States produce significantly toxic venom. After cleansing and disinfecting, apply an ice pack to reduce pain and retard the spread of the venom, then keep the bitten area lower than the heart. Young children and the elderly are at greatest risk for dangerous complications, but everyone should be alert to indications of severe reactions (rapid pulse, breathing difficulty, diarrhea, nausea, convulsions) that require immediate medical attention and an antivenin injection.

Jellyfish and Sea Anemones

With transparent tentacles that can trail invisibly for up to 60 feet, jellyfish and Portuguese man-of-war (actually a colorful colony of many jellyfish in various stages of development) are the most common stinging swimmers. Sea anemones, flowerlike creatures dwelling on the sea floor, have waving tentacles as hazardous as those of jellyfish. When the long tentacles encounter human skin, poisonous cells pierce it to inject venomous capsules. To avoid additional stings from broken-off tentacles adhering to the skin, carefully remove them with tweezers or a towel-protected hand; or cover the tentacles with a paste of sand or baking soda and sea water, then scrape them off with a knife or plastic credit card. Pressure or vigorous rubbing can activate any stinging cells that have not ruptured. Fresh water also activates the capsulated venom. Rinse the area with salt water before applying one of the following substances to deactivate the stinging cells.

- ○ Splash with vinegar, diluted lemon juice or ammonia, or alcohol (rubbing alcohol is preferred; wine or any liquor will suffice).
- ○ Coat with a paste of salt water mixed with papain-based meat tenderizer, alum, baking soda, flour, or talcum powder. Reapply once or twice, but if the pain does not subside within a few hours, or if severe symptoms such as muscle cramps, vomiting, or shortness of breath develop, obtain medical assistance.

Sources (see Bibliography)

2, 17, 20, 42, 45, 46, 49, 50, 57, 64, 65, 69, 72, 75, 87, 98, 104, 108, 109, 111, 135, 144, 149, 150, 169, 176, 186, 195, 202, 203, 207, 256, 281, 284, 285, 293, 300, 312, 313, 322

Stomach Flu (Acute Gastroenteritis)

A lso known as intestinal flu, intestinal grippe, 24-hour virus, or "the bug that's going around," acute gastroenteritis is commonly referred to as stomach flu. Viruses are responsible for 90 percent of the cases of inflammation of the stomach and intestinal tract that produce flulike aching and general malaise along with vomiting, abdominal cramping, and often, mild fever and episodes of diarrhea.[264] Occasional causes include bacterial infection from foods or beverages, overindulgence in alcohol, allergic reactions, and prescribed antibiotics or other medications that alter intestinal flora. Severity and duration of the symptoms depends on the irritant and the general health of the individual.[148] Norwalk virus infection, spread by contaminated water (including swimming pools) and foodstuffs, especially oysters and other shellfish, occurs in sporadic, local epidemics.[281]

Whatever the source, stomach flu appears suddenly and usually fades away within 12 to 48 hours. Bed rest is advisable until the vomiting and diarrhea subside (for specific remedies see "Diarrhea," "Nausea and Vomiting"). Since gastroenteritis can be contagious, the preventive measures of diligent hand washing and not sharing drinking or eating utensils helps avoid infecting other household members. A physician should be contacted if vomit or stools are bloody, if the vomiting cannot be stopped within a day, if severe pain is localized in the abdomen or rectum, or if symptoms persist longer than 4 days.

Diet and Supplements (see note on page xii)

Fluid replacement is important (particularly for children, the chronically ill, and the elderly) because vomiting and diarrhea can quickly lead to dehydration and loss of essential minerals. Sucking ice chips is helpful until other liquids will stay down. Then, a few tablespoons of ginger ale, cola, or other carbonated beverage; clear broth; savory vegetable juice; or diluted, sweetened fruit juice are often better tolerated than plain water and can be taken at frequent intervals. Ample amounts of liquids should be continued and bland solid foods attempted before returning to a normal diet.

Twenty-five years ago, pediatricians advised that youngsters with gastrointestinal upsets be allowed no food for 24 to 48 hours. Current recommendations call for one day of half-strength formula for infants who are not breast-fed (breast milk is well tolerated and contains natural antibiotics), and semisolid foods (applesauce, bananas, cereal, rice, soups, gelatin desserts) as soon as the child can tolerate them.[44]

Although Joey N. began to "feel funny" as soon as he sat down at his desk, the third-grader hesitated to ask permission to leave the room so soon after recess—and hesitated too long. He threw up just outside the door. His embarrassment eased when another boy in the nurse's office admitted he had done the same thing, and Joey felt better while he waited for his mother. The respite was only temporary. He dashed to the bathroom the moment they got home. Too miserable to complain about being put to bed in the middle of the day, Joey dutifully sucked a vitamin C lozenge, sipped ginger ale, and dozed all afternoon. The chicken soup he had for supper stayed down. So did his bedtime snack of gelatin with banana slices. The diarrhea did not recur, and by morning, Joey was ready for breakfast and another school day.

Stomach flu stages such brief encounters that special dietary supplements are seldom necessary. However, taking 100 to 250 milligrams of vitamin C every 3 or 4 hours during the siege (to discourage invading germs) and a few acidophilus capsules or servings of yogurt after the bout is over (to help restore normal intestinal flora) may be beneficial.

Sources (see Bibliography)

41, 44, 75, 87, 98, 148, 201, 234, 254, 255, 264, 279, 281, 283, 294, 300

Sunburn

Burns from the sun can be as serious as those from flames or hot objects, and require up to 3 months for skin recovery.[312] Repeated sunburns are a shortcut to the premature facial aging, brown spots, and skin-cancer risks engendered by accumulated ultraviolet-ray damage from everyday exposure and suntans. Sunscreens and other preventives described in "Sun Exposure" would make sunburn an extinct ailment if it were not for "operator error," underestimation of the power of UVB rays, and contributory factors.

Staying out of the sun between 10 A.M. and 3 P.M. is not always feasible. Hats blow off. Sunglasses get stepped on. Sunscreen can be forgotten or fall overboard when the boat motor malfunctions a mile from shore. And nature's apparent protection is fallible. Sven E. discovered this when he succumbed to sleepiness under a sheltering tree and awoke in blazing sunshine, with the shade several feet away. Lorna C., who was aware that over 80 percent of the burning rays could creep through cloud cover, did not realize that fog, smog, and a cool breeze would not deter UVB rays. She got burned while huddling on a California beach waiting for the sun to break through so she could get a start on a tan.

Water is Sol's participating partner. Whether frozen on a ski slope or shimmering in a pool, water reflects sunlight to increase its intensity. If not protected by sunglasses, the clear, outer layer of the eyes can be sunburned and require days of light-free recovery time. Besides permitting the penetration of UV rays to sunburn swimmers, water can act as a prism to concentrate the sun's heat on stationary body parts in the same way that a magnifying glass can be used to start a fire. Jon R. couldn't walk for a week after he "cooked" his feet by dangling them in the lake while he sat on the bank and fished all one afternoon. The pain and pinkness began that evening; by morning, each foot had a puffy scarlet circle 2 inches in diameter on the instep, another the size of a dime on the sole.

Shaving immediately before sun exposure exaggerates the sun-sensitivity of male faces or female legs. Certain after-shave products, colognes, cosmetics, and soaps sometimes instigate a burnlike rash after only a few minutes in the sun. Medications such as antibiotics, antihistamines, diuretics, oral contraceptives, and tranquilizers can increase and amplify sunlight's harmful effects for some individuals.

First-Aid Tips Taking two aspirin tablets at the first hint of overexposure and repeating the dosage six times at 4-hour intervals helps reduce redness, pain, and swelling. Prompt cooling, maintained for 15 minutes, not only relieves pain but may lessen the severity of a sunburn by conducting heat away from the skin. Cloth-covered ice packs or cool-water compresses may be used for small areas. A physician should be consulted if nausea, chills, or fever accompany a severe sunburn.

Baths

Soaking in a tub of cool water dissipates heat and helps rehydrate sun-parched skin. To soothe sun-sore eyes at the same time, cover them with slices of raw apple, cucumber, or potato, or with tea bags squeezed out of cold water. These old-fashioned additives may boost the benefits of plain bath water:

- One-half to 2 cups of baking soda, cornstarch, or colloidal oatmeal (a commercial blend of powdered oatmeal, lanolin, and mineral oil); or a handful of instant oatmeal scattered in the tub; or a cup of regular oatmeal or dried camomile flowers secured in cheesecloth with a rubber band and squished in the water.

- Two cups of fluid milk or ⅔ cup of instant dry milk, or 2 cups of vinegar swished in the water.

Cooling Applications

When tub bathing is impractical, any of these liquids can be utilized as cooling compresses or can be sprayed, splashed, or smoothed on sunburned skin: milk, vinegar, or witch hazel—full strength or diluted with water; 2 tablespoons of salt dissolved in 2 cups *each* milk and water; a quart of cool water with 3 tablespoons of baking soda or 2 tablespoons of rubbing alcohol; triple-strength burdock, pekoe, or sage tea cooled with ice cubes; or raw cucumber or potato juice prepared in an electric blender or juicer.

After-Cooling Soothers

Air-excluding substances should not be immediately applied to sun-burned skin—they can seal in the heat. Used after the initial cooling, however, they moisturize, help relieve pain, and may encourage the redness to turn into a tan. Aloe vera gel, reapplied every hour, is the oldest burn remedy. Mayonnaise, petroleum jelly, vegetable oil, and white vegetable shortening are other time-tested favorites.

Lotions To cool and soothe, lotions can be concocted from an egg white beaten with a teaspoon of castor oil; a mixture of ½ cup vinegar, 3 tablespoons yogurt, 2 tablespoons salt, and 1 tablespoon aloe vera gel; ¼ cup commercial moisturizer, 2 tablespoons aloe vera gel, and 2 drops of *either* oil of cloves or oil of peppermint; or by whirring half a peeled cucumber with ¼ cup *each* oatmeal and yogurt in an electric blender.

Pastes To be applied and rinsed off after half an hour, pastes can be prepared from baking soda or cornstarch and water; laundry starch, cooked as for starching shirt collars; a raw cucumber blended with 1 tablespoon witch hazel and 1 teaspoon honey; raw tomato, peeled and pureed with a little buttermilk; stirred egg yolks; or plain yogurt or heavy cream.

Blisters

To relieve discomfort, one edge of a blister may be punctured with a sterilized needle and the top gently pressed to force out the fluid,[293] but the upper layer should not be peeled off. To guard against infection, blistered areas should be washed with mild soap and water and carefully blotted dry. Applying a protective coating of aloe vera gel, or a half-and-half mixture of honey and wheat germ oil, or vitamin E oil, or vitamin E from snipped capsules may hasten healing. Sprinkling talcum powder on the sheets minimizes nighttime friction and irritation.

Diet and Supplements (see note on page xii)

Taking 25,000 IU of beta carotene, extra vitamins C and D, and the B-complex vitamins PABA and pantothenic acid have corrected some cases of abnormal sun-sensitivity.[224] Many individuals react adversely to PABA (a UVB shield used in the first sunscreens), but for those who do not, taking

1,000 milligrams of PABA daily may speed sunburn healing—especially when PABA ointment, or a lotion made by dissolving 1 teaspoon of the crushed tablets in ¼ cup of water is applied to sunburned areas.

Drinking eight or more glasses of water or nonalcoholic beverages daily helps counteract the dehydrating effects of a sunburn. A balanced diet with ample protein provides nutrients needed for skin and tissue repair. Supplements of the antioxidant vitamins A (25,000 IU of beta carotene), C with bioflavonoids (1,000 to 10,000 milligrams in divided doses), E (100 to 600 IU), plus 15 to 50 milligrams of zinc help neutralize the damaging free radicals released when skin is sunburned and assist the healing process.

Sources (see Bibliography)

6, 16, 17, 32, 45, 46, 47, 53, 85, 87, 92, 98, 108, 124, 135, 149, 150, 159, 184, 186, 224, 231, 254, 276, 293, 294, 300, 304, 312, 313, 322

Sun Exposure and Pigment Spots

Dermatologists agree that sun exposure can prematurely age skin by as much as 20 years, and as reported in *Health After 50* (July 1991), 90 percent of the skin changes associated with aging—pigment spots, wrinkles, rough or leathery texture—are due to accumulated damage from ultraviolet light. The short, "burning" rays (UVB), which are strongest during midday hours when the sun is overhead, activate pigment cells in the skin's outer layer to produce the melanin that thickens and darkens the epidermis as a defense against sunburning. The longer ultraviolet rays (UVA) are present from sunup to sundown, penetrate more deeply, decimate supportive tissue, and hasten the development of sags and wrinkles.

Ultraviolet radiation is also a health hazard. Besides destroying protective antibodies in the skin and increasing the incidence of skin disorders such as cold sores and warts,[108] UV rays can instigate cataracts and skin cancers from 5 to 20 years after the original exposure.[184] Recent research indicates that all ultraviolet exposure is cumulative and that long-term consequences of overexposure may include suppression of the immune system to increase susceptibility to all sorts of ailments, disruption of the genetic material (DNA) in skin cells to slow and distort cell renewal, and tissue damage that can lead to skin cancers on body areas that have never been exposed to the sun.[177, 254] Bronzing lotions are harmless, but an artificial tan cannot deter a sunburn. Sun lamps and tanning beds are not recommended—their UV rays are five to ten times more potent than natural sunlight.[300]

Dodging Sol's damaging rays is difficult. They penetrate cloud cover, smog, 3 feet of water, and loosely woven clothing, and can bounce back from concrete, sand, snow, or water to attack bodies sitting "safely" in the shade. Window glass stops UVB but does not shield skin from UVA radiation. With skin cancer escalating at an epidemic rate (over half a million new cases a year according to the May 1991 *FDA Consumer*) and the constantly dwindling ozone layer allowing more UV rays to reach the earth, "safe sun" requires self-protection.

Sunscreens

The rate at which sun damage is acquired and becomes evident depends on individual skin type as well as on the amount of exposure. People with dark or olive complexions are affected more slowly than the fair-skinned because skin-coloring pigment absorbs some of the UV rays, but the harmful effects are cumulative. The 1992 guidelines from the American Cancer Society and the Skin Cancer Foundation advise everyone, regardless of age or skin color, to use a broad-spectrum sunscreen with a sun protection factor (SPF) of at least 15 every day; a waterproof sunscreen of at least SPF 30 during outdoor activities.

SPF refers to the amount of protection from UVB rays. UVA protection (indicated by "broad spectrum" or a UVA listing on the label) also is essential to decrease the risk of skin cancer and prematurely aged skin. Waterproof products cling to the skin during swimming or sweating but must be renewed after being toweled off. To be effective, sunscreen should be smoothed on 30 minutes before going outside (20 minutes before covering with makeup) and lavished on vulnerable areas like the ears, nose, and hands. For convenience, there are sunscreen-containing cosmetics, hand lotions, and lip balms.

Experts estimate that the regular use of an SPF 15 sunscreen during the first 18 years of life would reduce the incidence of skin cancer by 80 percent.[300] By adhering to a year-round regimen of applying sunscreen under makeup or after shaving, adults can halt further harm and allow the body to repair some of the existing damage. When shielded from the sun for a year or so, skin-supporting collagen and elastin partially regenerate to reduce sags, lines, and wrinkles; age spots and pigment blotches begin to fade; the purple purpura patches and spidery red lines of sun-induced blood vessel hemorrhages develop less frequently; and even precancerous lesions may disappear.[294]

Sunglasses

Orientals wore tinted lenses 2,000 years ago, Nero is said to have watched the gladiators through genuine emerald lenses, and Eskimos peered through slits carved in ivory to shield their eyes from sun glare. Modern sunglasses are advised for every daytime encounter with the outdoors. Ultraviolet radiation not only etches wrinkles in delicate tissue around the eyes and encourages eyelid skin cancer, it can damage the eye's cornea, lens, and retina, and initiate or exacerbate cataract formation. Studies reported in the *Berkeley Wellness Letter* of June 1991, indicate that visible sunlight (called blue light) also can damage the retina and speed retinal degeneration, a major cause of blindness among the elderly. For adults and children, most ophthalmologists recommend sunglasses that filter out at least 95 percent of UVB rays, 60 percent of UVA rays, and 60 to 90 percent of blue light. Large lenses and massive frames or wraparounds protect the entire eye area and reduce side-entry light. Glasses that block 99 percent of UV radiation and 97 percent of blue light may be advisable for people who have had cataract surgery or are taking tetracycline (which increases sun sensitivity), or for anyone planning a trip to a tropical beach or a glaring ski slope.

Protective Clothing

Tests conducted by *Consumer Reports* (June 1992) show that hair sunscreens do not effectively prevent hair from becoming dry, brittle, and dull when exposed to ultraviolet rays. Wearing a headscarf or a baseball cap protects hair or a balding pate; a broad-brimmed hat offers bonuses. A visor provides an SPF of only 2 but doubles the SPF of sunscreen on nose and forehead.[186] As explained in *American Health* (March 1992) and *Longevity* (June 1992), a 3-inch-wide brim cuts eye exposure to UVB rays in half and shields the ears, sides of the face, and back of the neck. During prolonged periods in the sun, long sleeves and full-length pants are recommended. The SPF of any hat or garment can be gauged by holding it up to the light. Tightly woven, dark, synthetic material absorbs more radiation than light-colored cotton does; UV rays flow through loosely woven fabrics and open-weave straw hats. Harlan K., an elementary school physical education instructor, had enjoyed his year-round tan for 15 years and had given no thought to possible harm from the desert sun. When skin cancers began to appear, he considered early retirement with a sunless future. Then a dermatologist suggested skin-protecting alternatives, and Harlan adopted all of them. He slathers sunscreen on his face, hands, shoulders, and arms; wears long-sleeved shirts, a broad-brimmed "gambler's hat," and, by special dispensation from the school board, sports a neatly trimmed beard while he continues to conduct classes in the sunshine.

Supplements (see note on page xii)

Manufacturers are now incorporating vitamins A, C, D, and E in sunscreens to help protect the skin. Many nutritionists and holistic doctors recommend oral supplements of all the antioxidants (see Introduction) to neutralize the free radicals created by ultraviolet radiation (as well as by oxidation within the body) that can harm DNA and both internal and external cells—pigment spots are surface signs of free-radical damage.[17, 45]

Vitamin A In the form of beta carotene, 25,000 to 50,000 IU daily. Taking extra vitamin A before an anticipated outing helps prevent the temporary night blindness that often follows exposure to extremely bright light.

Vitamin C with Bioflavonoids 1,500 to 5,000 milligrams in divided daily doses to help prevent pigment clumping and skin sags by strengthening the supportive collagen.[276]

Vitamin D 400 IU if not provided by fortified milk or a daily multivitamin. Sunscreens as low as SPF 8 block the body's formation of natural vitamin D from sunlight on bare skin.[151, 231]

Vitamin E 200 to 600 IU daily. In one study, participants taking 200 IU of vitamin E each day for a year reduced their free-radical level by 26 percent.[45]

Selenium 50 to 200 micrograms daily.

Zinc 15 to 50 milligrams daily.

Pigment Spot Treatments

Age spots, medically termed senile lentigines or lentigo (from Latin words for "old" and "freckle"), are small, brownish patches of clumped pigment sometimes referred to as liver spots because of their color—the sun, not liver dysfunction, is responsible for their formation. Taking a daily B-complex supplement plus additional B2 may help lighten existing brown spots;[146] consistent treatment with home remedies may fade or even clear them.

○ Twice each day, smooth on aloe vera gel; or rub the spots for 2 or 3 minutes with the milky sap from crushed dandelion stems or with a slice of red onion.

○ Once a day, cover the spots with cotton saturated with fresh pineapple juice; with a paste of lemon juice and salt or sugar, or with a water-based paste of dry comfrey root tea—leave for 20 minutes, then rinse off with lemon juice.

Sources (see Bibliography)

17, 28, 45, 46, 49, 50, 51, 53, 98, 99, 108, 109, 111, 124, 146, 150, 151, 177, 184, 186, 206, 224, 231, 234, 254, 276, 283, 293, 294, 300, 312

Tinnitus

An estimated 36 million Americans are afflicted in one or both ears, either occasionally or constantly, by the buzzing, chirping, clanging, hissing, ringing, roaring, tinkling, or whistling sounds of tinnitus.[300] Although a symptom rather than a disease, and "all in your head," the noise is real in that acoustic nerves are transmitting impulses to the brain from internal stimuli. Temporary tinnitus may be due to hardened earwax, or to a loose ear hair or a fragment from a recent haircut, any of which can vibrate close to the eardrum and create thunderous noises. Tinnitus that usually disappears when the triggers are controlled, limited, or avoided can be instigated by sinus congestion, antibiotics, barbiturates, quinine-containing medications, exposure to chemicals such as carbon monoxide from gasoline fumes or the benzene used by dry cleaners, or by excessive consumption of aspirin, alcohol, or caffeine. According to the *New England Journal of Medicine* (February 1991), ringing in the ears may result from the jarring force of high-impact exercises, which can disrupt the auditory system's normal function. Persistent or recurrent tinnitus, frequently accompanied by hearing loss, may be caused by exposure to loud noise from blaring radios, gunshots, jackhammers, industrial machinery, rock concerts, or other sources. Professional diagnosis is advisable because disorders such as a perforated eardrum, inflammation or infection of the inner or middle ear, high blood pressure, high cholesterol, or other physical problems may be responsible for tinnitus. Until the condition is corrected, it may be possible to cover up the annoying noise by listening to a radio or television, or by using a cassette player with headphones. Tinnitus maskers, available without prescription, are worn like a hearing aid to produce a neutral white sound that has relieved 60 percent of patients with severe tinnitus.[300]

Diet and Supplements (see note on page xii)

Personal experimentation can determine if allergic reactions to certain foods aggravate the affliction. For some individuals, caffeine or other stimulants, excess salt, or the quinine in tonic water can trigger an episode of ear noise. Tinnitus support groups have found that proper nutrition helps reduce unwanted ear sounds. A high-fiber, low-fat diet including raw vegetables and their juices often improves blood flow and diminishes the distressing sounds.[108, 305] Increasing dietary magnesium and potassium (good sources are apricots, baked potatoes, bananas, beets, leafy greens, and nuts) and taking a daily multivitamin-mineral plus separate supplements may help compensate for the above-average nutrient needs of some tinnitus sufferers.

B Complex One comprehensive tablet daily. Taking an additional 50 milligrams of B_6 two or three times a day may help stabilize inner-ear fluids. Choline (provided by two lecithin capsules at each meal or 2 tablespoons of brewer's yeast daily) has cleared ear noises in less than 2 weeks for some patients with high blood pressure.[2] Della W.'s job entailed so much air travel that when the hissing and humming sounds started she attributed them to jet lag and assumed the problem was only temporary. It wasn't. A medical checkup disclosed no underlying disorder, and a lavage treatment to remove accumulated earwax failed to abolish the annoyance. During her next flight, Della mentioned the discomfort to a fellow passenger who had been researching tinnitus remedies and shared his notes with her. As soon as she arrived at her destination, Della bought a bottle of multivitamin-minerals plus some B-complex stress tablets and began taking them as directed. By the time she got home, the ear noises were lessening. Adding brewer's yeast to her morning tomato juice helped even more, and although eliminating caffeine from her diet was a sacrifice, the blissful silence that ensued was well worth the effort.

Tissue Salts Three tablets of 12X Kali. Sulph. may be taken every 2 hours during the evening to relieve nighttime tinnitus. Other tissue salts (3X or 6X potency) taken several times a day may help reduce specific sounds: Ferr. Phos., for noises like running water; Mag. Phos., for ringing in the ears with hearing loss; Nat. Mur., for humming or singing sounds.

Zinc—Studies show that high doses of zinc sulfate can reduce or eliminate the ear sounds suffered by older patients, but more than 80 milligrams daily should not be taken without medical supervision.[29, 109]

Folk Remedies

An old Chinese remedy calls for eating sunflower seeds and drinking a tea brewed from their hulls.[150] Drinking a cup of fenugreek seed tea each morning, noon, and night is reported to abolish disturbing ear noises.[312] Recent studies show that 40 milligrams of ginkgo biloba (an ancient remedy from China) taken three times daily improved all the tinnitus patients tested.[51, 61] As yet unsubstantiated folk remedies include putting three or four drops of castor oil in each ear once a day and inserting a cotton plug; or using 1 drop of onion juice three times a week until relieved, then once each week or 10 days for maintenance.

Nerve Pressure and Massage

○ Several times a day, hold the ears close to the head and use the thumbs and index fingers to massage the outer edges of both ears, including the earlobes. Or press and massage the area below the last two fingers on the palm of each hand, and/or the sole of each foot between the little toe and the middle toe.

○ For tinnitus with hearing impairment, once each day press and massage the hollows behind both earlobes and the jawbone directly beneath the ears; and/or press on the gums behind the wisdom teeth with a pencil eraser, or bite down on a wad of cotton in the same location for several minutes.

Relaxation and Guided Imagery

Some people are disturbed by ear noises only when they are fatigued or under pressure; for others, stressful situations aggravate existing tinnitus—and the affliction itself is stressful. Practicing deliberate relaxation as described in the Introduction may help alleviate the problem. Incorporating guided imagery for a mental return to a pleasant episode before the onset of tinnitus may provide at least temporary relief. By replaying the sights, sounds, and sensations in detail, and giving the original experience a name such as "peace" before ending the relaxation session, many sufferers are able to abolish the objectionable noises for minutes at a time just by repeating the clue-in name.[186] For nighttime ear noises that preclude or interfere with sleep, deliberately relaxing while listening to soft music (or a commercial "sleep tape" of rain on the roof or other sandman-summoning sounds) often controls tinnitus and in some cases completely eliminates it.[294]

Sources (see Bibliography)

2, 29, 48, 49, 51, 58, 59, 61, 64, 65, 75, 86, 87, 108, 109, 111, 135, 150, 164, 177, 186, 207, 213, 220, 234, 244, 254, 255, 281, 294, 300, 305, 312, 313

TMJ (Temporomandibular Joint Syndrome)

TMJ disorders occur when the jaw joints (the temporomandibular joints connecting the lower jaw to the skull) and the muscles and ligaments controlling and supporting them do not function together correctly. The most common symptoms are restricted jaw movement (which may be accompanied by clicking, grinding, or popping noises) and facial pain. Other TMJ problems can include earache, toothache, and pain or numbness in the shoulders, neck, and back.

Frequently caused by spasm of the chewing muscles due to excessive teeth clenching and grinding (see "Bruxism"), TMJ symptoms may also be initiated by yawning (which can be halted by ducking the head or pressing a fist under the chin), or by arthritis, physical injury, or malocclusion (irregular bite resulting from a lost tooth or an uneven crown or filling). Persistent or recurrent TMJ that does not respond to home remedies should be professionally diagnosed and the underlying dysfunction treated.

Diet

Caffeine-containing beverages (coffee, tea, chocolate, soft drinks) are not advised for TMJ victims because caffeine can increase muscle tension and sensitivity to pain.[47] Herbalists suggest teas of hops, passion flower, skullcap, or valerian root. When jaw movement is painful, the necessary soft-food diet need not be blandly boring.

During the year Myles L. suffered from TMJ while having its instigators (impacted wisdom teeth and an infected salivary gland) diagnosed and removed, his wife concocted appetizing easy-chew meals. An innovative dietitian, Ardis made super soups by pureeing stew, chili, or ham and beans. For eye-appealing salads, she prepared the "bed of greens" by stirring ½ cup of chicken broth into 2 teaspoons of unflavored gelatin and ½ teaspoon *each* salt and sugar, bringing it to a boil and pouring it into the blender over 3 cups of chopped lettuce, 1 tablespoon mayonnaise, and 1 teaspoon lemon juice; whirring the mixture until smooth, and then chilling it in a shallow pan. For fresh tomatoes, she substituted ⅓ cup of spicy tomato juice and 3 ripe tomatoes (peeled and seeded) for the broth and lettuce, and left out the mayonnaise. When Myles yearned for shrimp cocktail, she whirred a cup of cooked shrimp with the gelatin mixture and served it with cocktail sauce over cubes of the lettuce gelatin.

To augment casserole entrees, Ardis utilized her food processor to make melt-in-the-mouth meatloaf or salisbury steak. She processed ¼ cup *each* instant dry milk, quick-cooking oats, grated Parmesan cheese, and soy flour for 30 seconds with ½ teaspoon *each* salt and dried sage. Then she added ½ pound ground beef, ¼ cup *each* catsup and chopped onion, 1 egg, and, with the processor running, slowly poured ½ cup of beef broth through the feed tube. After the puree was baked at 350 degrees, either as a loaf or in a shallow pan so it could be cut into "steaks," it was served with barbecue sauce, catsup, mustard, or other toppings.

Supplements (see note on page xii)

Nutritionists suggest a daily multivitamin-mineral to compensate for possible deficiencies due to a limited diet. Additional supplements may help combat the stress that often accompanies TMJ.

B Complex One tablet with each meal, plus 100 milligrams of pantothenic acid twice a day.

Vitamin C 2,000 to 8,000 milligrams in divided daily doses. Taking 500 milligrams of vitamin C along with 500 milligrams of the amino acid L-tyrosine and 50 milligrams of B$_6$ at bedtime may help relieve anxiety and improve the quality of sleep.[17]

Calcium and Magnesium 2,000 milligrams of calcium and 1,500 milligrams of magnesium (some researchers advise 1,000 milligrams of calcium and 2,000 milligrams of magnesium) in divided doses with meals and before bed has a calming effect and helps regulate involuntary muscle movement.

Heat and Cold

Facial pain may be relieved by applications of moist heat (a washcloth wrung out of hot water), or cloth-covered ice (see "First-Aid Supplies" in the Introduction for homemade ice packs), or by following alternate hot and cold treatments with gentle massage. Holding a hot-water bottle over a wet compress will keep it warm for an extended period. Ice should be removed as soon as the joint feels numb. A 5-minute treatment that provides hours of relief for some cases calls for three repetitions of a cycle of 20 seconds of ice, 1 minute of heat, and 30 seconds of massage.

Nerve Pressure and Massage

To ease the tension that worsens TMJ, press and massage points on both temples an inch above the ears and an inch toward the center of the forehead for 10 seconds. Release for 10 seconds and repeat three times. Then use the same sequence to apply circular massage and pressure to each side of the back of the head at the hairline, halfway between the bottom of the earlobe and the spine.

Posture and Position

Anything that throws the upper body out of its natural alignment can contribute to the woes of TMJ and interfere with recovery. For ideal posture either sitting or standing, the back should be straight, the shoulders and chest in a relaxed position, the chin level, and the cheekbones in line with the collarbones. Extending the neck with the chin tilted while working at a desk or computer is a common cause of TMJ problems. Adjusting the back support and seat height of the chair may resolve the problem. Bifocal wearers may need to switch to single-vision reading glasses to avoid the strain of tipping the head back to read the computer screen.

When sleeping on one side, the pillow should be thick enough to hold the head and neck horizontally level. To reduce back and neck strain while lying on the back, place a rolled up towel instead of a pillow under the neck, then tuck the pillow under the knees.

Potentially harmful habits and positions to avoid include cradling a telephone between ear and shoulder, always carrying a shoulder bag on the same shoulder, lying down with the head propped up at a sharp angle to read or watch television, or painting or doing other work on ceilings or high walls.

Stress Management

Even when not evidenced by teeth clenching or grinding, emotional stress can be a predisposing factor in the development or recurrence of TMJ disorders. Taking time for enjoyable pursuits and exercise, and practicing some of the relaxation techniques described in the Introduction often relieve the tension that causes facial muscle spasm and discomfort—especially when the session includes mental imagery and an affirmation such as "my jaw is relaxed and comfortable." A positive approach to the problem may also be beneficial—a negative attitude has been found to increase the likelihood of painful symptoms.[111]

Sources (see Bibliography)

17, 43, 47, 49, 75, 80, 109, 111, 186, 255, 265, 281, 283, 293, 300

Toothache

Thanks to improved dental hygiene and fluoridated drinking water, half of all schoolchildren in the United States are cavity-free (20 years ago, 75 percent had decayed teeth) and periodontal disease and tooth loss are declining among Americans of all ages.[111, 300] Statistics, however, are of little comfort when the throbbing pain of a toothache strikes. Occasionally the discomfort is a side effect of temporomandibular joint syndrome (TMJ) or a sinus problem. If a food fragment trapped between two teeth is responsible, it may be dislodged by vigorously swishing warm water in the mouth or by gentle flossing. Most commonly, a toothache indicates inflammation of the soft tissue within the tooth. The irritation or infection may be caused by accidental injury, bruxism (tooth grinding), a cracked tooth, or decay under a cavity or a worn-out filling. Professional diagnosis should be obtained to avoid the possibility of abscesses and tooth loss. Until a dentist can be reached, home remedies may alleviate the pain.

First-Aid Tip To save an injured tooth, a dentist should be seen within 30 minutes; 2 to 3 hours at the most. Broken-tooth parts should be saved, then the mouth rinsed with warm water. A tooth that has been knocked out should be picked up by the crown (not the roots), and wrapped in wet cloth or placed in a container of whole milk (not skim milk) or water with a pinch of salt—not plain tap water, which contains minerals that could damage the tooth. If neither liquid is available, the tooth can be held inside the cheek or under the tongue.[300, 322]

Cold and Hot Treatments

A hot, moist compress applied to the cheek over the pain site may relieve discomfort if the tooth nerve is dead. If the tooth nerve is alive, cold packs are preferable because heat can worsen the problem by drawing the infection to the outside of the jaw.[293] A sliver of ice placed next to the aching tooth, or a cold compress or ice pack against the nearest cheek, reduces both pain and swelling and may be repeated four or five times a day. When continued for 5 minutes, rubbing a cloth-wrapped ice cube over the V-shaped area on the back of the hand where the bones of the thumb and forefinger meet has been found to short-circuit pain in the same manner as an acupuncture needle.[16] Folk therapists advise keeping the feet on a hot water bottle or heating pad while cold treatments are in progress.

Folk Remedies

Packing a cavity with cotton saturated with oil of cloves (oils of cayenne, cinnamon, primrose, or sassafras are sometimes substituted), or rubbing the oil on the gum, is a universal remedy. Sucking on whole cloves or softening them in hot water or honey then chewing and holding the cloves in the mouth next to the aching tooth is considered almost as effective. Aloe vera gel, the juice squeezed from a fresh fig, fresh lime juice, or vanilla extract can be applied directly to the source of the pain, but crushed aspirin is not advised because it may harm tender tissues. To hold pain-relieving powdered catnip, cayenne, or mustard against the tooth, folk healers sprinkle the dry herb on a bit of bread spread with peanut butter. Two teaspoons of dried yarrow can be moistened with boiling water and secured in a small piece of cheesecloth. A mixture of equal amounts of powdered alum and salt, wrapped in a tuft of moist cotton and placed over the tooth, is an alternative said to bring quick relief.

Holding every mouthful of a cup of double-strength sage tea for 30 seconds before swallowing—or holding (but not swallowing) vinegar warmed with a sprinkling of cayenne—may be helpful. Crushed garlic or grated fresh horse-radish can be placed on the tooth or, according to folklore, wrapped in muslin and held in the bend of each arm and leg to draw out the pain.

Poultices placed on the outside of the jaw are also believed to reduce pain. An egg yolk mixed with a teaspoon of honey—or a paste of bread crumbs and alcohol with a sprinkling of cayenne—can be spread on gauze. Cloths can be squeezed out of warm camomile tea or the water in which grated ginger root has been simmered. Or heavy brown paper can be soaked in vinegar, sprinkled with grated ginger, applied to the affected side of the face, and left in place overnight.

Nerve Pressure and Massage

○ Press a point on the temple, 1½ inches above the top of the ear, then press inward and upward in the depression in front of the center of the ear.

○ Place the first two fingers of each hand against the hollows at the base of the skull and massage in a clockwise direction.

○ Using three fingers, push on the cheek an inch above the aching tooth for 2 or 3 minutes.

○ Massage the hinge of the jaw and, if the aching tooth is in the lower jaw, rub the outer edge of the jawbone about 1½ inches below the earlobe.

○ On the same side as the aching tooth, press between the thumb and index finger— against the bone leading to the finger. If a front tooth on the left side is aching, massage the thumb and first finger of the left hand; if the painful tooth is a molar on the left side, massage the last three fingers of the left hand. Massage the same fingers of the right hand for pain on the right side.

Tissue Salts

Once each hour, for up to 8 hours, dissolve three 6X-potency tablets under the tongue; for toothache with sore, swollen gums, use Calc. Sulph. and/or Ferr. Phos.; for sharp, shooting, spasmodic pain, take Mag. Phos.; for deep-seated pain around the tooth, use Silicea. Eleven-year-old Adrianne A. had been allowed to bring her best friend along on a family camp-out vacation, and the girls had been having a wonderful time until Adrianne felt the stabbing pain of a toothache on their final day in the wilderness. Dutifully, she took the Mag. Phos. that her mother carried in their first-aid kit. Her father's suggestion that she try the folk remedy of holding a spoonful of his "medicinal" brandy in her mouth aroused more enthusiasm, and Adrianne winked at her friend as she swallowed a bit of the liquid before spitting it out. Her parents still debate the efficacy of each remedy, but three repetitions of the combination kept Adrianne pain-free until they reached the nearest dental office.

Sources (see Bibliography)

16, 17, 41, 42, 43, 46, 49, 57, 58, 59, 63, 64, 65, 85, 98, 109, 111, 112, 135, 148, 150, 151, 153, 164, 176, 187, 195, 202, 203, 250, 256, 275, 286, 293, 294, 300, 306, 311, 312, 313, 322

Traveler's Diarrhea (Tourista)

Humorously referred to as the Aztec two-step, Casablanca crud, Delhi belly, Montezuma's revenge, and Tokyo trot, tourista strikes up to 50 percent of world travelers with diarrhea that ranges in severity from an inconvenient episode to a 5-day, debilitating bout. The usual cause is the *E. coli* bacteria, which is part of normal intestinal flora but which exists in different forms in different geographical areas. When ingested with food or drink, unfamiliar variants of *E. coli* produce toxins that interfere with the intestine's ability to absorb fluids—and watery diarrhea results. Less common instigators are *Salmonella*, *Shigella*, and *Vibrio* bacteria; or assorted viruses and parasites that can add fever and vomiting to diarrheal discomfort. United States' campers, as well as globe trotters, should guard against *Giardia lamblia* (a protozoa acquired from fecal-contaminated streams) by purifying drinking water with iodine tablets or boiling it for 3 to five minutes.[281, 294] Medical attention should be obtained if traveler's diarrhea continues for more than 5 days; if stools are bloody; or if there is severe vomiting, fever, or abdominal pain—these symptoms could indicate amebic dysentery or other disorders requiring professional treatment.

Prevention

Bolstering the body's defenses before departure may pay off in enjoyable travel time. Taking a daily multivitamin-mineral reinforces the immune system. Drinking acidophilus milk or eating yogurt establishes invasion-resistant flora in the digestive system. To minimize the chances of contracting tourista while traveling:

○ Drink bottled carbonated water or boiled water, canned or bottled juices or soft drinks (acidic juices and colas help control the bac-

386

teria), beer, wine, or coffee or tea made with boiled water. Do not drink tap water, mixed alcoholic drinks, or beverages with ice cubes.

○ Eat only freshly prepared foods; forego salad bars, steam tables, and edibles from street vendors. Especially when in Africa, Asia, or Latin America, avoid dairy products, raw vegetables or uncooked shellfish, and fresh fruit that has been peeled before serving. Sipping a little fresh lemon or lime juice before meals, or taking three acidophilus capsules during each meal, sometimes wards off tourista's miseries. Corbin H. swears by garlic. His first trip to Mexico had been spoiled by a siege of Montezuma's revenge. So on his second south-of-the-border venture, he took all possible precautions plus two deodorized garlic capsules with three meals every day. After 2 problem-free weeks in Mazatlan and Acapulco, Corbin feels he has achieved his revenge against Montezuma's microbes.

○ Practice fastidious cleanliness. Wash hands before eating as well as after going to the rest room, and never share eating or drinking utensils—the tourista bug is contagious.

Treatment (see note on page xii)

Preventing dehydration and helping the body purge itself of unwanted organisms are the goals of tourista treatment. Taking 100 milligrams of vitamin C each waking hour during the first day or so helps battle the invaders. Three activated charcoal tablets or capsules taken every 2 hours can shorten diarrhea's duration by absorbing harmful bacteria and transporting them out of the body.[6, 313] Medical anthropologist John Heinerman[149] recommends six capsules of slippery elm bark, preferably taken with apple or pineapple juice in which a spoonful of cornstarch has been dissolved; or a tablespoon of kelp granules plus 1½ teaspoons black pepper stirred into a pint of freshly boiled water. Natural antibiotics in yogurt have antibacterial powers as effective as some pharmaceutical products—taking the lactobacillus in acidophilus capsules three times daily may alleviate the diarrhea and help prevent an attack of the wearies after recovery.[56, 293] Antidiarrheal drugs are seldom advised for traveler's diarrhea because they may make matters worse by prolonging the elimination of *E. coli* or other toxins.[201]

Diet

Replenishing the fluids and minerals being flushed out of the system avoids the serious problem of dehydration. The Mayo Clinic recommends a rehydrating beverage made by dissolving ¼ cup sugar and ½ teaspoon *each* salt and baking soda in a quart of carbonated water or water that has been boiled for 15 minutes.[109] A two-glass diarrhea cure recommended by worldwide health agencies calls for sipping alternately from one glass of distilled water with ¼ teaspoon baking soda, and another glass containing fruit juice plus a pinch of salt and ½ teaspoon honey.[312] Additional liquids can be provided by clear soups, fruit juices, gelatin desserts, weak tea (ginger tea helps relieve abdominal cramping),[17] bottled mineral water, and soft drinks. Salted crackers may be munched as desired. Eating "baby food" carrots may speed recovery—carrots contain substances that can destroy at least some of the diarrhea-producing microorganisms—adding a spoonful of carob powder hastens the process.[150, 234] As the condition subsides, solid foods like baked potatoes, rice, noodles, baked chicken or fish, applesauce, and bananas can be added gradually.

Sources (see Bibliography)

6, 17, 42, 50, 56, 75, 77, 98, 101, 109, 112, 148, 149, 150, 186, 201, 234, 254, 255, 279, 281, 283, 293, 294, 300, 312, 313

Ulcers

The gnawing pain or raging inferno of a peptic ulcer emanates from a craterlike sore in the lining of the digestive tract. Duodenal ulcers in the upper portion of the small intestine are the most common, developing in about one in eight Americans. Gastric ulcers erode the stomach linings of one person in thirty; esophageal ulcers (due to a reflux of stomach acid) are extremely rare. Peptic ulcers, which once beset only middle-aged males, are increasing by half-a-million cases a year and, according to the National Center for Health Statistics, now affect more women than men.[75, 186]

Genetic inheritance increases the risk of peptic ulcers caused by excessive secretion of digestive juices, weak digestive-tract linings or reduced secretion of the mucus that provides their protective coating, or by *Campylobacter* or *Helicobacter pylori* bacteria, which according to a report in the December 1990 issue of *Health After 50,* may also be infectious through personal contact. Factors that raise the risk of ulcer development and adversely affect treatment include continual use of aspirin and nonsteroidal anti-inflammatory drugs, cortisone therapy, emotional stress, dietary deficiencies, and overindulgence in alcohol, coffee, or tobacco—smoking inhibits the pancreatic release of the natural antacids.[46]

Peptic ulcers may respond to home remedies combined with removal of irritants, but professional diagnosis is advised if discomfort persists longer than 3 days and is imperative if symptoms include nausea and vomiting or black, tarry stools, because underlying problems may be involved. Prescription drugs can reduce stomach acid, apply an internal bandage over the ulcer, or by combining antibiotics with a bismuth preparation, destroy the destructive bacteria. Professional monitoring is important because unpleasant side effects sometimes negate the pleasure of pain relief, and even excessive use of over-the-counter antacids can accentuate heart problems, disrupt bowel habits, lead to mineral imbalances, and instigate the return of an apparently healed ulcer.[151, 254]

Diet

The previously ordained bland regimen has been abandoned and milk, once the mainstay of ulcer diets, is no longer recommended. It has been established that milk provides only temporary relief, then stimulates stomach acid secretions and actually retards the healing of ulcers.[147] Studies show that a diet rich in fiber from fruits, vegetables, and whole grains promotes ulcer healing and reduces their recurrence by buffering stomach acid.[46, 312] During acute attacks, it may be beneficial to puree fruits and vegetables, or eat bottled baby food, and supplement with a nonirritating fiber like psyllium.

Eating five or six small meals a day often relieves ulcer upsets because moderate amounts of food neutralize stomach acid. Allowing the stomach to remain empty for long periods or overloading it can increase the secretion of gastric juices. Extremely hot or cold foods may also disturb digestive function. Rather than prescribe a specific ulcer diet, gastroenterologists advise avoiding anything that provokes an individual's symptoms. Coffee (decaffeinated as well as regular), tea, beer, and wine may increase ulcer problems by stimulating the secretion of stomach acid—distilled liquors do not have this effect but may irritate tender tissue.[186] Chocolate; concentrated sweets; fried, salty, or highly spiced foods; and soft drinks are irritating for some people, innocuous for others.

Supplements (see note on page xii)

A daily multivitamin-mineral is usually recommended for ulcer patients. Additional supplements should be taken only with the consent of the attending physician.

Vitamin A In the form of beta carotene, 25,000 to 50,000 IU daily for a month to accelerate healing, then 10,000 to 25,000 IU a day to protect the mucous membranes of the gastrointestinal tract.

B Complex One comprehensive tablet daily plus extra B_2, B_6, and 50 to 100 milligrams of pantothenic acid three times a day to speed ulcer healing.[98]

Vitamin C with Bioflavonoids 100 to 2,000 milligrams of this combination in divided daily doses. Vitamin C promotes healing; bioflavonoids strengthen newly formed tissue covering the ulcer. If not taken with meals or in a buffered form, ⅛ teaspoon of baking soda may be stirred into the accompanying water to neutralize vitamin C's acidity.

Vitamin E 400 to 800 IU daily to reduce stomach acid and pain, hasten healing, and to preclude the formation of scar tissue.

L-glutamine 500 milligrams once daily on an empty stomach. Naturopathic physicians consider this amino acid important in the healing of peptic ulcers.

Tissue Salts At the onset of an ulcer attack, take one *each* Kali. Phos. and Nat. Phos in the 3X or 6X potency. Repeat each 30 minutes for several hours or until relieved.[64]

Zinc 50 milligrams taken once daily with food. Controlled studies show that zinc triples the healing rate of ulcers without creating any side effects, and in many cases, it effects a complete cure.[151]

Folk Remedies

One or 2 tablespoons of aloe vera juice or three capsules of bee propolis with meals, or portions of an egg white beaten with 2 tablespoons of olive oil and taken several times a day are said to bring relief and hasten ulcer healing.

Cabbage Juice As documented in the September 1950 *Journal of the American Dietetic Association,* drinking two to five glasses of fresh cabbage juice a day is credited with curing ulcers in less than a month. Celery juice (from stalks and leaves) is believed to contain a similar antiulcer substance and may be substituted for one-fourth of the cabbage juice.

Herbs Alfalfa (available in tablets, meal, or dried leaves for tea) contains vitamin K as well as other healing agents. Taking a capsule of cayenne pepper with each meal is believed to encourage ulcer healing.[312] Licorice root has been used as an ulcer treatment in China for at least 3,000 years. Other recommended herbs are camomile, catnip, comfrey, marshmallow and slippery elm.

Plantains Famed as an ulcer treatment in India, recent research indicates that large, unripe plantains (not common bananas) contain an antiulcer factor that strengthens the stomach lining and triggers the release of a protective film to seal the surface and prevent further damage by digestive acids. Green plantains may be boiled, baked, or fried and eaten like potatoes, or utilized as a concentrated powder.[56]

Nerve Pressure and Massage

○ Press or massage above the nose where the eyebrows would meet.

○ Press down on the back of the tongue with a popsicle stick.

○ Massage the pad at the base of each thumb, the webs between thumbs and index fingers, and the area below each middle finger, then massage the front or back of the wrists, whichever is tender.

○ Press four points in a square around the outer edge of the navel.

○ Massage the ball of each foot.

Stress Management and Guided Imagery

Varying with each individual's response to the situation, emotional stress can damage the body's defense of the stomach lining, increase the production of gastric acids, and instigate or aggravate a peptic ulcer. Practicing the relaxation techniques described in the Introduction may prevent or alleviate stomach-churning tension.[201] Excellent results have been reported from this 3-week series of three-times-a-day, 3-minute sessions of guided imagery: Following a few deep breaths with eyes closed, visualize healthy tissue growing over the open sore—or imagine a minuscule fairy godmother waving a healing wand. If necessary, repeat the series after a week's respite.[186]

Sources (see Bibliography)

6, 15, 17, 26, 28, 42, 45, 46, 50, 51, 56, 58, 59, 60, 64, 75, 98, 101, 109, 135, 147, 150, 151, 164, 171, 176, 186, 190, 201, 204, 207, 209, 244, 250, 254, 256, 293, 294, 304, 312, 313, 316, 317

Varicose Veins

Varicosities are not a side effect of modern lifestyles—bulging blue leg veins are described in a 3,400-year-old Egyptian papyrus. Their underlying cause is a genetic predisposition toward a malfunction in the body's circulatory system. Blood is pumped from the heart, with gravity's help, through the arteries to the legs, where it is collected by the veins. Then the blood is returned to the heart, against the pull of gravity, by leg-muscle contractions with the assistance of one-way venous valves. Either leaky valves or weak vein walls can lead to swollen, distorted surface veins. Deeper veins within the leg are rarely affected because they are supported by muscle and fat. Although experts estimate that heredity makes half the population susceptible to varicose veins, one or more aggravating factors must be present before the problem develops.[18, 177]

Hormonal fluctuations during pregnancy and menopause may be responsible for the high proportion of varicosities among women. Dietary deficiencies or the loss of skin elasticity due to aging are contributory factors. Prolonged standing or sitting, constipation, constrictive clothing, lack of exercise, obesity, or repeated heavy lifting can interfere with normal circulation to increase the likelihood that varicose veins will develop—and can worsen existing varicosities. In chronic cases, the distended veins may be accompanied by aching pain or itching, and if the stretched skin breaks down, open sores may form. Home remedies may be able to prevent, delay, alleviate, or even reverse varicose veins, but a doctor should be consulted if they are painful, appear to contain blood clots, or if they rupture and bleed.

Clothing

Tight garments can restrict venous blood flow to leave blood pooled in the legs. Particularly harmful are girdles or pantyhose too snug in the groin area, garters, calf-hugging boots, or waist-cinching belts. Support hose, however, exert graduated pressure on the legs to facilitate blood flow, delay the onset of varicosities for people prone to them, and provide relief from the discomfort of bulging veins. In severe cases, specially fitted knee-high elastic stockings may be prescribed.

Diet and Supplements (see note on page xii)

A diet low in fats and refined carbohydrates and high in fiber-rich fruits, vegetables, and whole grains promotes bowel regularity to avoid the constipation that can contribute to the development or worsening of varicose veins. One or two glasses daily of fresh fruit or vegetable juices—especially any combination of apple, beet, carrot, celery, citrus, parsley, or pineapple—and dietary supplements may be helpful in preventing and treating varicosities.

Vitamin A In the form of beta carotene, 25,000 IU for skin integrity and to speed varicose ulcer healing.

B Complex One comprehensive tablet plus a tablespoon of brewer's yeast daily to help maintain strong blood vessels.

Vitamin C and Bioflavonoids 1,000 to 5,000 milligrams of vitamin C and 100 to 1,000 milligrams of bioflavonoids in divided daily doses to aid circulation, promote the healing of sores, and strengthen vein walls to prevent dilation.

Vitamin E 300 to 800 IU in gradually increased dosages to improve circulation, reduce susceptibility to varicose veins, relieve pain, and, sometimes, correct varicosities. Topical applications of vitamin E squeezed from capsules often relieves localized irritation and speeds the healing of varicose ulcers.[17, 98]

Lecithin One tablespoon of granules daily (or two capsules with each meal) to emulsify fats and aid circulation.

Tissue Salts Two tablets of 6X Calc. Fluor. each morning and evening to improve the elasticity of blood vessel walls.

Zinc 50 milligrams daily to assist with healing and collagen formation and to help maintain the proper concentration of vitamin E in the blood.

Exercise and Leg Elevation

Any program of regular exercise stimulates circulation, improves muscle tone, and helps prevent varicosities. According to a report in *Berkeley Wellness Letter* (June 1992), however, high-impact aerobics, jogging, strenuous cycling, or any intense activity may increase blood pressure in the legs and accentuate varicose veins. Walking and swimming are considered excellent therapy, as are gentle leg-muscle stretches and utilizing a rocking chair while watching television.

Lying flat on the floor and resting the legs on a chair seat or straight up against a wall for 2 minutes immediately after donning support hose drains blood from swollen veins. Elevating the feet higher than the hips with a recliner or ottoman, and raising the foot of the bed a few inches, helps blood flow back to the heart from the legs. Muscular movement at frequent intervals is more beneficial than occasional, strenuous exercise sessions. When remaining stationary is essential, unobtrusive muscular movements help prevent blood pooling. If confined to a seat behind a computer, in a theater, or on an airplane, press down on the balls of the feet, rotate the ankles, and wiggle the toes. If standing in one spot, shift body weight from foot to foot; rock back and forth from heel to toe; and if possible, elevate one foot on a block, bar rail, or cabinet shelf under the kitchen sink.

Mark N.'s visibly distended leg veins presented no problems until he retired from his job as a building inspector and devoted full time to his hobby of constructing ornate wooden clocks and lamps. Accustomed to walking around all day, Mark was surprised when the varicosities began to throb and his feet and legs ached after a few hours of standing in front of his workbench. A rubber floor mat and shoes with cushioned insoles helped a little, but he eventually resolved the problem by taking a brisk 2-minute walk every hour, and several times a day, taking 20-minute "reclining breaks" with his feet propped up higher than his head.

Folk Remedies

Alternating 2-minute icy cold and very hot (preferably with 2 tablespoons of epsom salts per quart of water) compresses or leg baths for 10 minutes a day stimulates circulation to relieve and heal varicosities. Treatments said to bring noticeable improvement within a month are 30-minute applications twice a day of cloths saturated with apple cider vinegar accompanied by a drink of 2 teaspoons of the vinegar in a glass of water; or overnight bandaging of the legs over a coating of salve prepared by stirring 2 cups of chopped calendula flowers, leaves, and stems into an equal amount of melted lard, letting the mixture stand for 24 hours, then reheating and straining.[150, 172, 313] Steeping crushed, fresh violet leaves and flowers or marigold flowers in boiling water, and applying compresses of the liquid—plus eating a few fresh marigold petals every day—is believed to shrink varicosities and nourish the veins.

Herbal teas (one cup or two capsules daily) recommended for preventing or relieving varicose veins include butcher's broom, ginkgo biloba, horse chestnut, oatstraw, parsley, shave grass, yellow dock, and white oak bark. External applications of camomile, comfrey, oatstraw, white oak bark, or witch hazel are believed especially beneficial. Aloe vera gel can be used to soothe itchy or irritated varicosities. To speed the healing of varicose sores, folk practitioners suggest overnight poultices of bruised cabbage leaves, rotten apples, chopped brown onions, or a half-and-half blend of cod liver oil and raw honey.

Nerve Pressure and Massage

○ On the palm of the left hand, press and massage 1 inch down from the web between the last two fingers; then a 2-inch area on the back of each hand, from the wrist to the center and outer edge.

○ Press and massage the hinge of the jawbone just in front of each ear.

○ Massage the pad under the little toe on the right foot; then the sole of each foot from just above the heel pad to the center of the arch.

Sources (see Bibliography)

6, 17, 18, 26, 49, 51, 57, 60, 65, 75, 92, 98, 109, 111, 135, 150, 151, 164, 172, 176, 177, 186, 218, 233, 244, 252, 254, 255, 256, 281, 293, 300, 312, 313

Wrinkles

Living leaves facial mementos of expression lines and crinkly wrinkles. Men, because of their thicker skins and more productive oil glands, and dark-skinned people, with sun-protection provided by pigmentation cells, tend to wrinkle about 10 years later than fair females. With increasing age, cell renewal slows, supportive tissues (collagen and elastin) deteriorate, and less internal moisture reaches the surface. The skin becomes drier, thinner, less resilient, and wrinkle prone. Inadequate nourishment, inappropriate skin care, and environmental factors can accelerate this normally gradual process.

Many dermatologists believe that sunlight is primarily responsible for premature facial aging. Ultraviolet rays from the sun or tanning lamps cause photoaging by destroying the fortifying fibers that make skin spring back after being stretched into a smile or folded into a frown. Using sunscreen daily prevents additional damage and allows the skin to at least partially repair itself. Applying moisturizers (see "Dry Skin") helps preserve diminishing internal supplies and plumps up the epidermis so that fine lines seem to disappear.

Expression lines and creases—horizontal forehead furrows, vertical scowl lines, mirthful or squinty eye wrinkles, nose-to-chin arcs, pursed-lip sunburst grooves—result from years of habitual movements that are subject to personal control.

○ Keep a mirror by the telephone to provide clues to unconscious facial habits, an opportunity to practice relaxing tensed muscles, and a chance to rehearse the semblance of a smile as a permanent feature—slightly upturned lip corners make faces appear years younger than they are. When alone, flattening scowl lines with a strip of cellophane tape serves as a crinkling, crease-reducing reminder.

○ Wear sunglasses whenever outdoors and corrective lenses if needed to relieve eyestrain prevent squinting and crow's feet.

○ Avoid sleep-spawned wrinkles by not pushing the face into a pillow and by using satin pillowcases that do not cling to skin or absorb as much facial moisture as those made of cotton.

Diet and Supplements (see note on page xii)

Good nutrition is vital to wrinkle control. Skin cells perish and are replaced more rapidly than most body cells, so a constant supply of nutrients is essential for a smooth epidermis. Quick-loss reducing diets often deprive the skin of essential nourishment and cause it to lose elasticity. Yo-yo dieting fosters wrinkling by shrinking and stretching the skin to cover repeatedly lost and gained pounds. When losing weight, 2 pounds per week is considered a sensible limit. A daily multivitamin-mineral plus optional supplements help maintain skin integrity and prevent or slow the loss of elasticity.[206]

Vitamin A—In the form of beta carotene, 25,000 IU daily to delay wrinkles by helping preserve the supportive tissues as well as the surface.

B Complex One comprehensive tablet daily to benefit both collagen and elastin by helping counteract the detrimental effects of stress.

Vitamin C with Bioflavonoids 1,000 to 3,000 milligrams in divided daily doses to preserve collagen and increase its production. Smoking not only decreases nourishing blood flow to the skin but also burns up from 500 to 5,000 milligrams of vitamin C per pack of cigarettes.[273] Other vitamin C destroyers that call for additional supplementation are alcohol, antibiotics, barbiturates, and over-the-counter pain relievers.[189]

Vitamin E 200 to 400 IU daily to maintain cell membranes and help protect the skin from environmental substances that promote premature wrinkling.[276]

Minerals Especially magnesium, manganese, selenium, and zinc—are important in cell building and in the production of collagen.[40, 206]

Tissue Salts Three 3X tablets daily of Calc. Phos. to help restore tone to weakened tissues, and of Kali. Sulph. to promote the tissue assimilation of oxygen from the blood stream.[65]

Exercise

Studies show that a program of regular aerobic exercise (walking, swimming, cycling) helps retard wrinkling by improving blood circulation to supply more nutrients to the skin and encouraging the production of supportive elastic fibers.[108, 294]

Facial Massage

The value of facial exercise is debatable. Muscles of the face attach to skin rather than bone as they do in the rest of the body, and deliberate exercise may reinforce the existing lines created by repetitive movements.[45] Gentle massage, however, helps stimulate blood flow and relax facial muscles to augment other relaxation techniques (see Introduction) in minimizing stress-induced wrinkling. On a clean face (lightly coated with vegetable oil, if desired) use fingertips or knuckles to massage tiny circles in the following locations:

- Two spots directly above the center of the eyes at the hairline, then straight down in the middle of the forehead.
- The bones under the end of the eyebrows next to the nose, then the bones at the outer edge of the eyes.
- The central depression between nose and upper lip, ½ inch out from the corners of the mouth, and halfway between the lower lip and the center of the tip of the chin.

Home Remedies

An Egyptian papyrus dating from 2900 B.C. tells of a potion that removes all facial lines, but it fails to furnish the formula. Modern-day wrinkle erasers, Retin A (a derivative of vitamin A) and fruit acids (alpha-hydroxy acids from apples, citrus fruits, grapes, sour milk, and sugar cane), are available without prescription. Several months of treatment with Retin A is reported to reduce fine wrinkles but increases sun sensitivity and sometimes causes skin inflammation. Alpha-hydroxy acids, which act as a natural face-peel and also work beneath the surface, may be more effective for deep creases.[151,184]

Cosmetic promoters promise eternally young skin from external applications of products containing collagen and elastin; scientists argue that molecular structure prohibits their absorption. Seventy-year-old Ursula O.

is not interested in the debate. She credits her lack of wrinkles to pampering her always-dry skin with everything possible, and includes plain collagen and elastin (from a health food store) in her face-saving program. Each morning Ursula smooths on elastin gel between cleansing and moisturizing; at night, she uses collagen gel before applying her moisturizer. Mother Nature's larder is amply supplied with other wrinkle regulators.

Brewer's Yeast Besides being an excellent source of B vitamins when ingested, brewer's yeast has been found to increase collagen production and help smooth out wrinkles when mixed with water, wheat germ oil, or yogurt, patted over the lines, and allowed to dry before being rinsed off.[151, 184, 312]

Castor Oil Smooth the oil over the delicate area around the eyes.

Cocoa Butter or Avocado Oil Gently massaged into freshly washed wrinkles every day, these are said to make lines less noticeable within 2 weeks.[151]

Eggs To make fine lines vanish for a few hours, coat them with a film of stirred egg white, or use a pointed paintbrush to fill in tiny wrinkles, then let dry before carefully covering with makeup. A mask of stiffly beaten egg white allowed to harden before being rinsed off also disguises wrinkles. For a skin-rejuvenating mask: whisk an egg yolk with a tablespoon of olive oil, brush or pat over the face, and let dry for 10 minutes before applying the egg-white meringue.

Grapes To tone and tighten skin, seedless white grapes can be cut in half, smoothed around eyes and mouth, and the juice allowed to dry before makeup is applied. For a firming facial, whir a handful of grapes in a blender, pat over the face, and rinse off after 20 minutes. Good champagne, swished on with a cotton ball and allowed to dry, is a French favorite for tightening loose skin beneath the eyes or on the throat.

Honey Soften skin and help smooth away wrinkles with honey. Each morning, splash warm water over face and throat, then cover with honey and wait 5 minutes before washing off. To increase the benefits, mix apple cider vinegar, bee pollen grains, or heavy whipping cream with the honey.

Light Cream and Lemon Juice After dinner, mix 2 tablespoons warm light cream with ½ teaspoon lemon juice, cover, and let stand for 2 or

3 hours. At bedtime, massage into freshly cleansed skin and let dry, then remove with warm water and smooth on a film of olive oil. Use the remainder of the mixture in the morning. When repeated daily, this treatment is reputed to make wrinkles less noticeable within a few weeks.[150, 313]

Mayonnaise Enriched with one egg yolk per ¼ cup and applied several times a day for several months, mayonnaise is reported to remove "prune face" wrinkles.[74]

Vitamin E Squeezed from snipped capsules, vitamin E can penetrate skin and when patted under the eyes and smoothed across sunburst-lined lips every day has resulted in wrinkle reduction within a month.[266, 267]

Sources (see Bibliography)

40, 45, 53, 65, 74, 98, 99, 108, 109, 111, 112, 150, 151, 177, 184, 189, 206, 218, 254, 266, 267, 273, 276, 293, 294, 302, 312, 313

Yeast Infections (Vaginal Candidiasis)

Formerly called vaginal thrush or moniliasis, yeast infections result from an overgrowth of *Candida albicans*, a normally harmless yeastlike fungus that exists in many parts of the body and is held in check by beneficial bacteria, the immune system, and the acidic pH of the vagina. Candidiasis can be precipitated by anything that alters body chemistry: drugs used to treat arthritis, chemotherapy, nutritional deficiencies, oral contraceptives, or pregnancy. Chemical douches, feminine hygiene sprays, spermicides, and alkaline bubble baths or soaps may upset the pH of vaginal walls and allow yeast organisms to flourish in the alkaline environment.[186, 281] Antibiotic treatment often instigates Candida overgrowth because the yeast feeds on the antibiotic as well as on the friendly flora killed along with the harmful bacteria, then rapidly multiplies in the vagina's moist warmth to cause itching, burning, swelling, pain, and the characteristic white discharge.[318]

Medical diagnosis is advised (it is essential if pregnant or lactating) before attempting self-medication. Although over-the-counter, prescription-strength fungicidal products are available, other disorders such as chlamydia, gardnerella vaginalis, or trichomoniasis can mimic a yeast infection but require different treatment.

Recurrent Candidiasis

Three out of four adult females suffer at least one attack of candidiasis; most of them have recurring episodes.[296] A woman whose infection has been cured can be reinfected by her sexual partner. Gynecologists recommend that intercourse be avoided during a yeast infection, and if the vaginitis recurs, that the male partner also be examined and treated to prevent passing the infection back and forth.[108] Men can harbor *Candida albicans* on their hands and in their mouths without evidencing any symptoms—only rarely is there inflammation or infection of the head of the penis.[75]

Precautionary measures include:

○ Practicing "safe sex" by using a condom and cleansing hands and genitals before and after intercourse. Egg white, mineral oil, and plain yogurt are nonirritating lubricants.

○ Drying thoroughly after the daily bath (with a hair dryer, if desired) but not dusting with powder containing cornstarch, which is believed to encourage yeast growth.

○ Allowing air circulation by wearing cotton-crotch panties or pantyhose and loose, "breathable" clothing, promptly changing out of a wet swimsuit, and sleeping in a nightgown or nothing.

○ Destroying the yeast spores deposited on panties during an infection by boiling, soaking in bleach for 24 hours, or pressing the crotch with a hot iron. Researchers have found that Candida survives normal laundering and can reinfect the wearer.[293]

○ Alternating cotton tampons with sanitary napkins to permit natural vaginal flushing.

○ Using unscented personal products and plain white toilet tissue to avoid possible irritation from chemicals, and wiping from front to back after defecation to prevent intestinal microorganisms from migrating to the vagina.

Diet

Acidophilus yogurt can be both a preventive and a remedy for yeast infections. Eating yogurt or taking acidophilus supplements with each meal during and for 2 weeks after treatment with antibiotic or steroid drugs helps halt Candida overgrowth and replenish friendly flora. Clinical studies noted in the March 1992 issues of *Annals of Internal Medicine* and *Science News* show that a cup of yogurt daily can clear some cases of chronic candidiasis and reduce the frequency of recurrence by two-thirds for others. The remedial ingredient is the *Lactobacillus acidophilus* bacteria contained in yogurt made at home from live cultures or acidophilus milk, or in commercial brands labeled "acidophilus." Research reported in *Health*

World (May/June 1991) indicates that nondairy yogurt is the most effective for relieving vaginal candidiasis.

Candida thrives on sugar. Studies show that high sugar intake from the lactose (milk sugar) in dairy products and artificial sweeteners as well as from table sugar, fruit sugar, and other sweets can precipitate or aggravate yeast infections. Diabetics are at especially high risk because of fluctuating blood sugar levels.[186, 192, 293] Besides providing sugar (fructose), citrus fruits, pineapples, and tomatoes are alkaline-forming encouragers of Candida. Eliminating all of them for a month, then limiting consumption to one or two servings each week may bring relief from chronic conditions.[17] Candida overgrowth often creates allergic sensitivity to foods and beverages containing other yeasts, fungi, and molds. Women who have frequently recurring episodes may benefit from avoiding or at least minimizing ingestion of aged cheeses, beer and wine, cured meats, raw mushrooms, sauerkraut and other fermented foods, and yeast-leavened flour products. Although there is no evidence that brewer's yeast increases susceptibility to or exacerbates yeast infections, some experts advise avoiding it and using only yeast-free supplements.[151]

Supplements (see note on page xii)

Studies have noted that many women with recurrent candidiasis are deficient in iron, selenium, and zinc, and that supplementation often corrects the condition.[17, 151, 204] Nutritionists recommend a daily multivitamin-mineral plus optional individual supplements to counteract these and other deficiencies apparent in most patients with chronic yeast problems.

Vitamin A In the form of beta carotene, 25,000 IU daily to stimulate yeast-inhibiting vaginal secretions and reinforce the body's defenses.

B Complex One comprehensive tablet three times daily during an infection; once daily as maintenance to compensate for the malabsorption common in candidiasis. Biotin, in particular, has been found to suppress Candida.[318]

Vitamin C with Bioflavonoids 500 to 5,000 milligrams in divided daily doses to speed healing and forestall future infections by increasing tissue strength and reducing the reaction to allergens.

Vitamin E 100 to 400 IU daily to assist the body's defenses. A pierced vitamin E capsule may be used as a vaginal suppository for more immediate relief.[98]

Tissue Salts Three tablets of 6X Nat. Phos. dissolved under the tongue three times a day may help relieve yeast-infection discomfort.

Folk Remedies

Although some physicians recommend that home remedies be used only to augment yeast-killing drugs, self-treatment, if commenced at the onset, may be able to reverse Candida overgrowth and halt recurrences[16, 204] but should not be attempted without medical approval if pregnant or under doctor's care for other ailments. The four major folk remedies—yogurt, garlic, herbs, and vinegar—are often used in combination.

Acidophilus Yogurt Intravaginal applications enhance the effectiveness of oral acidophilus and help restore pH balance. Blend ¼ cup yogurt with the contents of four acidophilus capsules (¼ to ½ teaspoon ground cinnamon may be included—studies show that it may help thwart Candida).[16] On each of 5 consecutive nights, insert 2 teaspoons of the mixture with a medicine applicator or clean, bulb-type poultry baster. Each morning, douche with a vinegar-and-water solution.[317] As alternatives, use a douche of diluted yogurt or a blend of two acidophilus capsules and a pint of water, or insert a punctured acidophilus capsule at night.[17, 176]

Garlic Recent research has reinforced garlic's reputation as a Candida killer.[318] For a douche, the contents of two garlic capsules can be mixed with a pint of water, or a small clove of garlic can be blended with the water and strained before using. For a vaginal suppository, a peeled garlic clove can be wrapped in sterile gauze and inserted for 12 hours. Capsules of odorless garlic may be taken orally. Estelle V. had battled yeast infections for years, with only temporary victories. The itching and discharge returned a few weeks after each apparent cure. By taking two garlic capsules three times a day along with the next round of fungicidal medication, and by using daily vinegar douches, Estelle won the war. She maintains supremacy by continuing to take garlic capsules with two of her daily meals and by douching only after each menstrual period to assure vaginal acidity.

Herbs Douching with slippery elm tea is an old remedy for irritated vaginal membranes. Chaparral, comfrey, garlic, goldenseal, thyme, or white oak bark tea, or an infusion prepared from witch hazel leaves are suggested douches for yeast infections. These two herbal remedies have proven successful in recent clinical studies, but neither should be used without a physician's approval.

○ Echinacea, when combined with antifungal medication, reduced recurrence by 44 percent and completely cleared many cases of chronic yeast infection.[50] Available in capsules or powder, echinacea is believed especially effective when one to three cups daily of the tea (enhanced, if desired, by the addition of half as much myrrh as echinacea) are augmented with nightly garlic suppositories for 2 weeks.[16, 256] An ointment made from echinacea and vitamin E has resolved some cases of recurrent candidiasis.[111, 296]

○ Pau d'arco (also known as ipe roxo, lapacho, and taheebo) has produced dramatic results in some cases but had no effect in others. The tea can be used as a douche twice daily, or one to six cups may be sipped each day for 2 weeks, with part of the brew used as a douche if desired. Drinking a cup of clove tea instead of the pau d'arco every other day may be beneficial.[17, 192, 256, 312]

Vinegar When begun at the first sign of itching and discharge, vinegar douches plus other home remedies are credited with clearing yeast infections. Vinegar has approximately the same Ph as a healthy vagina. Douching with four teaspoons vinegar in 2 cups of water (or sitting for 15 minutes in a tub of hip-deep water with 1 cup of vinegar) helps restore normal acid/alkaline balance and speed healing. A suggested combination treatment to follow the vinegar douche or sitz bath each morning and evening for 3 days calls for drying the genital area, wiping with pure olive oil, then inserting a tampon coated with acidophilus yogurt.[201]

Sources (see Bibliography)

2, 16, 17, 50, 65, 75, 87, 98, 108, 109, 111, 150, 151, 176, 186, 190, 192, 201, 202, 204, 254, 255, 256, 281, 293, 294, 296, 312, 317, 318

Bibliography

1. Abrahamson, E.M., and A.W. Pezet. *Body, Mind and Sugar*. New York: Pyramid, 1971.

2. Adams, Rex. *Miracle Medicine Foods*. West Nyack, NY: Parker, 1977.

3. Adams, Ruth, and Frank Murray. *Complete Home Guide to Vitamins*. New York: Larchmont, 1978.

4. ———. *Is Low Blood Sugar Making You a Nutritional Cripple?* New York: Larchmont, 1975.

5. Airola, Paavo. *Health Secrets from Europe*. West Nyack, NY: Parker, 1970.

6. ———. *How to Get Well*. Phoenix, AZ: Health Plus, 1974.

7. ———. *Stop Hair Loss*. Phoenix, AZ: Health Plus, 1965.

8. Albright, Peter, and Elizabeth Albright. *Body, Mind and Spirit*. Lexington, MA: Stephen Greene, 1980.

9. Alexander, Dale. *Arthritis and Common Sense*. New York: Simon & Schuster, 1954.

10. Allen, Oliver E., and eds. of Time-Life Books. *Secrets of Good Digestion*. Alexandria, VA: Time-Life Books, 1982.

11. Anderson, James W. *Diabetes: A Practical New Guide to Healthy Living*. New York: Arco, 1981.

12. Andron, Michael. *Reflex Balance: A Foot and Hand Book for Health*. New York, 1980.

13. Ashmead, DeWayne, ed. *Chelated Mineral Nutrition in Plants, Animals and Man*. Springfield, IL: Charles C. Thomas, 1982.

14. Atkins, Robert C. *Dr. Atkins' Nutrition Breakthrough*. New York: Perigord, 1981.

15. Bailey, Herbert. *Vitamin E, Your Key to a Healthy Heart*. New York: ARC Books, 1971.

16. Bakule, Paula Dreifus, ed. *Rodale's Book of Practical Formulas*. Emmaus, PA: Rodale, 1991.

17. Balch, James F., and Phyllis A. Balch. *Prescription for Nutritional Healing*. Garden City Park, NY: Avery, 1990.

18. Baron, Howard C., with Edward Gorin. *Varicose Veins*. New York: William Morrow, 1979.

19. Bauer, Cathryn. *Acupressure for Everybody*. New York: Henry Holt, 1991

20. Beeton, Isabella. *Book of Household Management*. London: S.O. Beeton, 1861.

21. Benham, Jack, and Sarah Benham. *Rocky Mountains Receipts and Remedies*. Reporter Printing, 1966. Revised edition. Bear Creek Pub. Ouray, CO.

22. Bennet, Hal Zina. *Cold Comfort*. New York: Clarkson N. Potter, 1979.

23. ———. *The Doctor Within*. New York: Clarkson N. Potter, 1981.

24. Benson, Herbert, with Miriam Z. Klipper. *The Relaxation Response*. New York: William Morrow, 1975.

25. Benson, Herbert, Eileen Stuart, and Associates of Mind/Body Medical Institute. *The Wellness Book*. New York: Birch Lane Press, 1991

26. Bergson, Anika, and Vladimir Tuchak. *Zone Therapy*. Los Angeles: Pinnacle Books, 1974.

27. Berkley, George. *Arthritis Without Aspirin*. Englewood Cliffs, NJ: Prentice Hall, 1982.

28. Beverly, Cal, ed. *New Natural Healing Encyclopedia*. Peachtree City, GA: FC&A, 1990.

29. Beverly, Cal, and June Gunden, eds. *New Health Tips Encyclopedia*. Peachtree City, GA: FC&A, 1989.

30. Bieler, Henry G. *Food Is Your Best Medicine*. New York: Random House, 1965.

31. Biermann, June, and Barbara Toohey. *The Diabetic's Book*. Boston: Houghton Mifflin, 1981.

32. Birnes, Nancy. *Cheaper and Better*. New York: Harper & Row, 1987.

33. Blaine, Tom R. *Goodby Allergies*. Secaucus, NJ: Citadel, 1968.

34. Bland, Jeffery. *Your Health Under Siege*. Lexington, MA: Stephen Greene, 1981.

35. Blauer, Stephen. *Rejuvenation*. West Palm Beach, FL: Hippocrates Health Institute, 1980.

36. Blaurock-Busch, Eleanor, with Bernd W. Busch. *The No-Drugs Guide to Better Health*. West Nyack, NY: Parker, 1984.

37. Boericke, William, and Willis Dewey. *The Twelve Tissue Remedies of Schuessler.* Harjeet.

38. Brady, William. *An Eighty-Year-Old Doctor's Secrets of Positive Health.* Englewood Cliffs, NJ: Prentice Hall, 1961.

39. Brennan, R.O., with William C. Mulligan. *Nutrigenics: New Concepts for Relieving Hypoglycemia.* New York: Signet, 1977.

40. Brenton, Myron. *Aging Slowly.* Emmaus, PA: Rodale, 1983.

41. Bricklin, Mark. *The Practical Encyclopedia of Natural Healing.* Emmaus, PA: Rodale, 1976.

42. ———. *Rodale's Encyclopedia of Natural Home Remedies.* Emmaus, PA: Rodale, 1982.

43. Bricklin, Mark, ed. *The Natural Healing Annual, 1986.* Emmaus, PA: Rodale, 1986.

44. ———. *The Natural Healing Annual, 1987.* Emmaus, PA: Rodale, 1987.

45. ———. *The Natural Healing and Nutrition Annual, 1988.* Emmaus, PA: Rodale, 1988.

46. Bricklin, Mark, and Sharon Stocker Ferguson, eds. *The Natural Healing and Nutrition Annual, 1989.* Emmaus, PA: Rodale, 1989.

47. ———. *The Natural Healing and Nutrition Annual, 1990.* Emmaus, PA: Rodale, 1990.

48. Bricklin, Mark, Mark Golin, Deborah Grandinetti, and Alexis Lieberman. *Positive Living and Health.* Emmaus, PA: Rodale, 1990.

49. Bricklin, Mark, and Matthew Hoffman, eds. *The Natural Healing and Nutrition Annual, 1993.* Emmaus, PA: Rodale, 1993.

50. Bricklin, Mark, and Heidi Rodale, eds. *The Natural Healing and Nutrition Annual, 1991.* Emmaus, PA: Rodale, 1991.

51. Bricklin, Mark, and Sharon Stocker, eds. *The Natural Healing and Nutrition Annual, 1992.* Emmaus, PA: Rodale, 1992.

52. Brody, Jane. *Jane Brody's Nutrition Book.* New York: Bantam, 1982.

53. Cameron, Myra. *Mother Nature's Guide to Vibrant Beauty and Health.* Englewood Cliffs, NJ: Prentice Hall, 1990.

54. Carey, G.W. *The Biochemic System of Medicine.* Biochemic Publications.

55. ———. *The Twelve Cell Salts of the Zodiac.* Health Research.

56. Carper, Jean. *The Food Pharmacy.* New York: Bantam, 1988.

57. Carroll, David. *The Complete Book of Natural Medicines.* New York: Summit, 1980.

58. Carter, Mildred. *Body Reflexology*. West Nyack: Parker, 1983.

59. ———. *Hand Reflexology: Key to Perfect Health*. West Nyack: Parker, 1975.

60. ———. *Helping Yourself with Foot Reflexology*. West Nyack: Parker, 1969.

61. Castleton, Michael. *The Healing Herbs*. Emmaus, PA: Rodale, 1992.

62. Challem, Jack Joseph. *Vitamin C Updated*. New Canaan, CT: Keats, 1982.

63. Chan, Pedro. *Finger Acupressure*. New York: Ballantine, 1974.

64. Chapman, Esther. *How to Use the Twelve Tissue Salts*. New York: Pyramid, 1971.

65. Chapman, J.B., and Edward L. Perry. *The Biochemic Handbook*. St. Louis, MO: Formur, Inc., 1976.

66. Chase, A.W. *Dr. Chase's Recipes or Information for Everybody*. Ann Arbor, MI: Published by the author. 1866.

67. Cheraskin, E., W.M. Ringsdorf, and Arline Brecher. *Psychodietics*. New York: Stein & Day, 1974.

68. Cheraskin, E., W.M. Ringsdorf, and Emily L. Sisley. *The Vitamin C Connection*. New York: Harper & Row, 1983.

69. Child, Mrs. Lydia Marie. *The American Frugal Housewife*. 20th ed. Boston: American Stationers' Co., 1836. Facsimile edition. New York: Harper & Row, 1972.

70. Cilentro, Lady. *You Don't Have to Live with Chronic Ill Health*. Australia: Whitcombe & Tombs, 1977.

71. Clark, Linda. *Get Well Naturally*. New York: Arco, 1968.

72. ———. *Handbook of Natural Remedies for Common Ailments*. Old Greenwich, CT: Devin-Adir, 1976.

73. ———. *How to Improve Your Health*. New Canaan, CT: Keats, 1977.

74. ———. *Secrets of Health & Beauty*. New York: Pyramid, 1974.

75. Clayman, Charles B., ed. *The AMA Home Medical Encyclopedia*. New York: Random House, 1989.

76. ———. *The AMA Home Medical Library, Know Your Drugs and Medications*. Pleasantville, NY: Reader's Digest Association, 1991.

77. ———. *The AMA Home Medical Library, Monitoring Your Health*, Reader's Digest, 1991

78. ———. *The AMA Home Medical Library: Your Heart*. Pleasantville, NY: Reader's Digest, 1989.

79. Cleave, T.L. *The Saccharine Disease.* New Canaan, CT: Keats, 1978.

80. Coleman, Lester D. *All Your Medical Questions Answered.* New York: Good Housekeeping Books. 1977.

81. Collins, R. Douglas. *What Every Patient Should Know About His Health and His Doctor.* Smithtown, NY: Exposition Press, 1973.

82. Cooley, Donald G. *After-Forty Health and Medical Guide.* New York: Meredith. 1980.

83. Coon, Nelson. *Using Plants for Healing.* rev. ed. Emmaus, PA: Rodale. 1979.

84. Crane, Eva. *A Book of Honey.* New York: Charles Scribner's Sons, 1980.

85. Cross, Jean. *In Grandmother's Day.* Englewood Cliffs, NJ: Prentice-Hall, 1980.

86. Davis, Adelle. *Let's Eat Right to Keep Fit.* New York: Signet, 1970.

87. ———. *Let's Get Well.* New York: Signet, 1972.

88. ———. *Let's Stay Healthy.* New York: Harcourt Brace Jovanovich, 1981.

89. ———. *You Can Get Well.* New York: Benedict Lust, 1975.

90. Davis, Francyne. *The Low Blood Sugar Cookbook.* New York: Grosset & Dunlap, 1973.

91. Dawson, Adele. *Health, Happiness and the Pursuit of Herbs.* Lexington, MA: Stephen Greene, 1980.

92. Dick, William B. *Dick's Encyclopedia of Practical Receipts and Processes; or, How They Did It in the 1870's.* New York: Funk & Wagnalls.

93. Di Cyan, Erwin. *Vitamins in Your Life.* New York: Simon & Schuster, 1972.

94. Dolinar, Richard O., and Betty Page Brackenridge. *Diabetes 101.* Wayzota, MN: DCI, 1989.

95. Dong, Collin H., and Jane Banks. *New Hope for the Arthritic.* New York: Thomas Y. Crowell, 1975.

96. Donsbach, Kurt W. *Menopause.* Huntington Beach, CA: International Institute of Natural Health Sciences, 1977.

97. Dufty, William. *Sugar Blues.* New York: Warner Books, 1976.

98. Dunne, Lavon J. *Nutrition Almanac.* 3rd ed. New York: McGraw-Hill, 1990.

99. Dychtwald, Ken, and Joe Flower. *Age Wave.* Los Angeles: Jeremy P. Tarcher, 1988.

100. Ehret, Charles F., and Lynn Waller Scanlon. *Overcoming Jet Lag.* New York: Berkley Books, 1983.

101. Ehrlich, David with George Wolf. *The Bowel Book*. New York: Schocken Books, 1981.

102. Ehrmantraut, Harry C. *Headaches: The Drugless Way to Lasting Relief*. New York: Autumn Press, 1977.

103. Eichenlaub, John E. *A Minnesota Doctor's Home Remedies for Common and Uncommon Ailments*. Englewood Cliffs, NJ: Prentice-Hall, 1980.

104. Emery, Carla. *Old-Fashioned Recipe Book*. New York: Bantam, 1977.

105. Evans, William, and Irwin H. Rosenberg, with Jacqueline Thompson. *Biomarkers*. New York: Simon & Schuster, 1991.

106. Faelton, Sharon, and Prevention Magazine, eds. *The Complete Book of Minerals for Health*. Emmaus, PA: Rodale, 1981.

107. ———. *Vitamins for Better Health*. Emmaus, PA: Rodale, 1982.

108. Failes, Janice McCall, and Frank W. Cawood. *Encyclopedia of Natural Health Secrets and Cures*. Peachtree City, GA: FC&A, 1988.

109. ———. *Natural Healing Encyclopedia*. Peachtree City, GA: FC&A, 1987.

110. Farb, Stanley M. *The Ear, Nose, and Throat Book: A Doctor's Guide to Better Health*. New York: Appleton-Century Crofts, 1980.

111. Feinstein, Alice, ed. *The Visual Encyclopedia of Natural Healing*. Emmaus, PA: Rodale, 1991.

112. Feltman, John, ed. *Giant Book of Health Facts*. Emmaus, PA: Rodale, 1991.

113. ———. *The Prevention How-To Dictionary of Healing Remedies and Techniques*. Emmaus, PA: Rodale, 1992.

114. Finley, K. Thomas. *Mental Dynamics*. Englewood Cliffs, NJ: Prentice Hall, 1991.

115. Finneson, Bernard E., and Arthur S. Freese. *Dr. Finneson on Low Back Pain*. New York: Putnam's Sons, 1975.

116. Fisher, M.F.K. *A Cordiall Water*. San Fransisco: North Point Press, 1981.

117. Flaxman, Ruth. *Home Remedies for Common Ailments*. New York: Putnam's Sons, 1982.

118. Ford, Norman D. *Eighteen Natural Ways to Beat the Common Cold*. New Canaan, CT: Keats, 1987.

119. Fredericks, Carlton. *Arthritis: Don't Learn to Live with It*. New York: Grosset & Dunlap, 1981.

120. ———. *Eat Well, Get Well, Stay Well.* New York: Grosset & Dunlap, 1980.

121. ———. *Look Younger, Feel Healthier.* New York: Simon & Schuster, 1982.

122. Fredericks, Carlton, and Herbert Bailey. *Food Facts and Fallacies.* New York: Arco, 1965.

123. Fredericks, Carlton, and Herman Goodman. *Low Blood Sugar and You.* New York: Constellation International, 1969.

124. Friedlaender, Mitchell H., and Stef Donev. *20/20: A Total Guide to Improving Your Vision and Preventing Eye Disease.* Emmaus, PA: Rodale, 1991.

125. Gach, Michael Reed. *Acupressure's Potent Points: A Guide to Self-care for Common Ailments.* New York: Bantam, 1990.

126. Galton, Lawrence. *The Disguised Disease: Anemia.* New York: Crown, 1975.

127. ———. *The Silent Disease: Hypertension.* New York: Crown, 1973.

128. Garten, M.O. *The Health Secrets of a Naturopathic Doctor.* West Nyack, NY: Parker, 1967.

129. Gaylean, Dorothy. *Grandma's Remedies.* Springdale, UT: Press Publishing, 1987.

130. Gebhardt, Susan F., and Ruth H. Matthews. *Nutritive Value of Foods (Bulletin #72).* Washington D.C.. U.S. Dept. of Agriculture, 1981

131. Gibbons, Euell. *Feast on a Diabetic Diet.* New York: McKay, 1969.

132. Gillespie, Larrian. *You Don't Have to Live with Cystitis.* New York: Rawson, 1986.

133. Gilmore, C.P., and Time–Life, eds. *Exercising for Fitness.* Alexandria, VA: Time–Life Books, 1981.

134. Goldberg, Phillip, and Daniel Kaufman. *Natural Sleep: How to Get Your Share.* Emmaus, PA: Rodale, 1978.

135. Goodenough, Josephus. *Dr. Goodenough's Home Cures and Herbal Remedies of 1904.* rev. ed. New York: Crown, 1982.

136. Green, Bernard, and Ted Schwarz. *Goodbye Blues.* New York: McGraw-Hill, 1981.

137. Grossbart, Ted, and Carl Sherman. *Skin Deep: A Mind/Body Program for Healthy Skin.* New York: William Morrow, 1985.

138. Haggard, Howard D. *Devils, Drugs and Doctors.* New York: Harper & Brothers, 1929.

139. Hales, Dianne. *The Complete Book of Sleep.* Reading, MA: Addison-Wesley, 1981.

140. Hall, Dorothy. *The Herb Tea Book.* New Canaan, CT: Keats, 1980.

141. Hamilton, Richard. *The Herpes Book*. New York: St. Martin's Press, 1980.

142. *Handbook for Home Growing and History of the Ornamental and Exotic Aloe Vera Plant*. Nurserymen's Exchange, 1977.

143. Harris, Ben Charles. *The Compleat Herbal*. New York: Larchmont, 1972.

144. ———. *Kitchen Medicines*. New York: Weathervane Books, 1968.

145. Hauri, Peter, and Shirley Linde. *No More Sleepless Nights: The Complete Program for Ending Insomnia*. New York: John Wiley, 1990.

146. Hauser, Gayelord. *Gayelord Hauser's Treasury of Secrets*. New York: Farrar-Straus, 1963.

147. Hausman, Patricia, and Judith Benn Hurley. *The Healing Foods*. New York: Dell, 1989.

148. Heimlich, Henry J. with Lawrence Galton. *Home Guide to Emergency Situations*. New York: Simon & Schuster, 1980.

149. Heinerman, John. *First Aid with Herbs*. New Canaan, CT: Keats, 1983.

150. ———. *Heinerman's Encyclopedia of Fruits, Vegetables and Herbs*. West Nyack, NY: Parker, 1988.

151. Hendler, Sheldon Saul. *The Doctors' Vitamin and Mineral Encyclopedia*. New York: Simon & Schuster, 1990.

152. Herter, George Leonard, and Berthe E. Herter. *Bull Cook and Authentic Historical Recipes and Practices, vol. 2*. Waseca, MN: Herter's, 1973.

153. ———. *Bull Cook and Authentic Historical Recipes and Practices, vol. 3*. Waseca, MN: Herter's, 1974.

154. Hess, Mary Abbott, and Anne Elise Hunt. *Pickles and Ice Cream*. New York: McGraw-Hill, 1982.

155. Hewitt, Edward R. *Lecithin and Health*. San Fransisco: Health Publishing, 1977.

156. Hill, Ann, ed. *Visual Encyclopedia of Unconventional Medicine*. New York: Crown, 1979.

157. Hill, Howard E. *Introduction to Lecithin*. New York: Pyramid, 1972.

158. Hills, Hilda Cherry. *Good Food to Fight Migraine*. New Canaan, CT: Keats, 1978.

159. Hirschhorn, Howard H. *Pain-Free Living: How to Prevent and Eliminate Pain All Over the Body*. West Nyack, NY: Parker, 1977.

160. Hochschuler, Stephen. *Back in Shape*. New York: Houghton Mifflin, 1991.

161. Hoehn, Gustave. *Acne Can Be Cured*. New York: Arco, 1977.

162. Hoffer, Abram, and Morton Walker. *Orthomolecular Nutrition: New Lifestyle for Super Good Health*. New Canaan, CT: Keats, 1978.

163. Hoffman, Joyce, and Prevention Magazine eds. *Here's to Your Good Health*. Emmaus, PA: Rodale, 1980.

164. Houston, F.M. *The Healing Benefits of Acupressure*. New Canaan, CT: Keats, 1974.

165. Hupping, Carol, Cheryl Winters Tetreau, and Roger B. Yepson, Jr. *Hints, Tips and Everyday Wisdom*. Emmaus, PA: Rodale, 1985.

166. Hurdle, J. Frank. *A Country Doctor's Common Sense Health Manual*. West Nyack, NY: Parker, 1975.

167. ———. *Low Blood Sugar: A Doctor's Guide to Its Effective Control*. West Nyack, NY: Parker, 1969.

168. Hutchinson, E. *Ladies' Indispensable Assistant*. New York: Published by the Author, 1852.

169. Huxley, Alyson, and Philippa Back. *The Two-in-One Herb Book*. New Canaan, CT: Keats, 1982.

170. Jacobson, E. *Progressive Relaxation*. Chicago: University of Chicago Press, 1938.

171. Jarvis, D.C. *Arthritis and Folk Medicine*. Greenwich, CT: Fawcett, 1960.

172. ———. *Folk Medicine*. New York: Holt, Rinehart & Winston, 1958.

173. Kadans, Joseph M. *Encyclopedia of Fruits, Vegetables, Nuts and Seeds for Healthful Living*. West Nyack, NY: Parker, 1973.

174. Kantrowitz, Fred G. *Taking Control of Arthritis*. New York: Harper-Collins, 1990.

175. Keim, Hugo A. *How to Care for Your Back*. Englewood Cliffs, NJ: Prentice-Hall, 1981.

176. Keith, Velma J., and Monteen Gordon. *The How To Herb Book*. Pleasant Grove, UT: Mayfield, 1991.

177. Keough, Carol, ed. *Future Youth*. Emmaus, PA: Rodale, 1987.

178. Kindler, Herbert K., and Marilyn C. Ginsburn. *Stress Training for Life*. New York: Nichols, 1990.

179. Kloss, Jethro. *Back to Eden*. Santa Barbara, CA: Woodbridge Press, 1975.

180. Kordel, Lelord. *Natural Folk Remedies*. New York: Putnam's Sons, 1974.

181. Kunin, Richard. *Mega-Nutrition*. New York: McGraw-Hill, 1980.

182. Lang, George. *Lang's Compendium of Culinary Nonsense and Trivia*. New York: Crown, 1980.

183. Law, Donald. *A Guide to Alternative Medicine*. New York: Doubleday Dolphin, 1976.

184. Lawson, Donna. *Looking Fit & Fabulous at Forty Plus*. Emmaus, PA: Rodale, 1987.

185. Lee, William. *Bee Pollen: Nature's Energizer*. New Canaan, CT: Keats, 1983.

186. LeGro, William, ed. *High-Speed Healing*. Emmaus, PA: Rodale, 1991.

187. Lehner, Ernst, and Johanna Lehner. *Folklore and Odysseys of Food and Medicinal Plants*. New York: Tudor, 1962.

188. Lenz, Frederick P. *Total Relaxation*. New York: Bobbs-Merrill, 1980.

189. Lesser, Gershon M. *Growing Younger*. Los Angeles: Jeremy P. Tarcher, 1987.

190. Lieberman, Shari, and Nancy Bruning. *The Real Vitamin and Mineral Book*. Garden City Park, NY: Avery, 1990.

191. Light, Marilyn. *Hypoglycemia: One of Man's Most Widespread and Misdiagnosed Diseases*. New Canaan, CT: Keats, 1983.

192. Lorenzani, Shirley S. *Candida: A Twentieth Century Disease*. New Canaan, Ct: Keats, 1986.

193. Lowenfeld, Claire, and Philippa Back. *Herbs, Health and Cookery*. New York: Grammercy, 1965.

194. Lubowe, Irwin I. *A Teenage Guide to Healthy Skin and Hair*. New York: E.P. Dutton, 1979.

195. Lucas, Richard. *The Magic of Herbs in Daily Living*. West Nyack, NY: Parker, 1972.

196. ———. *Nature's Medicines*. West Nyack, NY: Parker, 1966.

197. Maltz, Maxwell. *Psycho-Cybernetics*. Englewood Cliffs, NJ: Prentice-Hall, 1960.

198. Margo. *Growing New Hair*. New York: Autumn Press, 1980.

199. McGuire, Thomas L. *The Tooth Trip*. New York: Random House/Bookworks, 1972.

200. McIlwain, Harris H., Joel C. Silverfield, Michael C. Burnette, and Debra Fulghum Bruce. *Winning with Arthritis*. New York: John Wiley & Sons, 1991.

201. Melville, Arabella, and Colin Johnson. *Health Without Drugs*. New York: Fireside/Simon & Schuster, 1990.

202. Meyer, Clarence. *American Folk Medicine*. New York: New American Library, 1973.

203. ———. *Vegetarian Medicines*. Glenwood, IL: Meyerbooks, 1980.

204. Michaud, Ellen, Alice Feinstein, and Prevention Magazine eds. *Fighting Disease*. Emmaus, PA: Rodale, 1989.

205. Mindell, Earl. *Earl Mindell's Quick and Easy Guide to Better Health*. New Canaan, CT: Keats, 1982.

206. ———. *Earl Mindell's Shaping Up With Vitamins*. New York: Warner Books, 1985.

207. ———. *Earl Mindell's Vitamin Bible*. New York: Warner Books, 1979.

208. Mirsky, Stanley, and Joan Rattner Heilman. *Diabetes: Controlling It the Easy Way*. New York: Random House, 1981.

209. Morales, Betty Lee. *Aloe Vera: The Miracle Plant*. Health in Mind & Body, 1977.

210. Murphy, Joseph. *The Power of Your Subconscious Mind*. New York: Bantam, 1982.

211. Murphy, Wendy. *Coping with the Common Cold*. Alexandria, VA: Time–Life Books, 1981.

212. ———. *Dealing with Headaches*. Alexandria, VA: Time–Life Books, 1982.

213. ———. *Touch, Taste, Smell, Sight and Hearing*. Alexandria, VA: Time–Life Books, 1982

214. Mylander, Maureen. *The Great American Stomach Book*. New York: Ticknor & Fields, 1982.

215. Newbold, H.L. *Mega-Nutrients for Your Nerves*. New York: Berkley, 1978.

216. Norfolk, Donald. *The Habits of Health*. New York: St. Martin's Press, 1976.

217. Notelovitz, Morris. *Stand Tall: The Informed Woman's Guide to Preventing Osteoporosis*. Gainesville, FL: Triad, 1982.

218. Null, Gary and Steve Null. *Complete Handbook of Nutrition*. New York: Dell, 1972.

219. Padus, Emrika. *Woman's Encyclopedia of Health and Natural Healing*. Emmaus, PA: Rodale, 1981.

220. Page, Robin. *Cures and Remedies the Country Way*. New York: Summit Books, 1978.

221. Passwater, Richard A. *Selenium as Food and Medicine*. New Canaan, CT: Keats, 1980.

222. ———. *Super-Nutrition*. New York: Simon & Schuster/Pocket Books, 1975.

223. Pauling, Linus. *Vitamin C, the Common Cold and the Flu*. New York: W.H. Freeman, 1970.

224. Pearson, Durk, and Sandy Shaw. *Life Extension*. New York: Warner Books, 1983.

225. Pelletier, Kenneth R. *Holistic Medicine: From Stress to Optimum Health*. New York: Delecorte/Seymour, 1979.

226. Pelstring, Linda, and Jo Ann Hauck. *Food to Improve Your Health*. New York: Walker, 1974.

227. Pfieffer, Carl C. *Mental and Elemental Nutrients*. New Canaan, CT: Keats, 1975.

228. ———. *Zinc and Other Micro-Nutrients*. New Canaan, CT: Keats, 1978.

229. Pfeiffer, Carl, and Jane Banks. *Total Nutrition*. New York: Simon & Schuster, 1980.

230. Plaut, Martin E. *The Doctor's Guide to You and Your Colon*. New York: Harper & Row, 1982.

231. Prevention Magazine eds. *Lifespan-Plus*. Emmaus, PA: Rodale, 1990.

232. ———. *Natural Pain Relief*. Emmaus, PA: Rodale, 1979.

233. Prevention Magazine staff. *The Complete Book of Vitamins*. Emmaus, PA: Rodale, 1977, 1984.

234. ———. *The Encyclopedia of Common Diseases*. Emmaus, PA: Rodale, 1976.

235. ———. *No More Headaches*. Emmaus, PA: Rodale, 1982.

236. ———. *Rub Your Headache Away*. Emmaus, PA: Rodale, 1979.

237. Pritikin, Nathan, and Patrick McGrady, Jr. *The Pritikin Program*. New York: Grosset & Dunlap, 1978.

238. Rapoport, Alan, and Fred Sheftel. *Headache Relief*. New York: Simon & Schuster, 1990.

239. Rapp, Doris. *Allergies and Your Family*. New York: Sterling, 1981.

240. Reader's Digest. *Eat Better, Live Better*. Pleasantville, NY: Reader's Digest, 1982.

241. Reilly, Harold H., and Ruth Hagy Brod. *The Edgar Cayce Handbook for Health Through Drugless Therapy*. New York: Macmillan, 1975.

242. Reuben, David. *Everything You Always Wanted to Know About Nutrition*. New York: Simon & Schuster, 1978.

243. Revell, Dorothy. *Hypoglycemia Control Cookery*. New York: Berkley, 1973.

244. Rick, Stephanie. *The Reflexology Workout*. New York: Harmony Books, 1986.

245. Riedman, Sarah. *The Good Looks Skin Book*. New York: Julian Messner, 1983.

246. Riker, Tom, and Richard Robert. *Directory of Natural and Health Foods*. New York: Paragon, 1979.

247. Rinzler, Carol Ann. *The Dictionary of Medical Folklore*. New York: Ballantine, 1975.

248. Rodale, J.I., and Prevention Magazine staff. *Complete Book of Minerals for Health*. Emmaus, PA: Rodale, 1972.

249. Rodale Press eds. *The Fiber Revolution*. Emmaus, PA: Rodale, 1990.

250. ———. *Guide to Instant Pain Relief*. Emmaus, PA: Rodale, 1990.

251. ———. *Vitamins, Your Memory and Your Mental Attitude*. Emmaus, PA: Rodale, 1977.

252. Rose, Jeanne. *Herbs and Things*. New York: Grosset & Dunlap, 1972.

253. Rose, Louisa. *The Menopause Book*. New York: Hawthorn/E.P. Dutton, 1977.

254. Rosenfeld, Isadore. *The Best Treatment*. New York: Simon & Schuster, 1991.

255. ———. *Symptoms*. New York: Simon & Schuster, 1989.

256. Royal, Penny C. *Herbally Yours*. Payson, UT: Sound Nutrition, 1982.

257. Schneider, L.L., with Robert B. Stone. *Old-Fashioned Health Remedies That Work Best*. West Nyack: Parker, 1977.

258. Schoen, Linda Allen, ed. *AMA Book of Skin and Hair Care*. Philadelphia, PA: J.B. Lippincott, 1976.

259. Schulman, Brian, and Bruce Smoller. *Pain Control*. New York: Doubleday, 1982.

260. Schultz, William. *Shiatsu*. New York: Bell Publishing, 1976.

261. Schwartz, Alice Kuhn, and Norma S. Aaron. *Somniquest*. New York: Harmony Books, 1979.

262. Scott, Cyril. *Cider Vinegar, Nature's Great Health-Promoter*. rev. ed. England: Athene, 1982.

263. Seegmiller, J.P. *Gout*. Philadelphia, PA: Grune & Stratton, 1967.

264. Sehnert, Keith W., with Howard Eisenberg. *How to Be Your Own Doctor (Sometimes)*. New York: Grosset & Dunlap, 1981.

265. Shaw, Eva. *60-Second Shiatzu*. Bedford, MA: Mills & Sanderson, 1986.

266. Shute, Evan V. *Common Questions on Vitamin E and Their Answers*. New Canaan, CT: Keats, 1979.

267. Shute, Wilfrid E. *Health Preserver*. Emmaus, PA: Rodale, 1977.

268. ———. *Vitamin E Book*. New Canaan, CT: Keats, 1978.

269. Siegel, Bernie S. *Love, Medicine and Miracles*. New York: Harper & Row, 1986.

270. ———. *Peace, Love & Healing*. New York: Harper & Row, 1989.

271. Silva, José, and Robert B. Stone. *You the Healer*. New York: Instant Improvement, 1991.

272. Sobel, Dava, and Arthur C. Klein. *Arthritis: What Works*. New York: St. Martin's Press, 1989.

273. Stone, Irwin. *The Healing Factor: Vitamin C Against Disease*. New York: Grosset & Dunlap, 1972.

274. Stoppard, Miriam. *Healthcare*. London: Weidenfeld & Nicolson, 1980.

275. Svensson, Jon-Erik. *Folk Remedies, Receipts and Advice*. New York: Berkley, 1977.

276. Swarth, Judith. *Skin, Hair, Nails, and Nutrition*. San Diego, CA: Health Media of America, 1986.

277. ———. *Stress and Nutrition*. San Diego, CA: Health Media of America, 1986.

278. Swartout, Hubert O. *Modern Medical Counselor*. Takoma Park, Washington D.C.: Review & Herald, 1943.

279. Swartz, Harry. *Intelligent Layman's Medical Dictionary*. New York: Frederick Ungar, 1955.

280. Tanner, Ogden. *The Prudent Use of Medicines*. Alexandria, VA: Time–Life Books, 1981.

281. Tapley, Donald F., Robert J. Weiss, and Thomas Q. Morris, eds. *Complete Home Medical Guide*. New York: Crown, 1985.

282. Taylor, Robert B. *Dr. Taylor's Self-help Medical Guide*. New Rochelle, NY: Arlington House, 1977.

283. Thomas, Clayton L., ed. *Taber's Cyclopedic Medical Dictionary*. Philadelphia, PA: F.A. Davis, 1977.

284. Thomas, Mai. *Grannies' Remedies*. New York: Gramercy, 1965.

285. Thompson, William A.R. *Herbs That Heal*. New York: Charles Scribner's Sons, 1976.

286. Tierra, Michael. *The Way of Herbs*. New York: Simon & Schuster/Pocket Books, 1990.

287. Tilden, J.H. *The Pocket Dietitian*. Denver, CO: Brock-Haffner Press, 1918.

288. Time–Life consultants. *Eating Right*. Alexandria, VA: Time–Life Books, 1987.

289. ———. *The Fit Body*. Alexandria, VA: Time–Life Books, 1987.

290. ———. *Managing Stress*. Alexandria, VA: Time–Life Books, 1987.

291. ———. *Restoring the Body*. Alexandria, VA: Time–Life Books, 1987.

292. ———. *Staying Flexible*. Alexandria, VA: Time–Life Books, 1987.

293. Tkac, Debora, ed. *The Doctors Book of Home Remedies*. Emmaus, PA: Rodale, 1990.

294. ———. *Everyday Health Tips*. Emmaus, PA: Rodale, 1988.

295. Tobias, Maxine, and Mary Stewart. *Stretch and Relax*. Tuscon, AZ: Body Press/HPBooks, 1985.

296. Trowbridge, John Parks, and Morton Walker. *The Yeast Syndrome*. New York: Bantam, 1986.

297. Turin, Alan C. *No More Headaches*. Boston: Houghton Mifflin, 1981.

298. Tyler, Varro E. *The New Honest Herbal*. Philadelphia, PA: J.B. Lippincott, 1987.

299. Tyree, Marion Cabell, ed. *Housekeeping in Old Virginia*. Louisville, KY: John P. Morton, 1879.

300. University of California, Berkeley, Wellness Letter eds. *The Wellness Encyclopedia*. Boston: Houghton Mifflin, 1991.

301. Van Fleet, James K. *Extraordinary Healing Secrets from a Doctor's Private Files*. West Nyack, NY: Parker, 1977.

302. Wade, Carlson. *Bee Pollen and Your Health*. New Canaan, CT: Keats, 1978.

303. ———. *Carlson Wade's Lecithin Book*. New Canaan, CT: Keats, 1980.

304. ———. *Health Secrets from the Orient*. West Nyack, NY: Parker, 1973.

305. ———. *Helping Yourself with New Enzyme Catalyst Health Secrets*. West Nyack, NY: Parker, 1981.

306. ———. *Natural Folk Remedies*. Greenwich, CT: Globe, 1979.

307. Warner, Rebecca, Sidney M. Wolfe, and Rebecca Rich. *Off Diabetes Pills*. Washington D.C.: Public Citizens Health Research Group, 1978.

308. Weil, Andrew. *Natural Health, Natural Medicine*. Boston: Houghton Mifflin, 1990.

309. Wentzler, Rich. *The Vitamin Book*. New York: Gramercy, 1980.

310. White, Ellen G. *Healthful Living*. Medical Missionary Board, 1898.

311. Wigginton, Eliot, ed. *The Foxfire Book*. New York: Doubleday/Anchor Books, 1972.

312. Wilen, Joan, and Lydia Wilen. *Live and Be Well*. New York: HarperCollins, 1992.

313. ———. *More Chicken Soup and Other Folk Remedies*. New York: Fawcett-Columbine, 1986.

314. Willliams, Roger J. *Nutrition Against Disease*. New York: Pitman, 1971.

315. ———. *Nutrition in a Nutshell*. New York: Doubleday, 1962.

316. Williams, Roger J., and Dwight K. Kalita. *Physician's Handbook on Ortho-Molecular Medicine*. New Canaan, CT: Keats, 1977.

317. Wright, Jonathan V. *Dr. Wright's Book of Nutritional Therapy*. Emmaus, PA: Rodale, 1979.

318. Wunderlich, Ray C., Jr., and Dwight K. Kalita. *Candida Albicans*. New Canaan, CT: Keats, 1984.

319. Wurtman, Judith J. *Managing Your Mind and Mood Through Food*. New York: Rawson Associates, 1986.

320. Yudkin, John. *Sweet and Dangerous*. New York: Bantam, 1973.

321. Zi, Nancy. *The Art of Breathing*. New York: Bantam, 1986.

322. Zydlo, Stanley M., Jr., and James A. Hill, eds. *Handbook of First Aid & Emergency Care*. New York: Random House, 1990.

INDEX